Textbook of Ocular Trauma

Stephen C. Kaufman, MD, Ph.D.
Douglas R. Lazzaro, MD, FACS, FAAO
Editors

Textbook of Ocular Trauma

Evaluation and Treatment

Springer

Editors
Stephen C. Kaufman, MD, Ph.D.
Department of Ophthalmology
The State University of New York (SUNY)
Downstate Medical Center
Brooklyn, NY
USA

Douglas R. Lazzaro, MD, FACS, FAAO
Department of Ophthalmology
The State University of New York (SUNY)
Downstate Medical Center
Brooklyn, NY
USA

and

Kings County Hospital Center
Brooklyn, NY
USA

and

NYU Medical Center
New York, NY
USA

ISBN 978-3-319-47631-5 ISBN 978-3-319-47633-9 (eBook)
DOI 10.1007/978-3-319-47633-9

Library of Congress Control Number: 2016956637

Printed on acid-free paper

This Springer imprint is published by Springer Nature
The registered company is Springer International Publishing AG
The registered company address is: Gewerbestrasse 11, 6330 Cham, Switzerland

This book is dedicated to my family, my fellows, my mentors and my teachers, especially the great ones.

—Stephen C. Kaufman, MD, Ph.D.

This is dedicated to my wife and three sons who share me with work, my mentors E. Clifford Lazzaro and Richard C. Troutman, my residents, faculty, students, and colleagues, from whom I learn every day.

—Douglas R. Lazzaro, MD, FACS, FAAO

Foreword

I am happy and honored to have been asked to write the Foreword to this unique new volume the "Textbook of Ocular Trauma". As co-edited by Drs. Douglas R. Lazzaro and Stephen C. Kaufman, both extremely experienced anterior segment clinicians and surgeons in their own right, it brings together under one heading the combined clinical expertise of the faculty, residents and students at the SUNY Downstate Medical Center and Kings County Hospital Center Departments of Ophthalmology, among the most experienced in the New York Metropolitan area. The co-editors have done a magnificent work. I am proud they are representing the department I served as Chief for 27 years from 1956 to 1983 in this important academic endeavor.

Dr. Lazzaro serves as the Richard C. Troutman, MD Distinguished Chair of Ophthalmology and Ophthalmic Microsurgery and Professor and Chairman while Dr. Kaufman serves as the Director of the Division of Cornea, External Diseases, and Refractive Surgery and also as Vice-Chair. Both come from illustrious fathers in ophthalmology, and have succeeded in achieving high academic success. I commend them on this valuable scientific work which will add significantly to the ophthalmic literature in this important area.

Miami, FL — Richard C. Troutman, MD

The original version of the book frontmatter was revised: Volume editor name has been included in the Frontmatter. The erratum to the book frontmatter is available at 10.1007/978-3-319-47633-9_15

Contents

Contributors

Marib Akanda, BA Department of Ophthalmology, The State University of New York (SUNY) Downstate Medical Center, Brooklyn, NY, USA

Pasquale Aragona, MD, Ph.D. Department of Biomedical, Dental Sciences and Morphofunctional Imaging, University of Messina, Messina, Italy

Jay Arora, MD Department of Ophthalmology, The State University of New York (SUNY) Downstate Medical Center, Brooklyn, NY, USA; Kings County Hospital Center, Brooklyn, NY, USA

Alessandro Arrigo, MD Department of Biomedical, Dental Sciences and Morphofunctional Imaging, University of Messina, Messina, Italy

Edward Chay, MD Department of Ophthalmology, The State University of New York (SUNY) Downstate Medical Center, Brooklyn, NY, USA

Albert Y. Cheung, MD Department of Ophthalmology, William Beaumont Hospital, William Beaumont School of Medicine, Royal Oak, MI, USA

Inci Dersu, MD Department of Ophthalmology, The State University of New York (SUNY) Downstate Medical Center, Brooklyn, NY, USA

James A. Deutsch, MD Department of Ophthalmology, The State University of New York (SUNY) Downstate Medical Center, Brooklyn, NY, USA; Kings County Hospital Center, Brooklyn, NY, USA

Prachi Dua, MD Department of Ophthalmology, The State University of New York (SUNY) Downstate Medical Center, Brooklyn, NY, USA

Valerie I. Elmalem, MD Department of Ophthalmology, The State University of New York (SUNY) Downstate Medical Center, Brooklyn, NY, USA

Ilan Epstein, MD Department of Ophthalmology, The State University of New York (SUNY) Downstate Medical Center, Brooklyn, NY, USA

Samuel T. Gamsky, BA, BS Department of Ophthalmology, William Beaumont Hospital, William Beaumont School of Medicine, Royal Oak, MI, USA

Chirag K. Gupta, MD Department of Ophthalmology, William Beaumont Hospital, William Beaumont School of Medicine, Royal Oak, MI, USA

Andrew Hou, BS, MD Department of Ophthalmology, The State University of New York (SUNY) Downstate College of Medicine, Brooklyn, NY, USA

Stephen C. Kaufman, MD, Ph.D. Department of Ophthalmology, The State University of New York (SUNY) Downstate Medical Center, Brooklyn, NY, USA

E. Clifford Lazzaro, MD Department of Ophthalmology, The State University of New York (SUNY) Downstate Medical Center, Brooklyn, USA

Douglas R. Lazzaro, MD, FACS, FAAO Department of Ophthalmology, The State University of New York (SUNY) Downstate Medical Center, Brooklyn, USA; Kings County Hospital Center, Brooklyn, NY, USA; NYU Medical Center, New York, NY, USA

Jewel Liao, MD Department of Ophthalmology, The State University of New York (SUNY) Downstate Medical Center, Brooklyn, NY, USA; Kings County Hospital Center, Brooklyn, NY, USA

Charles D. McCanna, MD Department of Ophthalmology, The State University of New York (SUNY) Downstate Medical Center, Brooklyn, NY, USA; Kings County Hospital Center, Brooklyn, NY, USA

Alessandro Meduri, MD, Ph.D. Department of Biomedical, Dental Sciences and Morphofunctional Imaging, University of Messina, Messina, Italy

Reshma Mehendale, MD Department of Ophthalmology, The State University of New York (SUNY) Downstate Medical Center, Brooklyn, NY, USA

Laura Palazzolo, BA Department of Ophthalmology, The State University of New York (SUNY) Downstate Medical Center, Brooklyn, NY, USA

Jade M. Price, MD Department of Ophthalmology, William Beaumont Hospital, Royal Oak, MI, USA

Leon Rafailov, MD Department of Ophthalmology, The State University of New York (SUNY) Downstate Medical Center, Brooklyn, NY, USA

Allison E. Rizzuti, MD Department of Ophthalmology, The State University of New York (SUNY) Downstate Medical Center, Brooklyn, NY, USA; Kings County Hospital Center, Brooklyn, NY, USA

Mark A. Rolain, MD Department of Ophthalmology, William Beaumont Hospital, Royal Oak, MI, USA

Mamta Shah, MD Department of Ophthalmology, The State University of New York (SUNY) Downstate Medical Center, Brooklyn, NY, USA

Neha Shaik, MD Department of Ophthalmology, The State University of New York (SUNY) Downstate Medical Center, Brooklyn, NY, USA; Kings County Hospital Center, Brooklyn, NY, USA

Roman Shinder, MD, FACS Department of Ophthalmology, The State University of New York (SUNY) Downstate Medical Center, Brooklyn, NY, USA; Kings County Hospital Center, Brooklyn, NY, USA

Eric M. Shrier, DO Department of Ophthalmology, The State University of New York (SUNY) Downstate College of Medicine, Brooklyn, NY, USA

Nora Silverman, MD, Ph.D. Departments of Ophthalmology, The State University of New York (SUNY) Downstate Medical Center, Brooklyn, NY, USA; Kings County Hospital Center, Brooklyn, NY, USA

Jenny Temnogorod, MD Department of Ophthalmology, The State University of New York (SUNY) Downstate Medical Center, Brooklyn, NY, USA

Mario Urso, MD Department of Biomedical, Dental Sciences and Morphofunctional Imaging, University of Messina, Messina, Italy

Marco Zagari, MD Clinic "Centro Europeo", Acicastello, Italy

Introduction

Stephen C. Kaufman and Douglas R. Lazzaro

The most common emergency room injury after the 9/11 World Trade Center tragedy involved the eyes of first responders and those who escaped the buildings before their collapse. The emergency rooms of New York City were filled with individuals who were temporarily blinded by corneal foreign bodies from the debris of the twin towers. The inability to see or open an eye due to pain can be debilitating. Prompt emergency care prevented significant corneal pain, infections, scarring and blindness. Whether minor or severe, any individual who works in an emergency room, a trauma center or who provides eye care; should be familiar with the basics of ocular trauma care.

No matter whether the trauma is minor or severe, in an urban or rural setting, or involving an adult or child; it is imperative that the patient be medically stabilized and the eye thoroughly assessed. This book is intended for a diverse group of individuals who take care of eye injuries from the initial assessment to the final treatment. These include those in the first line of patient care: trauma physicians, emergency room physicians, physician's assistant, nurses, medical students and residents; to the associated specialists outside of ophthalmology: ear, nose and throat (ENT), neurology, neurosurgery and others; and finally, the ophthalmologist, who is frequently the ultimate specialist that cares for the ocular trauma patient. To that end, this book contains basic information about how to conduct an initial assessment of the eye, without worsening the eye injury, while also describing detailed information about testing, radiographic and MRI studies, and finally how to medically and surgically treat the eye injury in the adult and child.

Traumatic eye injuries frequently fall into general patterns and categories of ocular trauma. For the reader who reads this book cover to cover, he/she will gain an appreciation of the differences, similarities and integration of the types of ocular injuries and the anatomic location of the injury. Alternatively, by using this textbook's table of contents and the index, the reader can use this book as a reference resource, to address a specific issue.

The level 1 trauma center emergency rooms that our State University of New York—Downstate (SUNY—Downstate) Medical Center, Department of Ophthalmology covers throughout the five boroughs of New York City, are among the busiest trauma centers in New York and the entire United States. More than two dozen of our specialists and associates representing all ophthalmic subspecialties have come together to help you provide the best care possible for your ocular trauma patient. Each author has written a concise chapter with emphasis on important aspects of the assessment and treatment of the ocular trauma patient. We hope that this book serves as a valuable resource in the fight to preserve vision.

The Ocular Trauma Patient Encounter

1

Jewel Liao

As in any medical examination, the ophthalmic examination begins with a detailed history [1–4]. The details of the trauma including mechanism, circumstances, participants, relation to work safety, and witnesses, if any, should be recorded for medico-legal purposes. The patient's prior ocular history, systemic diseases, medications, tetanus status, and the time the patient last ate or drank should also be noted. In the physical exam, the best corrected visual acuity should be obtained and a slit lamp or pen light examination should be performed along with a measurement of intraocular pressure if there is no frank perforation of the globe. The examination should be conducted carefully and bilaterally. A dilated retinal exam should be performed if possible but this requires pharmacologic dilation of the pupils, which may interfere with the pupillary light response for hours or days, depending on the type of dilating agent used. The neurologist or emergency room physician may determine that pupil dilating drops should not be used so that the pupillary light response can be assessed and followed. A B-scan ultrasound and/or CT orbits can be considered to rule out an intraocular foreign body, look for orbital bone fractures, and even to assess globe contour. An examination under general anesthesia must be considered for any uncooperative patient, especially in the pediatric population.

Ocular trauma cases account for 6–9% of all ophthalmology-related litigation [5, 6]. Any loss of vision is an emotionally charged injury that will likely negatively affect a patient's quality of life and may make him or her more likely to seek litigation. In dealing with such cases, it is imperative to document meticulously. It has been shown that prosecution of medical malpractice cases often does not occur until 2–5 years after the injury [7]. Thorough documentation is frequently the best defense and can actually prevent frivolous litigation. It is very important to document visual acuity before and after any procedure in an affected trauma eye, while also documenting the exam of the unaffected eye. Any over-the-phone consultations and plans for follow-up should also have a note in the patient's chart. Once a claim has been brought, the medical record should not be altered.

It is imperative to provide a clear explanation of the prognosis of the eye injury to the patient, and the parents of pediatric patients. Sustaining ocular trauma can have a dramatic impact on a patient's life and their families' lives. Communication with the patient and the patient's family is crucial and it is important that the patient's condition be explained clearly. To that end, it is recommended to follow Dr. Baile's SPIKES protocol (Table 1.1) in delivering somber news [8].

The first step in the SPIKES protocol is setting up the interview [8]. One can mentally review the dialogue approach to broach the

J. Liao (✉)
Department of Ophthalmology, The State University of New York (SUNY) Downstate Medical Center, 450 Clarkson Avenue, MSC Box # 58, Brooklyn, NY, USA
e-mail: jewelliaomd@gmail.com

S.C. Kaufman and D.R. Lazzaro (eds.), *Textbook of Ocular Trauma*,
DOI 10.1007/978-3-319-47633-9_1

Table 1.1 Dr. Baile's SPIKES protocol

S—Setting • Arrange for privacy • Involve significant others • Sit down • Establish rapport • Manage interruptions
P—Perception • Determine what the patient knows already • Listen and offer information to the patient's level of comprehension
I—Invitation from Patient to give Information • Ask the patient if they want to know details about their condition • Accept patient's right not to know • Offer to answer questions
K—Knowledge • Use intelligible language • Parcel the information • Check for understanding • Respond to reactions • Give positive facts first, and give accurate information
E—Explore Emotions • Empathize • Allow the patient time to express their feelings
S—Strategy and Summary • Close the interview • Ask if they want any clarification • Offer agenda for next meeting

subject and be prepared for difficult questions. Negative feelings and feelings of frustration and responsibility may come up and are normal. However, it is ultimately your responsibility to communicate the prognosis to the patient. The key to setting up a good interview is arranging for privacy, involving significant others, having a place to sit down, and maintaining good eye contact.

The second step is to assess the patient's perception and the third step is obtaining the patient's invitation [8]. These steps are important when discussing the patient's condition because they may have misperceptions about their condition and they may not want to know their prognosis. Obtaining permission is important because the patient may not be in the mindset for discussion. You can start using open-ended questions to ascertain the patient's level of understanding and willingness to discuss the issue further. You can also provide a warning of bad news so that the patient can be prepared, and it is important to avoid medical jargon so that the patient can comprehend.

Step four involves giving the medical information to the patient [8]. The discussion of medical conditions can be improved if the conversation starts at the level of comprehension of the patient. For example, the vitreous can be explained as a "clear jelly" inside the eye. The use of analogies may be useful in certain situations. For example, if the patient has a severe dry eye due to trauma resulting in corneal surface irregularity, the surface can be compared to concrete rather than marble. It is important to confirm an understanding before proceeding to avoid miscommunication. Allow the patient to express questions and emotions. It is imperative to be supportive and empathetic of the patient's emotions as part of the fifth step of the protocol [8]. At the end of this session, the diagnosis and plan should be summarized so that both doctor and patient are all on the same page. Needless to say, any discussions should be documented in detail in the chart.

Numerous retrospective studies have been conducted to assess prognostic factors in predicting visual outcomes after ocular trauma. The most widely used system is the Ocular trauma score (OTS) system suggested by Kuhn et al. (Table 1.2). The OTS is based on an analysis of

Table 1.2 OTS raw score calculation [9]

Initial visual factor	Raw points
A. Initial raw score	NLP = 60, LP/HM = 70 1/200 to 19/200 = 80 20/200 to 20/50 = 90 $\geq$ 20/40 = 100
B. Globe rupture	−23
C. Endophthalmitis	−17
D. Perforating injury	−14
E. Retinal detachment	−11
F. Relative afferent pupillary defect	−10
Raw score sum = sum of raw points	

Table 1.3 Estimated Visual Prognosis [9]

Raw score	OTS score	NLP (%)	LP/HM (%)	1/200–19/200 (%)	20/200–20/50 (%)	≥ 20/40 (%)
0–44	1	73	17	7	2	1
45–65	2	28	26	18	13	15
66–80	3	2	11	15	28	44
81–91	4	1	2	2	21	74
92–100	5	0	1	2	5	92

about 2500 eye injuries and calculated by assigned raw points to six variables: initial visual acuity, globe rupture, endophthalmitis, perforating injury, retinal detachment, and relative afferent pupillary defect (RAPD) [9]. The scores are then stratified into five categories that give the probabilities of attaining a range of visual acuities post-injury (Table 1.3) [9].

Based on the current literature, the statistically significant prognostic factors include mechanism or type of injury, preoperative visual acuity (VA), time lag between injury and surgery, RAPD, size and location of the wound, retinal detachment, uveal or retinal tissue prolapse, vitreous hemorrhage, lens damage, hyphema, and number of operative procedures [10]. Of all these factors, however, preoperative visual acuity is most prognostic, followed by the presence of an RAPD, followed by vitreous loss [10]. These three factors were found to be statistically significant for poor visual outcome on a multivariate logistic regression analysis [10]. Hence, the importance of documenting initial visual acuity cannot be stressed enough.

The sequelae of ocular trauma are numerous and can be life long. They include glaucoma, cataract, retinal detachment, inflammation, tissue scarring, and/or sympathetic ophthalmia causing decreased vision of the unaffected eye, from the period of months to years after the injury. Close follow-up is recommended in all cases of significant trauma. Effective physician–patient communication is a key to ensure follow-up. The use of polycarbonate glasses or any other eye protection is recommended for monocular patients.

In summary, traumatic globe injuries are common and often result in permanent visual impairment and visual loss. Accurate diagnosis and management are crucial. The recommended practice worldwide is primary surgical closure of the open globe injury as soon as possible in order to restore the structural integrity. A key part in the management in every case is prompt, appropriate, and empathetic counseling of the trauma victim and family members. Recognizing the prognostic factors that affect final visual outcomes in risk assessment tools such as the OTS is an effective way for evidence-based counseling. And finally, meticulous documentation is vital against litigious actions in the future. In this text, details regarding all aspects of eye trauma will be discussed in significant detail.

In the ensuing chapters of this book, we will describe in detail the specific traumatic encounters seen in the periocular area, and within the eye. We hope this will help the reader appreciate the vast breadth of injuries that can be diagnosed and managed, with the ultimate goal of restoring normal integrity to the organ of sight and its surrounding structures.

References

1. Parver LM, et al. Characteristics and causes of penetrating eye injuries reported to the National Eye Trauma System Registry, 1985–1991. Public Health Rep. 1993;108:625–32.
2. National Society to Prevent Blindness. A guide for controlling eye injuries in industry. New York: National Society to Prevent Blindness; 1990.

3. Sastry SM, Paul BK, Bain L, et al. Ocular trauma among major trauma victims in a regional trauma center. J Trauma. 1993;34:223–6.
4. Duma SM, Kress TA, Porta DJ, et al. Airbag-induced eye injuries: a report of 25 cases. J Trauma. 1996;41:114–9.
5. Bettman JM. Seven hundred medicolegal cases in ophthalmology. Ophthalmology. 1990;97:1379–84.
6. Kraushar MF, Turner MF. Medical malpractice litigation in ophthalmology: the New Jersey experience. Ophthalmic Surg. 1986;17:671–4.
7. Shelton PA. Medicolegal concerns. In: Shingleton BJ, Hersh PS, Kenyon KR, editors. Eye trauma. St. Louis: Mosby-Year Book; 1991. p. 403–8.
8. Baile W, et al. SPIKES—a six-step protocol for delivering bad news: application to the patient with cancer. Oncol. 2000;5:302–311. Doi:10.1634/theoncologist.5-4-302
9. Kuhn F, Maisiak R, Mann L, Mester V, Morris R, Witherspoon CD. The ocular trauma score (OTS). Ophthalmol Clin North Am. 2002;15:163–5.
10. Rupesh A, et al. Prognostic factors for open globe injuries and correlation of ocular trauma score at a tertiary referral eye care centre in Singapore. Indian J Ophthalmol. 2013;61(9):502–6.

Corneal Trauma

2

Leon Rafailov and Douglas R. Lazzaro

Introduction

The cornea represents the anterior part of the outer tunic of the eye. It is clear in health and functions as a major refractive component of the eye as well as a protective surface for the anterior segment along with its extension, the sclera. The cornea is multilayered in dimension, and from anterior to posterior is composed of an epithelium, Bowman's layer (anterior condensation of stroma), the corneal stroma, Descemet's Membrane, and an endothelial layer responsible for keeping the cornea in a deturgesced state by virtue of its pump mechanism. In normal eyes, the central cornea is approximately 550 microns in thickness, and its overall diameter is between 11–12 mm. The cornea is a common site for traumatic eye injury, and in this chapter, we will look at the more common types of injury seen in the emergency setting.

L. Rafailov · D.R. Lazzaro (✉)
Department of Ophthalmology, The State University of New York (SUNY) Downstate Medical Center, 450 Clarkson Avenue, New York, NY 11203, USA
e-mail: douglas.lazzaro@downstate.edu

D.R. Lazzaro
Kings County Hospital Center, 541 Clarkson Avenue, New York, NY 11203, USA

D.R. Lazzaro
NYU Medical Center, 550 First Avenue, New York, NY 10016, USA

Burns of the Cornea

Thermal and UV Injury

Thermal injury can occur to the cornea when it comes into direct contact with a flame or with a hot object or liquid that is often projectile in nature. Thermal injuries from fires often happen in the context of other distracting large-scale burns to the rest of the body. Approximately 11% of patients admitted to burn units require ophthalmic consultation [1]. Prompt recognition of thermal injury to the eye is a key to successful management. Fortunately, burn injuries from flames are often limited by the ability of the eyelids to quickly close and provide insulation as well as a Bell's phenomenon if present. These burns often occur when there is an explosive thermal source or one that is projectile in nature when the patient does not have enough time to initiate a blink reflex [2]. In these cases, ruling out further injury from mechanical forces and foreign body is of utmost importance.

The etiology of contact burns to the cornea is either industrial in origin with use of soldering and hot iron particulates, or from home through cooking, curling irons and fireworks. These injuries are often unilateral. In a large study from New Delhi, 42% of patients with thermal burns had boiling fluids as a source [3]. In both this study and others, long-term sequelae were rare and seen in only 3% of patients with corneal burns, most often being symblepharon [4]. Amongst children, the sources of thermal injury are similar but with a greater incidence from

S.C. Kaufman and D.R. Lazzaro (eds.), *Textbook of Ocular Trauma*,
DOI 10.1007/978-3-319-47633-9_2

fireworks and superheated foods and liquids from microwaving, with eggs in particular being a common source [5]. Common household thermal items such as curling irons tend to disproportionately affect children as well [6]. These cases tend to be self-limiting with resolution of symptoms 48 h after onset with the use of debridement, topical antibiotics, cycloplegia, and pressure patching [7]. Limbal involvement is a key determinate of prognosis. Treatment for severe burns such as those with fireworks may require limbal stem cell transplantation combined with amniotic membrane transplantation [8]. A recent study by Sharifipour et al. demonstrated that using oxygen via face mask for one hour a day may speed up and improve recovery by improving limbal ischemia, accelerating epithelialization, increasing corneal transparency, and decreasing corneal vascularization [9]. Those patients with severe defects to the eyelids and at risk for exposure keratopathy may benefit from the use of a gas permeable scleral contact lens such as a Boston Ocular Surface Prosthesis [10].

UV light may also be a source of trauma and insult to the cornea, though the damage to the cornea is usually minor with rapid resolution. These injuries are often bilateral and occur from sunlight, tanning lamps, and welding arcs. Acute UV damage results in punctate keratitis and conjunctival chemosis usually 6–12 h after exposure. The de-epithelialization results in patients having pain, tearing, and blepharospasm, but is usually self-limited with re-epithelialization happening sooner than strict thermal or chemical injuries [11]. Patients may be treated symptomatically with lubricants and patching. A common comorbidity with this would be solar retinopathy, which can often have more severe consequences especially in cases of solar eclipse [12].

Chemical Injury

Chemical injury to the eye is a common source of acquired blindness. This type of injury affects men more often than women at a ratio of almost 5:1, often due to the fact that these injuries happen in an industrial setting [13]. These injuries tend to affect younger patients, such as ages 21–30, those who usually are inexperienced with using chemicals and do not use proper protective equipment. Given the young age of most of these patients, minimizing long-term disability is of paramount importance. Assaults, which represent approximately 11% of cases, tend to result in more severe injuries that have a poorer prognosis [14]. In all cases, immediate treatment with irrigation should precede any efforts to attain a history and complete physical exam. Studies indicate that 42% of injuries are bilateral so prompt treatment of the other eye should also be instituted if there is even minor suspicion of bilateral involvement [13]. Alkali injuries tend to be more severe than acid injuries because alkalis are hydrophilic and lipophilic, causing them to rapidly bind and penetrate through the ocular surface, as well as remain in the periocular area.

Acid Injury

Acid injury tends to occur in three major settings: laboratories, industry, and the home. The most common acids involved in injury in order of prevalence are sulphuric, nitric, hydrochloric, and oxalic acid [13]. The most severe of these acids is hydrofluoric acid due to its ability to penetrate the stroma and from additional damage of the fluoride ion [15]. Explosive car batteries are a large source of sulfuric acid injury in the population [14]. These explosive injuries tend to afflict those with increased exposure such as mechanics and engineers and can be complicated by blunt or penetrating trauma (See Fig. 2.1 below); these accidents are generally avoidable with use of proper safety precautions [16].

When acid comes in contact with the corneal surface, penetration is slowed in the stroma because the acid tends to bind the proteins of the corneal epithelium and collagen of the stroma causing protein precipitation and denaturation [17]. Experimental models in rabbits have demonstrated that this binding of collagen can cause shrinkage of the outer cornea and transiently increase intraocular pressure [18]. Further damage to the limbus and anterior chamber yields a worse prognosis. Damage that is severe

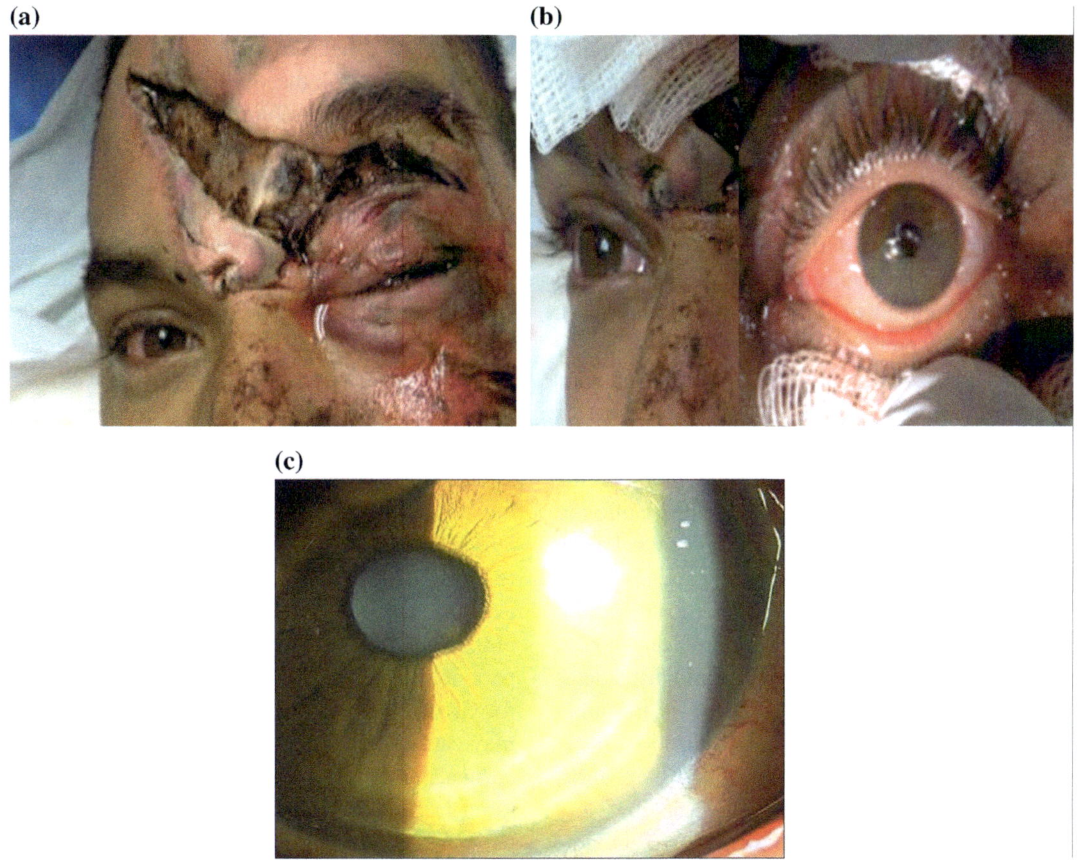

Fig. 2.1 Patient carrying a box with a car battery which exploded into his forehead. A mechanical and chemical acid injury resulted. In Fig. 2.1a, the extent of injury is noted. Figure 2.1b shows hazy inferior cornea which was flushed extensively and had an amniotic membrane (Prokera) placed. Figure 2.1c shows cornea after healing takes place

enough in nature to penetrate the cornea can result in secondary glaucoma and cataract [19]. Damage to the limbal stem cells does not allow the cornea to re-epithelialize and results in corneal conjunctivalization, vascularization, chronic inflammation, and epithelial defects [20].

Alkali Injury

Alkali injuries tend to be much more severe than acid injuries because of their lipophilic nature and their ability to penetrate through the eye. A saponification process also occurs when the dissociated hydroxyl ion acts on the cell membranes causing cellular destruction [21]. Alkalis tend to be a more common source of injury compared to acids. Among alkalis, sodium hydroxide, calcium hydroxide, and ammonium hydroxide are the most common in order of prevalence of injury [13]. Alkali injuries tend to come from plaster, lye, lime, cement, ammonia, and cleaning agents [14]. Magnesium hydroxide, which is the active ingredient in sparkler fireworks can cause both a thermal and alkali injury. Because these agents tend to be dry, using a cotton tip to initially brush the dry product out of the eye is preferred before irrigation.

Treatment

Treatment following chemical burns is similar in alkali and acid burns. Immediate management following chemical burns is of utmost importance and should theoretically start in the field of injury; variability in time before treatment can greatly determine the extent of damage [22]. Patients can become quickly disoriented due to the resultant blepharospasm, and often need assistance in guidance [23]. The patient should be made to lie down for irrigation of the affected eyes. Irrigant solutions differ in quality when comparing patient comfort and effectiveness in normalizing the pH. Water is not a preferred agent for flushing the eye in these injuries because it is hypotonic and may therefore diffuse across the cornea trapping or pushing the toxins instead of irrigating them [23]. That being said, water should be used in the absence of other irrigating solutions. Buffering capacity solutions when available are preferred; Previn, Diphoterine, or Cederroth Eye Wash solution are far superior in balancing intraocular pH based on testing with experimental models with rabbits eyes [24]. Irrigation should last at least 15 min with use of at least 1000 mls of irrigation solution with confirmation of normalization of pH with litmus strip. A Morgan lens can help direct the irrigation. Topical anesthesia can be very helpful if instilled prior to irrigation. Providers should irrigate the fornices, above and below the eyelids, as well as have the patient look in all directions during irrigation to make sure areas still containing or trapping the chemical are not missed. One should note that the use of ointments is not ideal after a chemical injury as this could potentially trap and prolong the noxious stimulus.

Following irrigation and immediate management the goals in the acute phase are to foster reepithelialization, decrease inflammation, prevent infection, reduce sequela, and prevent further damage [25]. There are different classification systems for chemical injury: Bagley, Dua [26], and Roper-Hall [27]. The median number of days for reepithelialization for patients with grade III–V injuries tends to be approximately 30 days using standard therapy [28]. During this time the cornea may be at risk for desiccation, increased friction from blinking, and exposure keratopathy from eyelid closure defects. While the cornea is rebuilding its epithelial layer, the provider must anticipate the functional deficits of this layer and treat proactively. Treatment in the early phase would include frequent preservative free artificial tears to prevent further erosion of the stroma. Mild chemical burns to the eye can be further managed with topical antibiotic.

Extensive damage, such as with Grade III–V chemical burns, require more substantial treatment and most likely require admission for intensive treatment and monitoring. Use of systemic ascorbic acid and ascorbate drops for chemical burns to the eye has been suggested for over 30 years because of their ability to help collagen production, but few studies exist to fully advocate its use for chemical burns to the eye [29]. Topical citrate has also been recommended as a means to reduce inflammation of the cornea by inhibiting polymorphonuclear leukocytes [30]. An 11-year retrospective review led by Brodovsky found that use of ascorbic acid, ascorbate drops, and citrate led to no benefit for Grade I–II burns, clinical benefit in patients with Grade III burns, and unclear effect for Grade IV burns [31]. Because chemical burns may cause shrinkage of the collagen fibers in the cornea, intraocular pressure must also be monitored in the early stages of treatment as 22% of patients with chemical burns develop secondary glaucoma, often requiring oral carbonic anhydrase inhibitors [19]. A study by Panda et al. found that using topical autologous platelet-rich plasma in the form of eyedrops for patients soon after injury can safely reduce the number of days needed for re-epithelialization due to the presence of growth factors in plasma [28].

Topical steroids are also used in the early stages of treatment to reduce inflammation and the release of collagenases and proteases. Steroids may be beneficial particularly in the early stages of treatment, though there is concern that prolonged and extensive use may prevent sufficient collagen production that can lead to cornea/scleral melting; concomitant use with topical vitamin C can help prevent this [32]. Cycloplegics such as homoatropine are also indicated for moderate-to-severe chemical burns, though cycloplegics with vasoconstrictive properties should be avoided. Cycloplegics will reduce pain and the risk of iris lens synechiae [33]. One experimental form of treatment not fully tested in humans is the use of oral tetracyclines during the recovery period due to their ability to inhibit metalloproteinases and collagenase activity [34].

Surgical management if required usually follows in the weeks following the insult. There are many relatively newer therapies available for treatment including amniotic membrane transplantation, limbal stem cell transplantation, corneal transplantation, and keratoprosthesis. Immediate therapy in the acute phase can include tenonplasty if warranted in severe burns. This is done by first removing necrotic conjunctiva and advancing Tenon's tissue from the orbital region to the limbus and securing it to the sclera to provide vascularization to the damaged region to help prevent perforation [35]. Amniotic membrane transplantation (AMT) for corneal chemical burns, first studied by Meller et al., found that the use of AMT within 2 weeks of injury for mild-to-moderate burns can rapidly restore corneal and conjunctival surfaces [36]. For severe burns, AMT was able to reduce limbal stromal inflammation and restore the conjunctival surface, and prevent symblepharon formation, it could not fully prevent limbal stem cell deficiency [36]. In these cases of severe burns, a limbal stem cell transplant may be necessary [37]. A recent study has shown that autologous limbal stem cells can be harvested from the contralateral eye and grown ex vivo on fibrin media, allowing transplantation that results in transparent self-renewing epithelium of the damaged eye in 76.6% of patients [38]. Usually these two modalities of treatment can be used together with superior results for severe burns when limbal stem cell deficiencies can be anticipated [39].

If the aforementioned therapies do not produce results allowing for meaningful recovery of vision, there are two options left for last resort, corneal transplantation and keratoprothesis. Corneal transplantation has a higher rate of rejection in chemical burns and requires large diameter transplants for limbal stem cell transfer [40]. If patients do not qualify for transplant or have repeatedly failed transplant, a Boston Type 1 keratoprothesis may ultimately be an option for therapy. A recent 7-year retrospective study shows that visual acuity of $\geq$ 20/200 using the prosthesis is achieved in 50% of patients and total device retention after 7 years is 67% [41]. The most common complications in order of prevalence were Retro-prosthetic membrane formation, glaucoma surgery, retinal detachment, and endophthalmitis [41] following keratoprosthesis. Further design and technological revisions may help reduce these complications in the years to come.

Corneal Abrasion

Corneal abrasion is one of the more common complaints of patients, representing approximately 24.3% of patients who present to the emergency room for ophthalmological complaints [42]. It occurs when the corneal epithelium is disrupted from a variety of injuries. As with other ocular injuries, these injuries tend to happen more often in the workplace or during sports activities. Common etiologies of corneal abrasions include fingernails, sports equipment, make-up brushes, and airbags. Children represent the most common source of fingernail injury, as patients are often parents who become injured while holding a small child [43]. Airbag deployment presents a particular challenge because it may also be associated with a high-energy blunt force as well as alkali injury [44]. In the hospital setting, corneal abrasion can happen more often in unconscious patients in the ICU or patients receiving non-ocular surgery as a complication of accidental injury during the surgery [45]. Patients often present with pain, tearing, blurred vision, photophobia, red eye, and foreign body sensation. Often times these injuries are associated with corneal lacerations and foreign bodies; and as with any mechanical injury, careful attention must be paid to the risk of an open globe. Prognosis is largely dependent on the size of the defect and depth of injury and involvement of Bowman's layer.

Work-up for such injuries includes careful investigation regarding the mechanism of the injury. High-energy forces such as with airbags, projectiles, and punches should alert the physician in seeking other sequelae of injury both ocular and non-ocular. Because of the severe pain and photophobia associated with abrasions, work-up must often begin with the use of anesthetic eye drops such as tetracaine or proparacaine. Topical anesthetics should never be given for outpatient use. Abrasions may be immediately visible to the naked eye as they may present with a haze due to the reduced light reflex. Using fluorescein dye will allow the examiner to see a more enhanced demarcation of the abrasion. All patients should have a full ophthalmologic exam to rule out other injuries, particularly to the anterior chamber and retina. A Seidel test can be used to determine if there is a leak from the anterior chamber indicating an open globe.

Treatment

Most patients with corneal abrasions require antimicrobial therapy to reduce the risk of microbial keratitis. Topical antibiotics, such as fluoroquinolones, should be broad-spectrum and anti-pseudomonal and should be initiated as soon as possible. Patching for corneal abrasions, once a standard of treatment, has been challenged as a practice in the 1990s. A meta-analysis review concluded that small abrasions do not need patching in the first day, and that patching may not reduce pain levels or speed healing [46]. Patching also causes monocular vision, which may become a cause of further injury and discomfort for the patient. A reasonable alternative may be the use of soft contact lenses. Topical NSAIDs such as diclofenac have been proven to be safe and effective in managing pain without slowing the healing process [47]. Topical NSAIDs may also help avoid the need for oral analgesics and narcotics. Cycloplegics may also be used for pain control, though should be reserved for larger defects. Most defects usually heal in 24 h while all defects are usually healed by 48 h. Recurrent corneal erosion can be an unfortunate consequence of corneal abrasion. Approximately 40% of recurrent corneal erosions are caused by trauma [48]. This can happen despite adequate initial treatment and can give the patient ocular pain upon awakening, tearing, discomfort, and foreign body sensation long after the initial injury [49].

Corneal Foreign Bodies

Corneal foreign bodies usually occur when the cornea comes in contact with a high-speed small projectile. These injuries therefore often occur in the workplace with metal workers and with patients who use power tools. Patients tend to be overwhelmingly male and often have a history of not using eye protection. Interestingly, a study from Australia found that 45% of patients presenting with metallic foreign bodies actually did use eye protection, but it is unclear if mechanism of injury occurred due to failure of the eye protector apparatus, or operator failure in using the proper eye protection needed for the job [50]. Broadly, foreign bodies can be divided into two classes, organic and inorganic. Prevalence between the two categories often depends on the location of the hospital or clinic in relation to the industry but foreign bodies tend to overwhelmingly be metal in nature [51]. Organic foreign bodies carry the increased risk of infection as they typically carry with them more bacteria and fungi. Inorganic foreign bodies such as glass, stone, plastic, and certain metals are frequently benign as they often do not induce inflammation. Of the metals, iron and copper tend to be the most troublesome due to their staining and ability to induce inflammation. Metal foreign bodies tend to have lower rates of infection as they are often heated when they become projectile. Overall, most foreign body injuries tend to be benign and not associated with significant morbidity. In a study of 288 patients with superficial corneal metallic foreign bodies, only 1 patient had concomitant corneal laceration [52]. Regardless, careful attention must be paid to the history and physical in determining the force of the projectile involved and the risk of an open globe (Fig. 2.2).

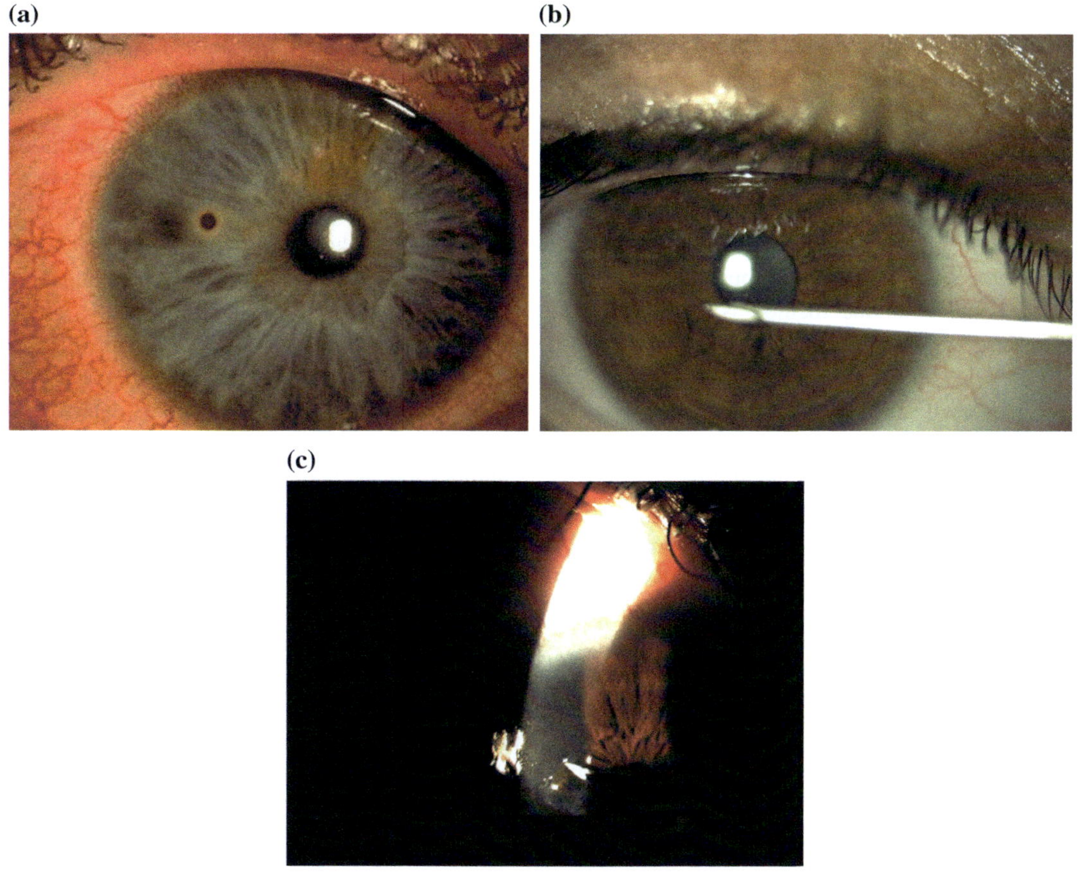

Fig. 2.2 Patient presented with corneal foreign body after metal grinding accident (Fig. 2.2a). It is important to view depth of foreign body at slit lamp before using sharp object to remove. It is the authors' preference to bend a 25 gauge needle so the needle is actually almost perpendicular to the cornea to avoid inadvertent damage to cornea (Fig. 2.2b, c). Some prefer to remove the rust ring with a rotating brush. Alternatively, the needle can be used to remove both the foreign body and rust. It is imperative to have patient seated at the slit lamp with the forehead pressed against band to avoid iatrogenic corneal perforation. If the foreign body is deep and against Descemet's membrane/endothelium, the removal should occur in the operating room

Patients with a corneal foreign body typically present with pain, foreign body sensation, tearing, red eye, and sometimes photophobia. Whether a patient presents with blurred vision is largely dependent on whether the foreign body is along the visual axis. The physical exam must focus on eliminating the possibility of intraocular injury and further ocular damage. If imaging is required, one should not use MRI if a metallic foreign body is suspected. As with corneal abrasions, fluorescein can help define the borders of the injury. A Seidel test can be used to determine if there is a leak from the anterior chamber. Topical anesthetics may have to be used early in the exam in order in increase patient comfort and compliance with the exam as well as to facilitate removal.

Treatment

Treatment should focus on removing the foreign body without damaging the surrounding structures. Oftentimes, certain inorganic foreign bodies may be safely left in if they are difficult to extract and do not cause visual disturbance and have low risk of inflammation and infection. Ferrous foreign bodies often need to removed as soon as possible due to their ability to create rust rings. Choice of intervention depends on the type of foreign body and depth of extension. Cotton applicators can be used to sweep foreign bodies if they are very superficial, though this may cause further corneal abrasion if not done carefully. Small gauge hypodermic needles can be bent at the bevel and used to dislodge and scoop foreign bodies. If a bent needle tip is preferred, it must be prepared in a sterile fashion; one method is by inserting a smaller gauge needle into the designated needle and bending the two at a 90° angle [53]. When using a needle, both the patient and the practitioner need to be optimally positioned in order to enhance stability through hand bracing and to reduce the risk of further injury. Rust rings can be treated as foreign bodies as well and can be removed using a powered burr or a needle, and care must be given to avoid creating a subsequent larger epithelial defect than what is necessary.

Patients should also receive antimicrobial therapy, approximately 14% of foreign bodies have been found to have positive culture results, with coagulase-negative *Staphylococcus* being the most common pathogen [51]. Antimicrobial therapy should be broad spectrum, such as fluoroquinolones. Fungal keratitis, though uncommon with foreign bodies, must be considered in cases where infection continues to occur despite antibacterial therapy, particularly with organic foreign bodies [54]. There is no current evidence to support the use of routine tetanus prophylaxis in nonperforating ocular injury [55]. As with corneal abrasions, the use of eye patches have been called into question as they have failed to demonstrate any advantage in healing [56]. In a study examining noncomplicated foreign body injury, defined as patients who are noncontact lens wearers and had foreign bodies outside the visual axis, the average length of time for resolution of the epithelial defect was approximately 4 days [57].

Corneal Laceration

A corneal laceration occurs when the cornea is cut, often with a sharp object, leaving a defect that can be partial or full thickness. Among corneal injuries, corneal laceration can often represent one of the more severe injuries due to comorbidities associated with further intraocular injury. For children, they represent a common cause of amblyopia and ocular morbidity. Approximately 86% of penetrating wounds to the eye occur in males [58]. Full thickness wounds present a particular challenge because of the increased risk of intraocular infection and often require early surgical repair.

A key part of the work-up for corneal lacerations includes determining whether the wound is partial or full thickness as well as determining the extent of other injuries. Depth of the anterior chamber can help determine whether there is a leak. A positive Seidel test can help rule in a full thickness laceration but a negative test cannot definitively rule it out due to the ability of full thickness wounds to self-seal. Once a full thickness laceration is discovered, CT of the orbits should be considered in order to rule out a retained intraocular foreign body. Full thickness injuries to the eye can be difficult to appreciate when the anatomy becomes significantly deformed [59].

Treatment

Patients often require thorough local and systemic pain control as well as an antiemetic in order to prevent vomiting and inadvertently increasing intraocular pressure. Nonpenetrating corneal lacerations can be treated the same way as a foreign body would. Topical antibiotics should be broad spectrum. Nonpenetrating lacerations also require thorough washout of the wound. Lacerations that are nonpenetrating and have some degree of avulsion should be re-approximated and fibrin glue can be placed on top to stabilize the defect. If this cannot be done without causing corneal deformity, then the wound should be closed surgically. Typically most smaller wounds, those 1–2 mm, can be closed with fibrin glue, as use of sutures can introduce further injury and points of infection [60, 61]. Typically if glue is used the patient can have a soft bandage contact lens applied after the glue is dried. If suturing is necessary, 10-0 nylon sutures are preferred and require very meticulous re-approximations of the cornea with attention to depth of layer sutured so as to avoid over-riding of the cornea and repeat leaks [62]. Patients who develop astigmatism from corneal deformity may eventually require rigid gas permeable contact lenses to correct astigmatism or a corneal transplant [63].

Corneal lacerations that are full thickness should be treated like an open globe (see section on ruptured globe for further detail). Careful inspection of the eye should focus on determining further intraocular injury including second points of extraocular communication that may cause further outflow or sources of infection. All interventions that put pressure on the eye such as applanation and B-scans should be minimized to avoid further spilling of intraocular contents. Patients with ruptured globes require admission and systemic and local broad-spectrum antibiotics with tetanus prophylaxis.

Surgical repair depends on the extent of damage. Studies have shown that laceration repair, traumatic cataract removal, and posterior chamber intraocular lens implantation can be attempted simultaneously with primary repair for those patients with stable injuries [64, 65]. Methods for repairing the corneal defect include use of amniotic membrane transplantation, lamellar transplantation, and use of autografts [66]. For children, particularly those under 7 years of age, focus should be on aggressive treatment to avoid amblyopia [67]. Treatments found to help prevent amblyopia include prompt traumatic cataract extraction with either primary or secondary IOL implantation, opening of a posterior capsular opacification with YAG laser, correction of refractive errors, and patching [68]. Initial visual acuity of 20/200 or better is usually a predictor of excellent outcome with 95% of patients having final visual acuity of 20/60 or better [58].

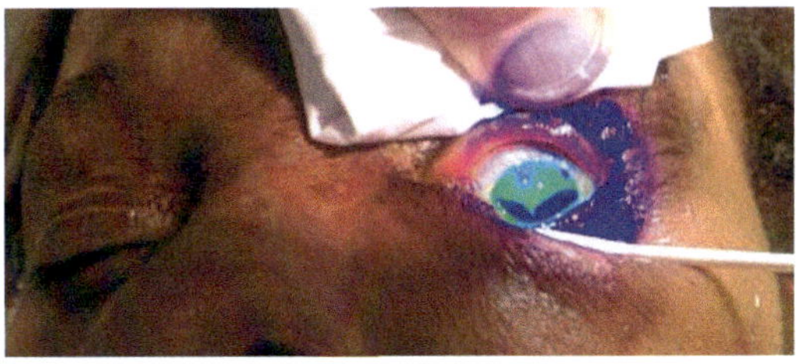

Corneal Case 1: A woman burned her cornea with hot oil while cooking

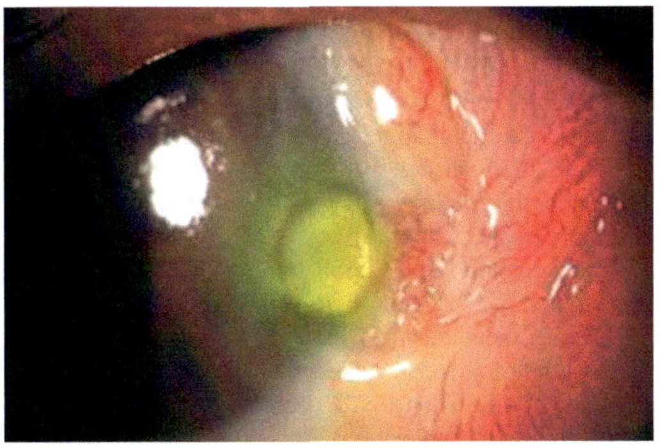

Corneal Case 2: Patient post pterygium surgery with large non-healing dellen

References

1. Bouchard CS, Morno K, Perkins J, et al. Ocular complications of thermal injury: a 3-year retrospective. J Trauma. 2001;50(1):79–82.
2. Boone KD, Boone DE, Lewis RW 2nd, Kealey GP. A retrospective study of the incidence and prevalence of thermal corneal injury in patients with burns. J Burn Care Rehabil. 1998;19(3):216–8.
3. Vajpayee RB, Gupta NK, Angra SK, et al. Contact thermal burns of the cornea. Can J Ophthalmol. 1991;26(4):215–8.
4. Boone KD, Boone DE, Lewis RW 2nd, Kealey GP. A retrospective study of the incidence and prevalence of thermal corneal injury in patients with burns. J Burn Care Rehabil. 1998;19(3):216–8.
5. Ratnapalan S, Das L. Causes of eye burns in children. Pediatr Emerg Care. 2011;27(2):151–6.
6. Qazi K, Gerson LW, Christopher NC, et al. Curling iron-related injuries presenting to U.S. emergency departments. Acad Emerg Med. 2001;8(4):395–7.

7. Mannis MJ, Miller RB, Krachmer JH. Contact thermal burns of the cornea from electric curling irons. Am J Ophthalmol. 1984;98(3):336–9.
8. Shimazaki J, Konomi K, Shimmura S, Tsubota K. Ocular surface reconstruction for thermal burns caused by fireworks. Cornea. 2006;25(2):139–45.
9. Sharifipour F, Baradaran-Rafii A, Idani E, et al. Oxygen therapy for acute ocular chemical or thermal burns: a pilot study. Am J Ophthalmol. 2011;151(5):823–8.
10. Kalwerisky K, Davies B, Mihora L, et al. Use of the boston ocular surface prosthesis in the management of severe periorbital thermal injuries: a case series of 10 patients. Ophthalmology. 2012;119(3):516–21.
11. Schein OD. Phototoxicity and the cornea. J Natl Med Assoc. 1992;84(7):579–83.
12. MacFaul PA. Visual prognosis after solar retinopathy. Br J Ophthalmol. 1969;53(8):534–41.
13. Saini JS, Sharma A. Ocular chemical burns–clinical and demographic profile. Burns. 1993;19(1):67–9.
14. Morgan SJ. Chemical burns of the eye: causes and management. Br J Ophthalmol. 1987;71(11):854–7.
15. McCulley JP. Ocular hydrofluoric acid burns: animal model, mechanism of injury and therapy. Trans Am Ophthalmol Soc. 1990;88:649–84.
16. Moore AT, Cheng H, Boase DL. Eye injuries from car battery explosions. Br J Ophthalmol. 1982;66 (2):141–4.
17. Dua HS, King AJ, Joseph A. A new classification of ocular surface burns. Br J Ophthalmol. 2001;85 (11):1379–83.
18. Paterson CA, Eakins KE, Paterson E, et al. The ocular hypertensive response following experimental acid burns in the rabbit eye. Invest Ophthalmol Vis Sci. 1979;18(1):67–74.
19. Kuckelkorn R, Kottek A, Reim M. Intraocular complications after severe chemical burns—incidence and surgical treatment. Klin Monbl Augenheilkd. 1994;205(2):86–92.
20. Arora R, Mehta D, Jain V. Amniotic membrane transplantation in acute chemical burns. Eye (Lond). 2005;19(3):273–8.
21. Wagoner MD. Chemical injuries of the eye: current concepts in pathophysiology and therapy. Surv Ophthalmol. 1997;41(4):275–313.
22. Schrage NF, Langefeld S, Zschocke J, et al. Eye burns: an emergency and continuing problem. Burns. 2000;26(8):689–99.
23. Kuckelkorn R, Schrage N, Keller G, Redbrake C. Emergency treatment of chemical and thermal eye burns. Acta Ophthalmol Scand. 2002;80(1):4–10.
24. Rihawi S, Frentz M, Schrage NF. Emergency treatment of eye burns: which rinsing solution should we choose? Graefe's Arch Clin Exp Ophthalmol. 2006;244(7):845–54.
25. Eslani M, Baradaran-Rafii A, Movahedan A, Djalilian AR. The ocular surface chemical burns. J Ophthalmol. 2014;2014:196827.
26. Dua HS, King AJ, Joseph A. A new classification of ocular surface burns. Br J Ophthalmol. 2001;85 (11):1379–83.
27. Gupta N, Kalaivani M, Tandon R. Comparison of prognostic value of Roper Hall and Dua classification systems in acute ocular burns. Br J Ophthalmol. 2011;95(2):194–8.
28. Panda A, Jain M, Vanathi M, et al. Topical autologous platelet-rich plasma eyedrops for acute corneal chemical injury. Cornea. 2012;31(9):989–93.
29. Pfister RR, Paterson CA. Ascorbic acid in the treatment of alkali burns of the eye. Ophthalmology. 1980;87:1050–7.
30. Pfister RR, Haddox JL, Paterson CA. The efficacy of sodium citrate in the treatment of severe alkali burns of the eye is influenced by the route of administration. Cornea. 1982;1:205–11.
31. Brodovsky SC, McCarty CA, Snibson G, et al. Management of alkali burns: an 11-year retrospective review. Ophthalmology. 2000;107(10):1829–35.
32. Davis AR, Ali QK, Aclimandos WA, Hunter PA. Topical steroid use in the treatment of ocular alkali burns. Br J Ophthalmol. 1997;81(9):732–4.
33. Gicquel JJ. Management of ocular surface chemical burns. Br J Ophthalmol. 2011;95(2):159–61.
34. Perry HD, Hodes LW, Seedor JA, et al. Effect of doxycycline hyclate on corneal epithelial wound healing in the rabbit alkali-burn model: preliminary observations. Cornea. 1993;12(5):379–82.
35. Kuckelkorn R, Kottek A, Schrage N, et al. Long-term results of Tenon-plasty in treatment of severe chemical eye burns. Ophthalmologe. 1995;92(4):445–51.
36. Meller D, Pires RT, Mack RJ, et al. Amniotic membrane transplantation for acute chemical or thermal burns. Ophthalmology 2000;107(5):980–9; discussion 90.
37. Tseng SC, Prabhasawat P, Barton K, et al. Amniotic membrane transplantation with or without limbal allografts for corneal surface reconstruction in patients with limbal stem cell deficiency. Arch Ophthalmol. 1998;116(4):431–41.
38. Rama P, Matuska S, Paganoni G, et al. Limbal stem-cell therapy and long-term corneal regeneration. N Engl J Med. 2010;363(2):147–55.
39. Shimazaki J, Yang HY, Tsubota K. Amniotic membrane transplantation for ocular surface reconstruction in patients with chemical and thermal burns. Ophthalmology. 1997;104(12):2068–76.
40. Maguire MG, Stark WJ, Gottsch JD, et al. Risk factors for corneal graft failure and rejection in the collaborative corneal transplantation studies. collaborative corneal transplantation studies research group. Ophthalmology. 1994;101(9):1536–47.
41. Srikumaran D, Munoz B, Aldave AJ, et al. Long-term outcomes of boston type 1 keratoprosthesis implantation: a retrospective multicenter cohort. Ophthalmology. 2014;121(11):2159–64.
42. Edwards RS. Ophthalmic emergencies in a district general hospital casualty department. Br J Ophthalmol. 1987;71(12):938–42.
43. Lin YB, Gardiner MF. Fingernail-induced corneal abrasions: case series from an ophthalmology emergency department. Cornea. 2014;33(7):691–5.

44. Ball DC, Bouchard CS. Ocular morbidity associated with airbag deployment: a report of seven cases and a review of the literature. Cornea. 2001;20(2):159–63.
45. Roth S, Thisted RA, Erickson JP, et al. Eye injuries after nonocular surgery. A study of 60,965 anesthetics from 1988 to 1992. Anesthesiology. 1996;85(5):1020–7.
46. Turner A, Rabiu M. Patching for corneal abrasion. Cochrane Database Syst Rev 2006(2):CD004764.
47. Jayamanne DG, Fitt AW, Dayan M, et al. The effectiveness of topical diclofenac in relieving discomfort following traumatic corneal abrasions. Eye (Lond). 1997;11(pt 1):79–83.
48. Diez-Feijoo E, Grau AE, Abusleme EI, Duran JA. Clinical presentation and causes of recurrent corneal erosion syndrome: review of 100 patients. Cornea. 2014;33(6):571–5.
49. Eke T, Morrison DA, Austin DJ. Recurrent symptoms following traumatic corneal abrasion: prevalence, severity, and the effect of a simple regimen of prophylaxis. Eye (Lond). 1999;13(Pt 3a):345–7.
50. Ramakrishnan T, Constantinou M, Jhanji V, Vajpayee RB. Corneal metallic foreign body injuries due to suboptimal ocular protection. Arch Environ Occup Health. 2012;67(1):48–50.
51. DeBroff BM, Donahue SP, Caputo BJ, et al. Clinical characteristics of corneal foreign bodies and their associated culture results. CLAO J. 1994;20(2):128–30.
52. Luo Z, Gardiner M. The incidence of intraocular foreign bodies and other intraocular findings in patients with corneal metal foreign bodies. Ophthalmology. 2010;117(11):2218–21.
53. Lim LT, Al-Ani A, Ramaesh K. Simple innovative measures for ease of corneal foreign body removal. Ann Acad Med Singapore. 2011;40(10):469–70.
54. Fahad B, McKellar M, Armstrong M, et al. Aspergillus keratitis following corneal foreign body. Br J Ophthalmol. 2004;88(6):847–8.
55. Benson WH, Snyder IS, Granus V, et al. Tetanus prophylaxis following ocular injuries. J Emerg Med. 1993;11(6):677–83.
56. Hulbert MF. Efficacy of eyepad in corneal healing after corneal foreign body removal. Lancet. 1991;337 (8742):643.
57. Brissette A, Mednick Z, Baxter S. Evaluating the need for close follow-up after removal of a noncomplicated corneal foreign body. Cornea. 2014;33 (11):1193–6.
58. Esmaeli B, Elner SG, Schork MA, Elner VM. Visual outcome and ocular survival after penetrating: a clinicopathologic studytrauma. Ophthalmology. 1995;102(3):393–400.
59. Hamill MB. Corneal and scleral trauma. Ophthalmol Clin North Am. 2002;15(2):185–94.
60. Nuhoglu F, Altiparmak UE, Hazirolan DO, et al. Comparison of sutures and cyanoacrylate tissue adhesives for wound repair in a rat model of corneal laceration. Ophthalmic Res. 2013;49 (4):199–204.
61. Siatiri H, Moghimi S, Malihi M, Khodabande A. Use of sealant (HFG) in corneal perforations. Cornea. 2008;27(9):988–91.
62. Rowsey JJ, Hays JC. Refractive reconstruction for acute eye injuries. Ophthalmic Surg. 1984;15 (7):569–74.
63. Zheng B, Shen L, Walker MK, et al. Clinical evaluation of rigid gas permeable contact lenses and visual outcome after repaired corneal laceration. Eye Contact Lens. 2015;41(1):34–9.
64. Lamkin JC, Azar DT, Mead MD, Volpe NJ. Simultaneous corneal laceration repair, cataract removal, and posterior chamber intraocular lens implantation. Am J Ophthalmol. 1992;113(6):626–31.
65. Rubsamen PE, Irvin WD, McCuen BW 2nd, et al. Primary intraocular lens implantation in the setting of penetrating ocular trauma. Ophthalmology. 1995;102 (1):101–7.
66. Vora GK, Haddadin R, Chodosh J. Management of corneal lacerations and perforations. Int Ophthalmol Clin. 2013;53(4):1–10.
67. Zaidman G, Ramirez T, Kaufman A, et al. Successful surgical rehabilitation of children with traumatic corneal laceration and cataract. Ophthalmology. 2001;108(2):338–42.
68. Segev F, Assia EI, Harizman N, et al. Corneal laceration by sharp objects in children seven years of age and younger. Cornea. 2007;26(3):319–23.

Trauma to the Anterior Chamber and Lens

3

Neha Shaik, Jay Arora, Jewel Liao and Allison E. Rizzuti

Anatomy of the Anterior Chamber and Lens

The anterior chamber of the eye is the fluid-filled space that is contained between the corneal endothelium and the iris. The anterior chamber angle lies at the junction of the cornea and the iris and contains Schwalbe's Line, Schlemm's canal, scleral spur, the trabecular meshwork, and the iris (Fig. 3.1). While the angle cannot be seen directly by the examiner, a *gonioscopy lens* can be used to view the angle structures at the slit lamp microscope. Anatomically, the anterior chamber measures on average 3.11 mm in depth [1], but it may be deeper in aphakia, pseudophakia and myopia, and shallower in hyperopia. A measurement of less than 2.5 mm is considered to be shallow, and may be a risk factor for angle closure glaucoma, or for the development of glaucoma after blunt injury to the eye. The volume of the anterior chamber is approximately 175 µl and is filled with aqueous humor, which is produced by the ciliary body. The fluid passes through the pupil aperture, into the anterior chamber, and drains primarily through the trabecular meshwork into Schlemms's canal. The aqueous humor helps to maintain the intraocular pressure of the eye, serves to offer nutrition and immunoprotection for the anterior chamber, and contributes to the refractive index of light entering the visual system.

The crystalline lens, which helps to refract light onto the retina, lies at the posterior border of the anterior chamber, behind the iris. It is suspended in position by delicate yet collectively strong fibers called the *zonules of Zinn*, which support the lens and attach it to the ciliary body. Trauma to these zonular fibers may lead to lens dislocation.

The lens can be divided into three main parts: the lens capsule, the lens epithelium, and the lens fibers. The lens capsule is a thin basement membrane that encompasses the lens in its entirety. It is made up primarily of Type IV collagen and glycosaminoglycans. One of the features of the lens capsule is to allow for stretching/contracting of the lens in order to refract light properly onto the retina. The capsule varies from 2 to 28 µm in thickness, and is thickest near the equator.

The lens epithelium comprises the anterior portion of the lens, and its primary purpose is to regulate homeostasis within the lens itself. It is very metabolically active and uses Na+/K+ -ATPase pumps to maintain osmotic concentration and lens volume. In addition, the lens epithelium serves to create new fibers and components to keep the lens growing over time.

The majority of the lens is composed of lens fibers. The lens fibers are long, densely packed cells that stretch from the posterior to anterior

N. Shaik · J. Arora · J. Liao · A.E. Rizzuti (✉)
Department of Ophthalmology, The State University of New York (SUNY) Downstate Medical Center, 541 Clarkson Avenue, E bldg, 8th Floor, Suite C, Brooklyn, NY, USA
e-mail: allison.rizzuti@downstate.edu

N. Shaik · J. Arora · J. Liao · A.E. Rizzuti
Kings County Hospital Center, Brooklyn, NY, USA

S.C. Kaufman and D.R. Lazzaro (eds.), *Textbook of Ocular Trauma*,
DOI 10.1007/978-3-319-47633-9_3

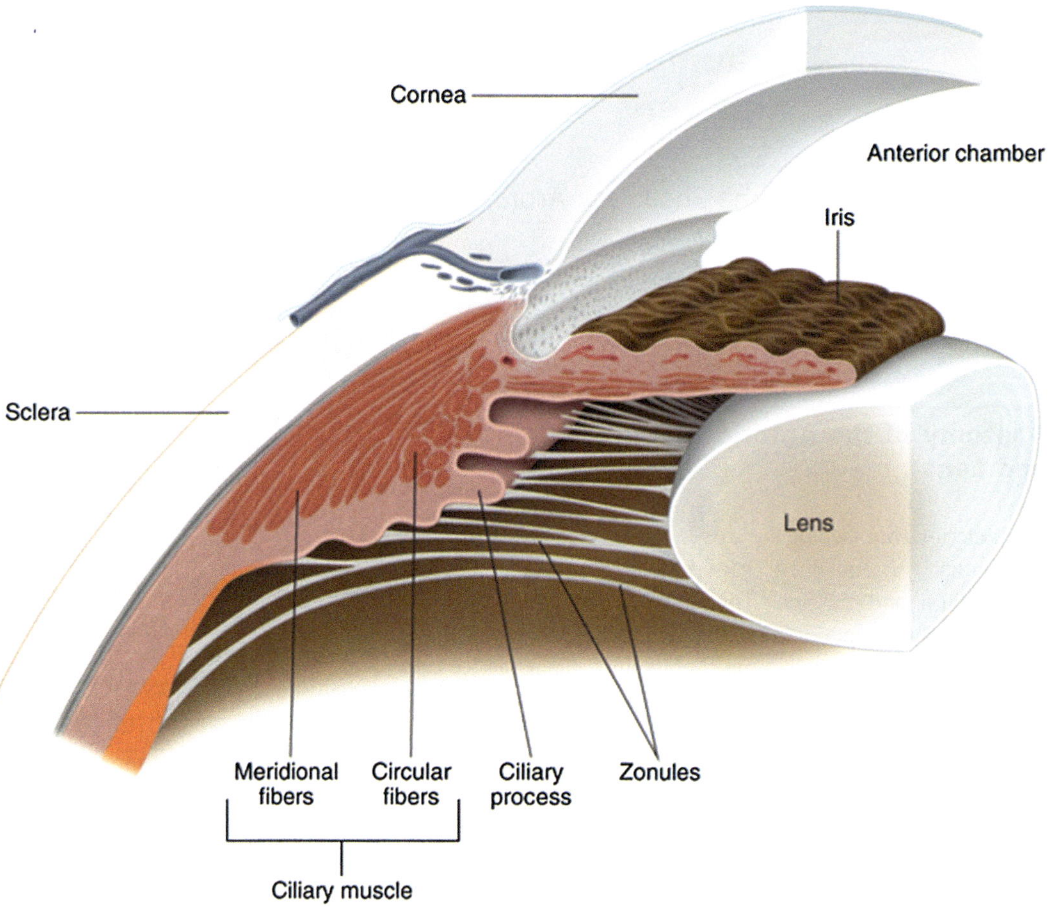

Fig. 3.1 Schematic representation of anterior chamber anatomy. *CB* Ciliary body. *S* Sclera. *SS* Scleral Spur. *SC* Schlemm canal. *I* Iris. *C* Cornea. *TM* Trabecular Meshwork. *IP* Iris Process. *SL* Schwalbe's line. *Z* Zonules. Photo courtesy of AAO.org BCSC Sect. 2: fundamentals and principles of ophthalmology

poles, and arranged in concentric layers to provide stability to the lens. As the lens fibers are generated, they attach to the outer cortex of the lens core, descending from the lens epithelium. As such, the central layers of the lens are composed of the oldest lens fibers, and extending outward, these layers become younger in age.

Anterior Chamber Trauma

Hyphema

Hyphema is defined as the presence of blood in the anterior chamber. It is one of the most common sequelae of blunt injury to the eye and its presence can signify major damage to the eye's blood vessels and intraocular structures. The blood may fill a portion of the anterior chamber, partially obstructing vision, or may entirely fill the anterior chamber and cause severe vision loss. A *microhyphema* occurs when there is no layering of blood, but red blood cells are seen within the anterior chamber. An *8-Ball Hyphema* is the result of a large amount of clotted, deoxygenated blood often giving a purple/black appearance [2].

Etiology and Pathogenesis

Hyphema is most commonly caused by blunt trauma, from a projectile or blunt trauma to the anterior portion of the eye. The hemorrhage is thought to be caused by a tear of the iris and/or ciliary body after the sudden posterior displacement of the lens and iris during injury [3]. A tear at the anterior aspect of the ciliary body is the most common site of bleeding and occurs in about 71% of cases [4]. As with most traumatic injuries to the eye, males are affected more than females. Non-traumatic causes of hyphema include surgery, hemodynamic abnormalities, and bleeding of abnormal vessels (neovascularization) in the iris or angle.

Signs and Symptoms

Patients with hyphema typically present after blunt trauma with complaints of pain, photophobia, and visual acuity changes. Hyphema is diagnosed by direct visualization of blood in the anterior chamber via penlight or slit lamp exam (Fig. 3.2). Because a hyphema may signify significant damage to the intraocular tissues, it is essential to perform a complete anterior and posterior examination in order to rule out the possibility of globe rupture. A B-scan ultrasound is often necessary, as the posterior segment may be obscured by blood, and a CT scan of the orbits may be indicated if the suspicion for open globe is high. Examination of the angle structures by gonioscopy is important to determine the severity of the blunt trauma that precipitated the hyphema. This is usually delayed until after the high-risk five-day rebleed period. Angle abnormalities and synechiae are commonly found. A useful way to grade the hyphema is by measuring its vertical height. This measurement can be repeated at each follow-up visit to monitor for resolution of the hyphema.

Increased intraocular pressure, as a result of red blood cells and fibrin clogging the trabecular meshwork, can occur in hyphemas of any size, and so tonometry must be performed on initial presentation and at each follow-up visit. It has been reported that a rise in intraocular pressure can occur in 32% of hyphemas, and patients with preexisting glaucoma are at higher risk [4]. For partial or microhyphemas, intraocular pressure is usually highest in the first 24 hours after injury and then normalizes after day 2. Larger or total hyphemas may cause intraocular pressure to be elevated for several days.

Secondary hemorrhage, or rebleeding after hyphema, may occur secondary to lysis of the clot which served to occlude the previously traumatized vessel. It can be seen in 25% of all patients with hyphema and typically occurs between 2 and 5 days after the initial trauma [5]. Studies have shown that rebleeds are seen more commonly in African American patients [6]. A rebleed is signified by an obvious increase in hyphema size during the follow-up period, and may result in vision threatening complications such as increased intraocular pressure, corneal

(a) (b)

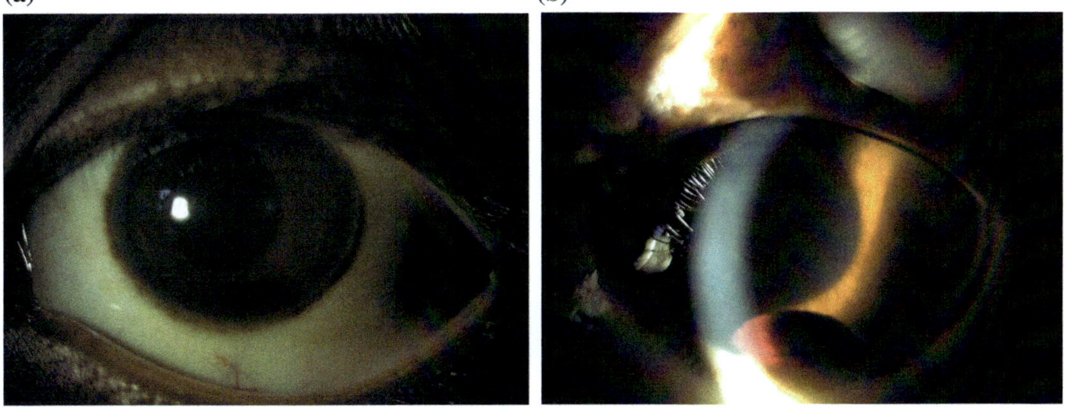

Fig. 3.2 **a** Anterior segment photo showing hyphema inferiorly in the anterior chamber of a sickle cell trait patient. **b** Slit lamp magnified view of hyphema settling inferiorly in anterior chamber. Kings County Hospital Center, Brooklyn, NY

blood staining, amblyopia and generally a worse visual prognosis [7].

Special consideration must be given to hyphema in the sickle cell patient, as the sickle-shaped red blood cells cannot effectively pass through the trabecular meshwork, leading to higher intraocular pressures for longer periods of time. These patients are also more prone to optic atrophy. Thus, it is important to obtain a sickle cell prep and hemoglobin electrophoresis in all patients with hyphema, and those positive for sickle cell disease or trait must be followed extremely closely.

Complications

The four complications of traumatic hyphema include: posterior synechiae, peripheral anterior synechiae, corneal blood staining, and optic atrophy.

Hyphema results in intraocular inflammation which may lead to the formation of posterior synechiae (iris adhesions to the lens), and/or peripheral anterior synechiae (iris adhesions to the cornea). Both situations can ultimately lead to angle closure glaucoma. Posterior synechiae, if substantial, may affect the movement of aqueous from the posterior to the anterior chamber causing secondary angle closure and iris bombe. Peripheral anterior synechiae may cause shallowing of the angle and blockage of outflow through the trabecular meshwork, also resulting in angle closure glaucoma.

Corneal blood staining is defined as the deposition of hemoglobin and its breakdown products into the cornea, and typically occurs in the setting of total hyphema with increased intraocular pressure. It has been reported that an IOP of 25 mm Hg or greater for more than 6–7 days increases the incidence of corneal blood staining. Patients with prior endothelial dysfunction are also at higher risk [4]. Corneal blood staining causes persistent reduction of vision, even after the hyphema has cleared, due to the presence of hemoglobin degradation products causing endothelial dysfunction. It is seen initially as a central yellow discoloration of the deep stroma which later spreads centrifugally to the periphery. The blood staining may extend to Bowman's layer and even the epithelium in severe cases. Clearance of the blood staining begins peripherally and progresses centrally, and can take up to 3 years.

Optic nerve atrophy is one of the most dreaded complications associated with hyphema as the damage caused is irreversible. Glaucomatous optic neuropathy may result from chronically elevated intraocular pressure while diffuse optic nerve pallor and atrophy may result from the acute transient rise in intraocular pressure, or from the initial direct trauma to the optic nerve. The risk for glaucomatous optic neuropathy is highest if the IOP remains 50 mm Hg or greater for 5 days or 35 mm Hg or greater for 7 days for the general healthy population [3]. However, in a sickle cell patient, the risk of developing optic nerve atrophy is much higher, even when the IOP is lower than 35 mm Hg [8].

Management

Management of hyphema is directed at reducing the incidence of rebleeding, and reducing the risk of corneal blood staining and optic atrophy. Traditionally, management included maintaining an atraumatic environment, which consisted of strict bed rest with the head in an upright position, bilateral patching, and sedation. More recent studies have shown that patients may remain ambulatory with a shield only on the injured eye, and achieve the same therapeutic results [9]. Medical treatment includes cycloplegic agents (such as atropine 1% solution, once daily) and topical steroids (prednisolone acetate 1%, four to six times daily) in order to control inflammation and prevent synechiae. If analgesics are needed, aspirin-containing products or NSAIDs are avoided as their antiplatelet effect can increase the risk of rebleeding [10]. Hospitalization may be considered in patients with severe trauma, or when noncompliance to the medical regimen is of concern.

Several studies have shown that systemic and topical aminocaproic acid (ACA) prevents rebleeding in patients with hyphema [11, 12]. ACA retards clot lysis by preventing plasmin from binding to lysine in the fibrin clot. The oral preparation, while effective, is not recommended for patients who are pregnant, or who have renal or hepatic insufficiency. The topical preparation appears to be just as effective in preventing rebleeds, with no systemic adverse effects [13].

Elevated intraocular pressure may be treated with topical IOP-lowering medications such as prostaglandin analogs, beta-blockers, or alpha-agonists. Oral carbonic anhydrase inhibitors may be needed if the intraocular pressure does not respond to topical therapy. In patients with sickle cell trait or sickle cell disease, where carbonic anhydrase inhibitors are contraindicated, methazolamide may be substituted.

While most hyphemas can be managed medically, some require surgical evacuation, or washout of the anterior chamber, in order to prevent severe vision loss. However, even total hyphemas can resolve spontaneously and it has been recommended to wait until after day 4 to surgically intervene. Surgery may be indicated in the following situations; microscopic corneal blood staining at any time, total hyphema with intraocular pressures of 50 mm Hg or more for 5 days (to prevent optic atrophy), total hyphemas or hyphemas filling greater than 75% of the anterior chamber present for 6 days with pressures of 25 mm Hg or more (to prevent corneal blood staining), hyphemas filling greater than 50% of the anterior chamber retained longer than 8–9 days (to prevent peripheral anterior synechiae), and patients with sickle cell trait or sickle cell disease who have hyphemas of ANY size that are associated with intraocular pressures of greater than 35 mm Hg for more than 24 hours. Surgery must also be considered in children who are at risk for developing amblyopia [6, 14].

The prognosis after hyphema resolution is mostly dependent on the associated injuries sustained from the initial trauma, and less so on the presence of rebleeding and the other described complications. Studies have shown that the majority of patients with decreased vision (<20/40) after hyphema are not the result of the hyphema itself, but from damage to the intraocular structures. This emphasizes the importance of hyphema as a marker for severe eye injury.

Traumatic Iritis

Traumatic Iritis, or Iridocyclitis, refers to inflammation of the iris and/or ciliary body secondary to blunt trauma to the eye. Trauma is one of the most common causes of anterior uveitis, especially in the pediatric population. It is most commonly seen in males between the ages of 20 and 50, and presents mostly unilaterally [15]. Traumatic iritis is thought to be caused by the inflammatory response to cell injury and necrosis following trauma. One study suggests that inflammation secondary to non-penetrating trauma may be similar to the dermatologic *Koebner phenomenon*, whereby minor skin trauma precipitates psoriasis flares in approximately 25% of patients [15].

Signs and Symptoms

Symptoms of traumatic iritis occur within 24 hours of injury and consist of ocular pain, photophobia, tearing, redness, and decreased vision [16]. Irritation of the iris and its attachment to the anterior ciliary body causes spasm of accommodation, sustained miosis and is often associated with a poorly dilating pupil. However, sometimes a larger mydriatic pupil can be seen when the iritis is associated with an iris sphincter muscle tear. The presence of cell and flare (i.e., white blood cells and proteins) in the anterior chamber will be seen on slit lamp examination (Fig. 3.3). These findings, with miosis and photophobia, are the hallmark findings of traumatic iritis. Cells and flare are seen due to intraocular inflammation causing the breakdown of the blood–aqueous barrier. However, the anterior chamber reaction may be surprisingly minimal. Intraocular pressure is often found to be low due to decreased aqueous production from ciliary body shock; however, it can sometimes be increased due to damage to the trabecular meshwork or from clogging of the trabecular meshwork by inflammatory debris. A rise in intraocular pressure can cause a secondary glaucoma, and if it goes unnoticed, can lead to optic neuropathy and vision loss. Other diseases that can be easily confused with traumatic iritis are infectious and noninfectious causes of

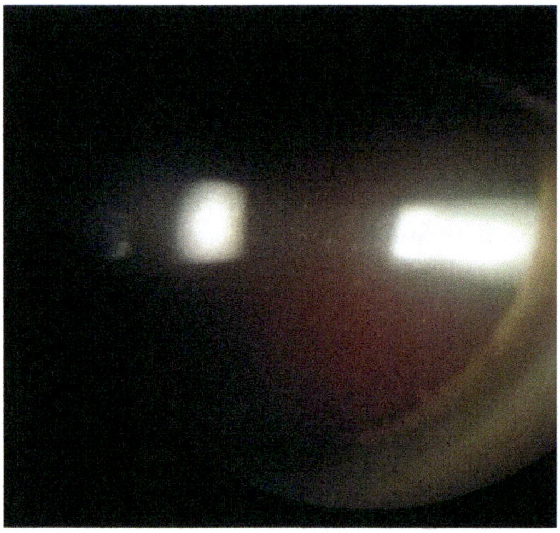

Fig. 3.3 Anterior segment photo showing traumatic iritis in a patient who sustained blunt trauma to the eye. Note the cell and flare in the anterior chamber. Kings County Hospital Center, Brooklyn, NY

anterior uveitis such as HLA B-27 related and HSV uveitis. Careful history and exam will help differentiate between these entities.

Treatment and Management

Traumatic iritis is a self-limiting entity and usually resolves on its own within 7–14 days [16]. Topical corticosteroid use has been the standard therapy since the 1950s, although the clinical evidence to support its use is sparsely documented in the literature [17, 18]. Currently, most practitioners chose to observe mild cases of traumatic iritis with close follow-ups. For moderate to severe cases, most physicians initiate topical steroid treatment to avoid complications associated with prolonged inflammation. If steroids are continued for more than approximately 2 weeks, it is important to look for a steroid induced rise in intraocular pressure. The treatment for moderate-to-severe cases includes cycloplegic agents (homatropine or cyclopentolate) to decrease ciliary spasm and relieve ocular pain and decrease the formation of posterior synechiae, and topical corticosteroids (prednisolone acetate) to control inflammation.

Rare complications from traumatic iritis include cataract, synechiae, and glaucoma. While these complications may be the result of prolonged inflammation, it is also important to note that cataract and increased intraocular pressure often result from the long-term use of topical corticosteroids. Because of this, it is important to start topical corticosteroids in appropriate cases and taper the dose accordingly.

Trauma to the Iris and Pupil

Injury to the iris can range from minor, temporary damage to its nerves and muscles to severe structural injury with partial or complete loss of iris tissue. Iris injury frequently results in pupillary abnormalities, and may cause *mydriasis* (a dilated pupil), *corectopia* (a displaced pupil), and even *polycoria* (more than one pupillary opening in the iris). An abnormal pupil will interfere with the eye's ability to focus light, leading to visual acuity changes and light sensitivity. If the injury involves the peripheral iris, the anterior chamber angle may be affected, and hypotony or glaucoma can result. In order to characterize the extent of iris injury, a slit lamp examination should be performed along with gonioscopy, and ultrasound biomicroscopy (UBM) or anterior segment ocular coherence tomography (OCT). The following entities are types of iris injury that are typically encountered.

Iris Sphincter Muscle Tears

Blunt trauma to the eye can cause tears of the iris sphincter muscle resulting in pupillary abnormalities, most notably traumatic mydriasis. While sphincter tears are the most common cause of anisocoria after trauma, it is crucial to rule out less common but more dangerous etiologies such as third nerve palsy or Horner's syndrome. It is also important to consider central nervous system pathology in the setting of bilateral mydriasis.

Signs and Symptoms

Classic clinical features associated with traumatic mydriasis include a fixed, dilated pupil with a diminished direct or consensual pupillary reaction to light and accommodative stimuli. The patient may complain of photophobia, as more light enters the pupil. The pupil may appear irregular and slit lamp examination may reveal small tears at the pupillary margin.

Treatment and Management

While sphincter tears and traumatic mydriasis can resolve after several weeks, they can often be permanent. Clinical and pathological studies have demonstrated failure of traumatic and surgical iris tears to heal spontaneously due to the absence of bridging iris stromal cells, fibroblasts, and pigmented cells to migrate between the wounded edges of iris, and to subsequently create a scar [19]. Treatment of mydriasis is largely dependent on symptoms of glare, diplopia, and rarely, on cosmesis. Medical management often includes use of miotics (i.e., pilocarpine or brimonidine), contact lenses, and sunglasses. However, due to the functional loss of the iris sphincter muscle, there is often minimal improvement with the use of miotic agents for traumatic mydriasis when compared to their use in paralytic or pharmacological causes of mydriasis. Colored contact lenses with a clear pupillary zone and opaque periphery are often used to hide iris defects and to artificially create a small iris pupillary diameter and minimize visual symptoms. The risks of contact lens wear can include infectious keratitis, and so these patients must be followed appropriately.

Surgical repair of traumatic mydriaisis is indicated when significant visual disturbance (glare, photophobia, and diplopia) is not correctable with medical management alone, when iris diaphragm support is needed for IOL placement, and rarely, for cosmetic reasons [19]. The standard and preferred surgical technique for permanent traumatic mydriaisis is Ogawa's iris suture cerclage using a 10–0 Prolene running suture technique [20].

Iridodalysis

Detachment of the iris root from its insertion site at the ciliary body results in iridodialysis. Iridodialysis frequently results in a central D-shaped pupil and a peripheral dark biconvex area near the limbus where the iris has detached (Fig. 3.4). Other associated findings include hyphema, damage to the trabecular meshwork and peripheral anterior synechiae (PAS). Patients may be asymptomatic and require no treatment, or in cases of a large iridodialysis, may complain of monocular diplopia, glare and photophobia [21]. The intraocular pressure can also be elevated many months after the injury, secondary to subsequent PAS formation or angle recession and fibrosis. In a recent study, traumatic iridodialysis, as one of the causes of posttraumatic glaucoma due to iridocorneal angle injuries, has been reported to be found in approximately 38% of cases [22].

Treatment

Management of Iridodialysis involves controlling associated symptoms. Sunglasses, tinted glasses, or colored contact lenses may help reduce symptoms of glare. If symptoms still persist and/or a large dialysis is present, then surgical

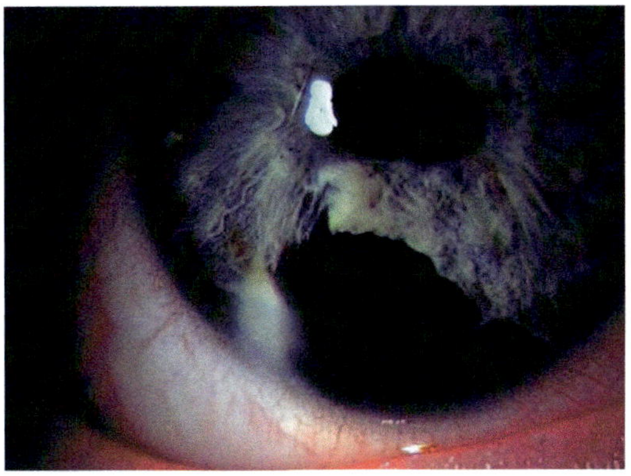

Fig. 3.4 Anterior segment photo showing inferior iridodialysis after injury with a projectile nail gun to the eye. (Photo courtesy of Minas Coroneo, MD. University of New South Wales, Sydney, Australia

repair should be considered. For sectoral iris defects or small iridodialysis (i.e., less than 3 clock hours), the McCannel Iris suturing method is the preferred technique [23]. This involves suturing the avulsed iris segment to the adjacent sclera and ciliary body junction using a 10-0 prolene or nylon suture. For larger iridodialyses and iris defects, prosthetic iris devices (PID) can be used. Burke et al., reported visual acuity improvement in 79% of patient using a PID. Although the use of such devices have been available in Europe for more than 15 years, they are still not FDA approved in the United States and are not widely available in other parts of the world [24].

Traumatic Aniridia

Traumatic aniridia, or complete loss of the iris tissue, can occur following severe eye injury and is usually accompanied by globe rupture and severe intraocular hemorrhage and hyphema. Frequently, the aniridia is only discovered after the absorption of blood from the anterior chamber, which can take days to weeks after the initial injury. Traumatic aniridia rarely occurs after blunt injury, and in these cases, the disinserted iris may be visible in the anterior chamber angle by gonioscopy. Cases of aniridia after blunt injury have also been described in eyes that have previously undergone cataract extraction, with the iris exiting a temporarily reopened surgical wound [25, 26]. Other causes of aniridia include congenital aniridia, and aniridia caused by ocular surgery.

Patients with traumatic aniridia universally complain of glare and photophobia because of a lack of the ability to regulate the amount of light entering the eye. The degree of photophobia can be severe and disabling. Vision changes may be mild secondary to spherical or chromatic aberration, or severe depending on the extent of ocular trauma. Patients also experience cosmesis-related problems, as the complete loss of iris is easily noted by the layperson. On slit lamp examination, complete loss of the iris is noted, and as with other cases of trauma to the anterior segment, a complete ocular examination must be performed in order to rule out globe rupture, and to assess for damage to the surrounding ocular structures.

There are various treatment options available to patients with aniridia that can restore pupil size and function. Cosmetic contact lenses are often utilized as they can relieve symptoms while providing a satisfactory cosmetic result. The risks of contact lens wear can include infectious keratitis, and lenses may be difficult to fit in cases of traumatic corneal scars. Corneal tattooing and intracorneal stromal implants have also been proposed with mixed results. In 1964, an anterior chamber intraocular lens (IOL) with a colored diaphragm was introduced for eyes with traumatic aniridia [27]. Various iris prosthetic devices have since been developed and have been used in Europe for the past 15 years including those by Morcher (Stuttgart, Germany), Ophtec (Groningen, the Netherlands), and HumanOptics (Erlangen, Germany). However, there are currently no FDA approved iris prosthetics available in the United States.

Cyclodialysis

Blunt ocular trauma can sometimes cause separation of the longitudinal fibers of the ciliary muscle from its attachment site at the scleral spur resulting in cyclodialysis [28]. A false passage is created where fluid flows from the anterior chamber into the suprachoroidal space. The direct connection between the anterior chamber and suprachoroidal space dramatically increases aqueous outflow resulting in very low intraocular pressures, and ocular hypotony (IOP $\leq$ 5 mmHg). Cyclodialysis clefts are viewed on gonioscopy as an abnormally widened ciliary body band, and may appear white, black, or gray. Other imaging studies that can aide in the diagnosis include ultrasound biomicroscopy (UBM) and anterior segment optical coherence tomography (AS-OCT). Cyclodialysis clefts often spontaneously resolve but can sometimes persist resulting in chronic hypotony and decreased vision secondary to maculopathy, optic disc edema, and corneal edema.

Cyclodialysis may be treated with topical cycloplegic agents (atropine sulfate 1% or cylcopentolate 1%). These agents cause relaxation of the ciliary muscle and help to oppose the detached ciliary muscle to the sclera. Corticosteroids should be avoided as the inflammatory reaction is beneficial to promote the adhesion of the ciliary muscle to the sclera.

When medical therapy fails, minimally invasive techniques such as argon laser photocoagulation or cryotherapy procedures are considered for small cyclodialysis clefts (less than 1.5 clock hours) to help reattach the detached ciliary muscle [29]. For large cyclodialysis clefts causing hypotony, direct surgical cyclopexy have been shown to be effective [30].

Trauma to the Crystalline Lens

Traumatic injury to the crystalline lens is a common occurrence following ocular trauma with 27–65% of civilian ocular injuries resulting in damage to the crystalline lens [31]. The injury may present as an acute, subacute, or late sequela of ocular trauma and is one of the major causes of acute or long-standing visual loss after injury to the eye. The estimated male: female ratio is 9:1 [21]. Traumatic injury to the lens and/or lens capsule have varied manifestations ranging from small focal opacifications, to complete cataract formation. Injury to the lens zonules, which maintain the anatomic lens position, can cause minimal lens displacement, or complete lens dislocation into the vitreous cavity. Traumatic *aphakia*, or expulsion of the lens from the eye, can occur in severe penetrating injuries.

Traumatic Cataract

Pathogenesis

Cataracts from blunt trauma are the result of *coup* (direct) and *contrecoup* (indirect) injury to the lens [32]. The resulting traumatic shockwave and equatorial expansion of the globe cause injury to both the anterior and posterior structures of the lens. Coup injury is also responsible for the imprint of pigment on the anterior lens capsule known as the *Vossius Ring* that is frequently seen in these cases. Blunt trauma may cause capsular disruption as well as cataracts that may be stable or progressive. Penetrating trauma or intraocular foreign bodies (IOFBs) can lacerate the anterior lens capsule, leading to focal cortical changes, or rapid lens opacification. The lens material that is released after both blunt and penetrating injury can lead to severe intraocular inflammation and a secondary elevation of IOP. Sometimes, the anterior hyaloid is also disrupted, and vitreous may enter the anterior chamber through disrupted lens zonules.

Signs and Symptoms

Patients with traumatic cataract usually complain of decreased vision, and sometimes glare and monocular diplopia. While a traumatic cataract may result immediately following the injury, it may also develop gradually over weeks, months, or years. Some traumatic cataracts remain localized and stable, while others may progress to total lens opacification. The traumatic cataract is seen on slit lamp examination classically as subcapsular and star-shaped, known as a *Rosette cataract* (Fig. 3.5). Other types of cataract, such as a mature white cataract can also be seen. Lens swelling and the integrity of the anterior and posterior capsule should be noted and, in the acute setting, the severity of lens-induced intraocular inflammation should be graded. The lens may or may not be dislocated as a result of trauma to the zonules and assessment of the lens stability should be performed (see section on lens subluxation). A complete ocular examination to rule out an open globe must be performed, especially in the case of penetrating ocular trauma. A B-scan may be necessary, as the cataract may obscure the view to the posterior segment. A CT scan may be indicated if the suspicion of open globe is high. Trauma to the surrounding structures in the anterior chamber should be noted, as these may guide the surgical plan if surgery is indicated. Gonioscopy and anterior segment optical coherence tomography may be useful for visualizing associated injury.

Lens Subluxation and Dislocation

In addition to lens opacities, blunt trauma to the eye can lead to zonular dehiscence, causing *ectopia lentis*, or displacement of the crystalline lens. The lens may be *subluxed* (partially displaced) while remaining in the pupillary space, or it may be *luxed* (completely dislocated) lying outside of the hyaloid fossa, free-floating in the vitreous, in the anterior chamber, or directly on the retina. Trauma is the most common cause of ectopia lentis. It is typically caused by a direct injury to the eye, but may also occur after blunt trauma to the head or orbit.

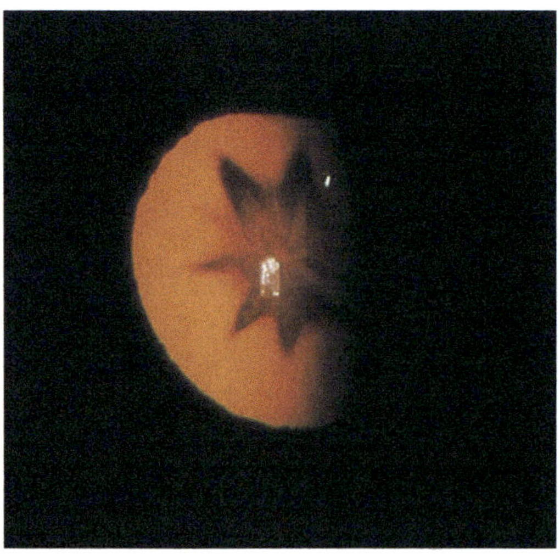

Fig. 3.5 Stellate cataract after contusion. Photo courtesy of AAO.org BCSC Sect. 11: lens and cataract. Chap. 4

Pathogenesis

In blunt ocular trauma, zonular dehiscence is thought to be caused by rapid expansion of the globe at the equatorial region immediately following globe compression [33]. Partial zonular injury (at least 25% of zonules) results in lens subluxation and complete zonular injury leads to lens dislocation. If a mild injury leads to subluxation, then systemic conditions that cause weak zonules should be considered, such as syphilis, Marfan's syndrome, Weill–Marchesani syndrome, Homocystinuria, and Pseudoexfoliation syndrome [34].

Signs and Symptoms

Symptoms of lens subluxation or dislocation depend on the degree of zonular injury and lens displacement. If the subluxation is minimal, visual acuity may not be affected or it may be mildly decreased secondary to lenticular astigmatism. Patients may complain of glare or monocular diplopia. Greater degrees of subluxation and dislocation out of the visual axis can cause a severe decrease in visual acuity. Slit lamp examination is necessary to examine the lens position. Iridodonesis (quivering of the iris) and/or phakodonesis (quivering of the lens) may be noted. The edge of a subluxed lens may still be visible through the dilated pupil (Fig. 3.6). The dislocated lens may be found in the anterior

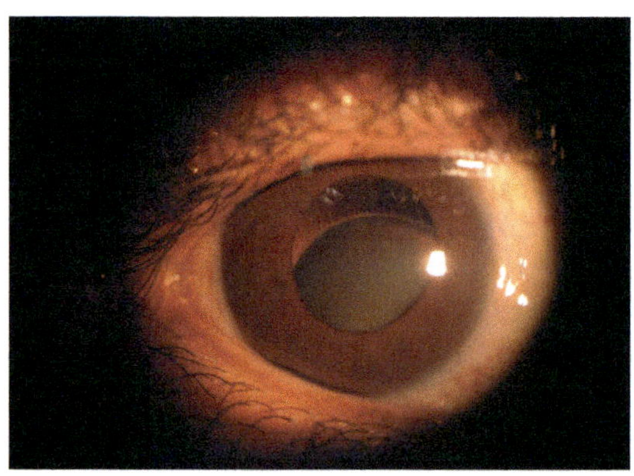

Fig. 3.6 Zonular dehiscence and inferior dislocation of the crystalline lens after blunt trauma. Kings County Hospital Center, Brooklyn, NY

chamber, floating in the vitreous, or laying on the retina. The location of the dislocated lens can also be visualized with B-scan or CT scan of the globes.

Complications of Lens Trauma

The most common vision threatening complication from lens injury is glaucoma, which can occur from a variety of different mechanisms. The release of macroscopic lens particles through a capsular rupture and into the anterior chamber can obstruct aqueous outflow and cause *lens-induced glaucoma*. Clinical findings include elevated IOP and visible lens material in the anterior chamber or angle. Anterior chamber inflammation is usually but not always present. *Phacoantigenic glaucoma* occurs when released lens material causes severe granulomatous immune reaction. Clinical findings include anterior chamber inflammation with keratic precipitates (KPs) in addition to elevated IOP. Pupillary block and subsequent angle closure glaucoma can occur when the lens dislocates into the anterior chamber. Other secondary causes of elevated IOP in the setting of lens injury include synechiae and other anterior chamber angle injuries.

Treatment and Management of Traumatic Lens Injury

Traumatic cataracts may be followed by observation if visual acuity is not compromised. Focal opacities of the peripheral lens causing glare and monocular diplopia may be managed with topical miotic agents. If the lens is dislocated into the anterior chamber, it may be managed initially with pharmacologic mydriasis and lens repositioning by placing the patient on his or her back and performing various head manipulations [35]. Once the lens is repositioned and the pupil is constricted, a prophylactic laser peripheral iridotomy is performed. In cases of dislocation into the vitreous cavity without inflammation or glaucoma, conservative management with aphakic correction may be appropriate. Surgery can be delayed for a later time if it becomes indicated [36]. In all cases of traumatic lens injury, a thorough eye examination is necessary to determine the need and timing of surgical intervention. Emergent or urgent surgical removal of the lens may be needed in the case of pupillary block glaucoma caused by the lens dislocating into the anterior chamber, or in cases of lens particle induced or phacoantigenic glaucoma [37]. Surgical timing is also important to consider in a child, in whom amblyopia is a concern [38].

In the setting of cataract associated with acute penetrating trauma, there is currently no consensus on whether the lens should be removed at the time of initial repair of the lacerated wound (primary procedure) or later, when the eye has recovered from the injury (secondary procedure). Studies have found adequate visual outcomes using both techniques [39]. If the lens is removed primarily, there is also no consensus on whether the intraocular lens implant should be implanted during the initial surgery, or at a later date in order to reduce the risk of infection. Despite the timing of lens extraction and lens implantation, management of traumatic cataracts and dislocated lenses is challenging, as they are often complicated by coexisting pathology, including zonular dialysis, posterior capsular tears, and iris trauma.

Surgical indications for traumatic cataract include: decrease in functional visual acuity, lens-induced inflammation and glaucoma, lens swelling from capsular rupture, and posterior segment injuries with poor visualization secondary to traumatic cataract [32, 40]. If the posterior lens capsule is grossly intact, and the lens is not dislocated, the cataract is removed via the anterior limbal approach. Visualization of the lens capsule may be poor during the surgery, and trypan blue can be useful in these cases. Care should be taken to avoid stress on possibly injured zonules and therefore, gentle hydrodissection or only hydrodelineation should be performed [41]. Surgeons should be prepared to manage zonular dehiscence and anterior vitreous prolapse. If the posterior capsule is found to be intact, the intraocular lens can be placed in the capsular bag. If localized zonular injury or weakness is found, then the intraocular lens can be implanted perpendicular to the area of weakness or a capsular tension ring can be placed prior to lens insertion [42]. If the capsule is significantly compromised, the intraocular lens may be placed in the ciliary sulcus or anterior chamber. Lastly, if the iris and capsule have both been significantly damaged from the injury, the intraocular lens may be sutured to the sclera, or a 3 piece posterior segment IOL can be placed in the sulcus and the haptics can be externalized into a scleral tract. Cases of mild lens subluxation may be managed with a similar anterior surgical approach using capsular tension rings and other support devices used to expand and stabilize the capsular bag before and during phacoemulsification [43].

If the lens is severely subluxed or dislocated posteriorly into the vitreous, and associated with inflammation, glaucoma, and/or posterior segment pathology, surgical intervention via pars plana vitrectomy and lensectomy is preferred [36]. An IOL is then placed in the anterior chamber or sutured to the iris or sclera.

Prognosis

The visual prognosis of patients with traumatic cataracts is guarded due to the frequently coexisting ocular pathology, and is generally worse than patients undergoing surgery for routine senile cataracts. Traumatic cataracts in children often lead to poor visual outcomes as a result of amblyopia and recurrent inflammation. Open globe injury has a more favorable prognosis than closed globe injury for satisfactory (>20/60) visual recovery after cataract surgery [44]. The ocular trauma score (OTS) was also found to be a reliable tool to predict visual outcome. Higher OTS scores tend to indicate a better prognosis [45].

The visual prognosis of patients with traumatic lens subluxation or dislocation is also guarded due to associated injury. Preferred management, surgical technique, and timing of surgical intervention vary from patient to patient, and is dependent on other associated ocular injuries, and hence, is still a topic of debate among surgeons. However, most surgeons agree that since the advancement of new closed surgical techniques since the 1970s (i.e., *limbal* and *pars plana* approaches), visual outcomes and long-term prognosis of these patients have been significantly improved with lower complication rates and better outcomes [46]. Alzuhairy et al., published a review of visual outcomes after lens subluxation surgery, comparing all etiologies, including genetic as well as traumatic causes. The authors found that visual outcomes of limbal and pars plana approach were similar, and that patients with genetic causes of lens subluxation had better visual outcomes compared to patients with traumatic subluxation [47].

Trauma to the Pseudophakic Patient

Special considerations must be taken into account when a pseudophakic patient sustains ocular trauma. Cataract surgery with successful posterior chamber intraocular lens (IOL) implantation is one of the most widely performed ophthalmic surgeries. Blunt force trauma can cause a malposition, dislocation and/or extrusion of the implant. Predisposing factors for lens dislocation include advanced age, pseudoexfoliation, uveitis, high myopia, previous vitrectomy, and inherited connective tissue diseases [48]. An intraocular lens malposition can range from a mild decentration to a complete dislocation.

A recent study by Gul et al. [48] found that surgical intervention is not essential in all cases of dislocated IOLs due to the fact that any manipulation of the anterior chamber may decrease the density of healthy endothelial cells. In some cases, the dislocation may not cause significant visual disability; and observation is appropriate. Surgery is indicated in cases of visual impairment, glaucoma, IOL dislocation into the vitreous cavity, cystoid macular edema, and retinal detachment. Surgical options include IOL repositioning, IOL replacement, suturing the IOL to the scleral wall or iris, and explantation of the IOL. Currently, there is no superior surgical technique regarding management of a dislocated IOL: [49–53].

Wound dehiscence following blunt trauma can occur in any patient who has had prior intraocular surgery and should be ruled out in any pseudophakic patient after ocular trauma. One study found that ruptured cataract surgery wounds account for approximately one-third of open globe injuries in the elderly population [54]. Dehiscence occurs because of a structural weakness at the site of the surgical incision and the risk decreases with a longer interval from surgery to trauma as the integrity of the wound strengthens. The risk is also increased with larger wounds and is much less common following modern cataract surgery in which the beveled surgical incision is self-sealing and may be as small as 2.2 mm. However, there remains a significant population of elderly patients who underwent cataract extraction via the extracapsular technique (ECCE) in which a large limbal incision or scleral tunnel was performed. These patients are particularly at risk, especially after sustaining a fall. The wound should be carefully examined in these patients, and a siedel test may be performed in less obvious cases when a dehiscence is suspected.

Traumatic wound dehiscence essentially constitutes an open globe, and must be managed expediantly in order to prevent infection. Primary wound closure is the preferred method of management unless additional procedures are required. In a study by Tseng et al., the incidence of traumatic wound dehiscence was 2.53% over a period of 9 years. About 56% of patients who had previous cataract surgery had IOL dislocations or extrusions and required a corrective procedure. Overall, the study found that prognosis is poor after a traumatic wound dehiscence but about 30% of eyes can recover useful vision [55]. In a more recent study that reviewed a large series of open globe injuries from 2000–2007, 83% of the 63 wound dehiscences were of extracapsular wounds and only 7% were phacoemulsification wounds. ECCE was associated with a worse visual prognosis with a best postoperative visual acuity of hand motions. Patients with phacoemulsification wounds did much better, with a median postoperative visual acuity of 20/60 [54]. As ECCE becomes more obsolete, the likelihood of wound dehiscence and subsequent vision loss after blunt trauma will be much lower, however, clinical suspicion should never wane.

References

1. Feng MT, Belin MW, Ambrosio R Jr, Grewal SP, Yan W, Shaheen MS, Steinmueller A. Anterior chamber depth in normal subjects by rotating scheimpflug imaging. Saudi J Ophthalmol. 2011;25(3):255–9.
2. Trattler WB, Kaiser PK, Friedman NJ. Chapter 10: anterior segment in review of ophthalmology. Edinburgh: Saunders Elsevier; 2012.
3. Hoskins HD. Secondary glaucoma. In: Heilman K, Richardson KT, editors. Glaucoma: conceptions of a disease, pathogenesis, diagnosis therapy. Philadelphia: WB Saunders; 1978. p. 376.
4. Read J, Goldberg MF. Comparison of medical treatment for traumatic hyphema. In: Transactions of the American Academy of Ophthalmology and Otolaryngology, vol. 78. 5 ed. 1974.
5. Walton W, Von Hagen S, Grigorian R, Zarbin M. Management of traumatic hyphema. Surv Ophthalmol. 2002;47(4):297–334.
6. Spoor TC, Kwitko GM, O'Grady JM, Ramocki JM. Traumatic hyphema in an urban population. Am J Ophthalmol. 1990;109(1):23–7.
7. Rahmani B, Jahadi HR, Rajaeefard A. An analysis of risk for secondary hemorrhage in traumatic hyphema. Ophthalmology. 1999;106(2):380–5.
8. Nasrullah A, Kerr NC. Sickle cell trait as a risk factor for secondary hemorrhage in children with traumatic hyphema. Am J Ophthalmol. 1997;123(6):783–90.
9. Gharaibeh A, Savage HI, Scherer RW, Goldberg MF, Lindsley K. Medical interventions for traumatic hyphema. Cochrane Database Syst Rev. 2013;12: Cd005431.
10. Crawford JS, Lewandowski RL, Chan W. The effect of aspirin on rebleeding in traumatic hyphema. Am J Ophthalmol. 1975;80(3 Pt 2):543–5.
11. Kutner B, Fourman S, Brein K, Hobson S, Mrvos D, Sheppard J, Weisman S. Aminocaproic acid reduces the risk of secondary hemorrhage in patients with traumatic hyphema. Arch Ophthalmol. 1987;105(2):206–8.
12. Pieramici DJ, Goldberg MF, Melia M, Fekrat S, Bradford CA, Faulkner A, Santander SH. A phase III, multicenter, randomized, placebo-controlled clinical trial of topical aminocaproic acid (Caprogel) in the management of traumatic hyphema. Ophthalmology. 2003;110(11):2106–12.
13. Crouch ER Jr, Williams PB, Gray MK, Crouch ER, Chames M. Topical aminocaproic acid in the treatment of traumatic hyphema. Arch Ophthalmol. 1997;115(9):1106–12.

14. Read J. Traumatic hyphema: surgical vs medical management. Ann Ophthalmol. 1975;7(5):659–662, 664–656, 668-670.
15. Rosenbaum JT, Tammaro J, Robertson JE Jr. Uveitis precipitated by nonpenetrating ocular trauma. Am J Ophthalmol. 1991;112(4):392–5.
16. Reidy JJ. Section 08: External disease and cornea. In: Basic and clinical science course. San Francisco, CA: American Academy of Ophthalmology; 2015. p. 363.
17. Islam, N., & Pavesio, C. (2010). Uveitis (acute anterior). BMJ Clin Evid. 2010.
18. Dunne JA, Travers JP. Double-blind clinical trial of topical steroids in anterior uveitis. Br J Ophthalmol. 1979;63(11):762–7.
19. Dunn SP, Stec L. Chapter 8: Iris reconstruction. Ophthalmic microsurgical suturing techniques. Berlin: Springer; 2007. p. 71–83.
20. Ogawa GS. The iris cerclage suture for permanent mydriasis: a running suture technique. Ophthalmic Surg Lasers. 1998;29(12):1001–9.
21. Canavan YM, Archer DB. Anterior segment consequences of blunt ocular injury. Br J Ophthalmol. 1982;66(9):549–55.
22. Ellong A, Ebana Mvogo C, Nyouma Moune E, Bella-Hiag A, Ngosso A, Njoh Litumbe C. Post-traumatic glaucoma with irido-corneal angle injuries in Cameroon. Bull Soc Belge Ophtalmol. 2005;(298):21–28.
23. Chang DF. Siepser slipknot for McCannel iris-suture fixation of subluxated intraocular lenses. J Cataract Refract Surg. 2004;30(6):1170–6.
24. Burk SE, Da Mata AP, Snyder ME, Cionni RJ, Cohen JS, Osher RH. Prosthetic iris implantation for congenital, traumatic, or functional iris deficiencies. J Cataract Refract Surg. 2001;27(11):1732–40.
25. Navon SE. Expulsive iridodialysis: an isolated injury after phacoemulsification. J Cataract Refract Surg. 1997;23(5):805–7.
26. Ball J, Caesar R, Choudhuri D. Mystery of the vanishing Iris. J Cataract Refract Surg. 2002;28 (1):180–1.
27. Choyce P. Intra-ocular lenses and implants HK Lewis. London: England p; 1964. p. 27–32.
28. Ioannidis AS, Barton K. Cyclodialysis cleft: causes and repair. Curr Opin Ophthalmol. 2010;21(2):150–4.
29. Han JC, Kwun YK, Cho SH, Kee C. Long-term outcomes of argon laser photocoagulation in small size cyclodialysis cleft. BMC Ophthalmol. 2015;15:123.
30. Ioannidis AS, Bunce C, Barton K. The evaluation and surgical management of cyclodialysis clefts that have failed to respond to conservative management. Br J Ophthalmol. 2014;98(4):544–9.
31. Smith MP, Colyer MH, Weichel ED, Stutzman RD. Traumatic cataracts secondary to combat ocular trauma. J Cataract Refract Surg. 2015;41(8):1693–8.
32. Wolter JR. Coup-contrecoup mechanism of ocular injuries. Am J Ophthalmol. 1963;56:785–96.
33. Weidenthal DT, Schepens CL. Peripheral fundus changes associated with ocular contusion. Am J Ophthalmol. 1966;62(3):465–77.
34. Bruce M, Zagelbaum PS. Anterior segment truama. In: Miller JW, Albert DM, editors. Albert & Jakobiec's principles & practice of ophthalmology. Philadelphia: Elsevier, 2008. p. 5093–5111.
35. Das Gupta BK, Basu RK. Bilateral dislocation of lens under complete voluntary control in Marfan's syndrome with cardiovascular anomaly. Br J Ophthalmol. 1955;39(9):566–8.
36. Oh J, Smiddy WE. Pars plana lensectomy combined with pars plana vitrectomy for dislocated cataract. J Cataract Refract Surg. 2010;36(7):1189–94.
37. Choi DY, Kim JG, Song BJ. Surgical management of crystalline lens dislocation into the anterior chamber with corneal touch and secondary glaucoma. J Cataract Refract Surg. 2004;30(3):718–21.
38. Magli A, Iovine A, Bruzzese D, Giani U, Fimiani F. Strabismus in developmental cataract. Eur J Ophthalmol. 2008;18(4):540–3.
39. Rumelt S, Rehany U. The influence of surgery and intraocular lens implantation timing on visual outcome in traumatic cataract. Graefes Arch Clin Exp Ophthalmol. 2010;248(9):1293–7.
40. Blum M, Tetz MR, Greiner C, Voelcker HE. Treatment of traumatic cataracts. J Cataract Refract Surg. 1996;22(3):342–6.
41. Irvine JA, Smith RF. Lens injuries. In: Shingleton BJ, Hersh PS, Kenyon KR, editors. Eye trauma. St Louis: MO, Mosby; 1991. p. 126–35.
42. Menapace R, Findl O, Georgopoulos M, Rainer G, Vass C, Schmetterer K. The capsular tension ring: designs, applications, and techniques. J Cataract Refract Surg. 2000;26(6):898–912.
43. Hoffman RS, Snyder ME, Devgan U, Allen QB, Yeoh R, Braga-Mele R. Management of the subluxated crystalline lens. J Cataract Refract Surg. 2013;39 (12):1904–15.
44. Shah MA, Shah SM, Shah SB, Patel CG, Patel UA, Appleware A, Gupta A. Comparative study of final visual outcome between open- and closed-globe injuries following surgical treatment of traumatic cataract. Graefes Arch Clin Exp Ophthalmol. 2011;249(12):1775–81.
45. Shah MA, Shah SM, Applewar A, Patel C, Shah S, Patel U. OcularTrauma score: a useful predictor of visual outcome at six weeks in patients with traumatic cataract. Ophthalmology. 2012;119(7):1336–41.
46. Olsen TW, Pribila JT. Pars plana vitrectomy with endoscope-guided sutured posterior chamber intraocular lens implantation in children and adults. Am J Ophthalmol. 2001;151(2):287–296.e282.
47. Alzuhairy SA, Bosley TM, Alotaibi AG. Retrospective review of visual outcome in operated lens subluxation. Saudi Med J. 2013;34(10):1030–4.
48. Gul A, Duran M, Can E, Yucel OE, Sullu Y. Surgical management of intraocular lens dislocations. Arq Bras Oftalmol. 2015;78(5):313–7.
49. Michaeli A, Soiberman U, Loewenstein A. Outcome of Iris fixation of subluxated intraocular lenses. Graefes Arch Clin Exp Ophthalmol. 2012;250 (9):1327–32.

50. Mello MO Jr, Scott IU, Smiddy WE, Flynn HW, Feuer W. Surgical management and outcomes of dislocated intraocular lenses. Ophthalmology. 2000;107(1):62–7.
51. Kim SS, Smiddy WE, Feuer W, Shi W. Management of dislocated intraocular lenses. Ophthalmology. 2008;115(10):1699–704.
52. Jakobsson G, Zetterberg M, Sundelin K, Stenevi U. Surgical repositioning of intraocular lenses after late dislocation: complications, effect on intraocular pressure, and visual outcomes. J Cataract Refract Surg. 2013;39(12):1879–85.
53. Gross JG, Kokame GT, Weinberg DV. In-the-bag intraocular lens dislocation. Am J Ophthalmol. 2004;137(4):630–5.
54. Kloek CE, Andreoli MT, Andreoli CM. Characteristics of traumatic cataract wound dehiscence. Am J Ophthalmol. 2011;152(2):229–33.
55. Tseng SH, Lin SC, Chen FK. Traumatic wound dehiscence after penetrating keratoplasty: clinical features and outcome in 21 cases. Cornea. 1999;18(5):553–8.

4 Post-refractive Surgery Trauma

Albert Y. Cheung, Jade M. Price, Samuel T. Gamsky, Chirag K. Gupta and Mark A. Rolain

Refractive Surgery: Introduction

Refractive surgery aims to alter the refractive state of the eye by means of various surgical techniques. In the human eye, the cornea accounts for approximately two-thirds of the eye's total optical/refracting power, while the crystalline lens accounts for the remaining one-third. Refractive surgery utilizes different modalities to modify the refractive power of the cornea, thereby correcting the refractive state of the eye, such as myopia, hyperopia, astigmatism, and presbyopia.

All of these procedures are either incisional, lamellar, photoablative laser, or intrastromal, and they all inherently weaken the native cornea. This inherent weakness may be exposed when the eye suffers a traumatic injury.

In patients with trauma, diagnosis and treatment of life-threatening injuries takes precedence over ophthalmic trauma. While a careful history regarding the nature of the inciting injury is important, even mild or benign appearing trauma may be more damaging in a post-refractive eye. Because of this, one must be more prepared to identify traumatic ophthalmic injuries in this population. In this chapter, we describe various types of refractive surgical procedures that one might encounter in an office, urgent care, and emergency room setting. We describe the types of traumatic injuries that each procedure would lend itself to as well as the management of such traumatic injuries.

A.Y. Cheung · J.M. Price · S.T. Gamsky · C.K. Gupta · M.A. Rolain (✉)
Department of Ophthalmology, William Beaumont Hospital, William Beaumont School of Medicine, Royal Oak, MI, USA
e-mail: m.rolain@universityeyecare.com

S.T. Gamsky
e-mail: stgamsky@oakland.edu

Incisional Refractive Surgery

Incisional Refractive Surgery: Procedures

Radial Keratotomy

Introduction

Radial keratotomy (RK) was pioneered by the Russian ophthalmologist Svyatoslav Fyodorov [1] in the 1970s. This procedure, performed for myopia, utilizes a series of radial incisions into the paracentral and peripheral anterior cornea to decrease the refractive power of the cornea (Fig. 4.1) [1]. This was the primary procedure for treating patients with −1.00 to −4.00 D of myopia until the mid-1990s when photorefractive keratectomy (PRK) and LASIK were approved in the United States. While this procedure is considered obsolete now, it was an important step in developing later refractive techniques.

Procedure

The surgeon makes a number of uniform microscopic cuts with a diamond-blade knife into the cornea to sever the collagen fibrils in the corneal stroma. These cuts are set to a specific

S.C. Kaufman and D.R. Lazzaro (eds.), *Textbook of Ocular Trauma*,
DOI 10.1007/978-3-319-47633-9_4

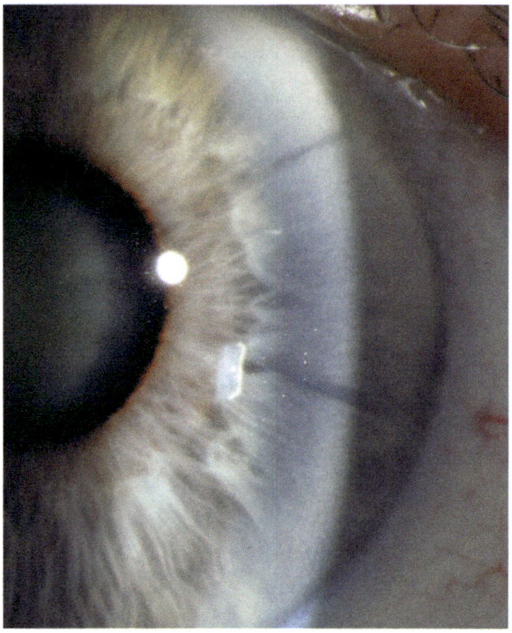

Fig. 4.1 Slit lamp photograph of normal radial keratotomy incisions

depth (ideal depth between 85–90%) and range between 4 and 32 in number. The incisions cause mid peripheral bulging of the cornea with a resultant flattening of the central cornea inducing a hyperopic shift. The diameter of the central optical clear zone is inversely related to the amount of refractive correction; for example, a 3 mm central clear zone yields a greater myopic correction than a 4 mm central clear zone.

Structural Effects of RK on the Cornea

Keratotomy wounds are partial thickness, unsutured, and typically not treated with prolonged topical corticosteroids. There are numerous studies looking at the structure and strength of these wounds in vitro, in both histologic studies and animal models. Histologically, RK incisions produce a sharp demarcated break in Bowman's layer and the stroma causing flattening and posterior bending of the corneal lamellae and Descemet's membrane toward the anterior chamber [2]. Additionally, when an incision exceeds 80% of the stromal thickness, there is loss of the endothelial cells in the areas of the incision [2].

With normal corneal wound healing, an epithelial plug, a bed of corneal epithelial cells that grow into the incision, forms but then regresses within 6–14 days. After 3–6 months, fibrocytes start to migrate to the wound resulting in a scar. The resultant scar, however, never regains its original tensile strength. Contrary to normal corneal wound healing, histological studies have shown that following RK the normal epithelial plug remains in the incision up to five and a half years and active fibroblasts have been shown to persist for many years as well. As a result of these wound changes, there is a wound gape which leads to refractive fluctuations due to changes in stromal wound healing and remodeling. This can be observed by slit lamp examination by observing a gray haze adjacent to the incisions. Due to a break in the continuity of the collagen fibrils once the wound is healed, the wound integrity is never the same as a normal cornea.

The reduced integrity of an RK incision is demonstrated by a case report by Jammal [3] who described multiple RK wound ruptures 20 years after surgery secondary to blunt trauma. Additionally, Glasgow wrote about a case of a 55-year-old male who sustained a traumatic dehiscence of a 7-year-old RK incision [4]. Upon microscopic examination of this patient's enucleation specimen, Glasgow et al. [4] observed persistent epithelial plugs in RK incisions. From this study, the authors hypothesized that the cornea may be susceptible to rupture from blunt trauma due to the presence of the epithelial plugs. Bryant et al. [5] studied human corneas 8 years after RK. They cut the cornea into strips and subjected various areas of the cornea with and without RK incisions to tensile testing by loading weights until rupture occurred. They concluded that indeed epithelial plugs cause a relative weakness in the RK wounds compared to the surrounding stroma.

The most common locations for globe rupture in the normal eye when subjected to blunt trauma are circumferential scleral arcs parallel to the limbus, just posterior to the muscle insertions, and at the equator. Luttrull et al. [6] studied enucleated porcine eyes and found that when incisional depths exceed 70%, there is an increased incidence of corneal rupture after blunt trauma; however, incisions that are 70% and less behaved more like normal globes, rupturing at the equator. Larson et al. [7] found that 98% of wound ruptures in rabbit eyes following 8-incision RK occurred in one or more of the incisions. Studies have also shown that in post-RK eyes, 54% less force was needed to cause a corneal rupture than in control eyes. Additionally, incisions traversing the limbus, microperforations during the surgery, and deeper incisions increased the incidence of a wound rupture. Fewer RK incisions, however, do not appear to be protective as the number of incisions does not appear to affect the likelihood of corneal rupture [8, 9].

Mini-radial keratomy (mini-RK) limits the extent of radial incisions from the 3 mm optical zone to the 7 mm optical zone, compared with "conventional" RK which extends to the 11 mm optical zone. Pinheiro et al. [10] showed that corneas that underwent mini-RK required significantly higher pressures to rupture than corneas that underwent regular RK. Steinmann [11], similarly, demonstrated that longer RK incisions require a lower force to rupture.

Trauma-Associated Complications with RK

Wound Rupture/Dehiscence

One of the worst trauma-related complications that occurs post-RK is a wound rupture. Even among the estimated 2–3 million eyes that have undergone RK [12], wound rupture appears to be relatively uncommon [12]. Based on animal models, the most common rupture pattern was a "cut-to-cut" rupture in which two RK incisions were connected by the rupture site (Fig. 4.2) [7]. The next most common rupture patterns by decreasing frequency are a radial corneoscleral laceration along an RK incision followed by a stellate rupture, in which 3 or more RK incisions rupture and connect to form a single laceration, followed by an "incision-opening" rupture involving a single RK incision without extension [13]. Examples of each of these rupture patterns have been described in case reports in human eyes [8].

Vinger et al. [14] studied the largest case series of 28 RK-related wound ruptures. They found that

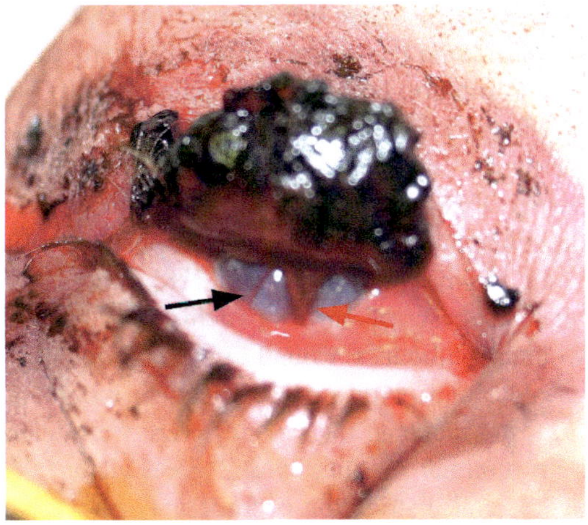

Fig. 4.2 External photograph of an expulsive hemorrhage through a radial keratotomy "cut-to-cut" rupture. Note the *black arrow* indicating an intact RK incision as well as the *red arrow* indicating the "cut-to-cut" rupture. Photograph courtesy of Lori Stec, MD

the rupture extended across the visual axis in over 70% of the eyes, which they suggested occurred due to the close proximity of the incisions to the visual axis. Another hypothesis is that a corneal dehiscence is more likely to propagate along the thinner central corneal tissue [12].

In terms of timing, half of all RK-related reported wound ruptures occur within 2 years of surgery, and about two-thirds within 3 years of surgery [14]. After 3–4 years, there appeared to be a decline in the risk for wound ruptures [14]. This is consistent with experimental models that have shown that the RK wounds are likely more susceptible to trauma earlier on due to abnormal wound healing and presence of epithelial plugs.

We know that some direct force is required to create a RK wound rupture; however, the threshold of force required to create a wound rupture is difficult to quantify. McKnight et al. [15] performed an experiment on adult cat eyes. The cat eyes underwent RK with incision depth set at 90% and were subjected to BB pellet trauma of different velocities. While control eyes, those without RK incisions, developed hyphemas without any corneal ruptures, about one-third of RK eyes that underwent impact with the highest velocity (240 ft/s) developed wound ruptures [15].

Conversely, there are examples of significant ocular trauma that did not result in a keratotomy wound rupture, because the remaining 5–10% of non-incised corneal stroma with Descemet's membrane appears to afford a relatively strong barrier to wound rupture [16]. Authors have described wound gapes that have resulted from blunt trauma [17]. Bouchard [18] described a bilateral case of anterior dehiscence of RK wounds without a wound rupture following a gasoline tank explosion injury. One month out from the incident, the wounds were well-healed with minimal irregularity and good vision. The degree and distribution of force may play a role in whether incisions rupture or just dehisce [18].

Epithelial Downgrowth

Epithelial downgrowth after RK is rare but can occur if deep radial incisions splay open during trauma [19]. The epithelial downgrowth may result from microperforation with implantation of epithelial cells into the anterior chamber from a preexisting epithelial plug that rapidly self-sealed [19]. If suspected, confocal microscopy allows noninvasive in vivo microscopic imaging to diagnose presumed epithelial downgrowth. Argon laser photocoagulation can only be used to confirm the diagnosis in cases with iris involvement.

Incisional Changes Without Dehiscence

Even without obvious trauma to the incisions on slit lamp examination, the incisions may still be affected. Forstot [20] reported a case of moderate, direct trauma that was significant enough to cause a subconjunctival hemorrhage and traumatic iritis. Although there was no opening of the RK incisions, they measured an increased keratometric cylinder of 1.5 diopters, which regressed spontaneously.

Incisional Infectious Keratitis

While relatively rare, infectious keratitis following RK may occur in the early or late postoperative period. Trauma has been found to be a risk factor for late-onset incisional keratitis as a source of microorganisms. Incisional keratitis may present with an infiltrate along the incision, conjunctival injection, surrounding corneal edema, with or without an anterior chamber reaction or hypopyon (Fig. 4.3). Pseudocysts within keratotomy wounds may be predisposing factors as they can lead to easier access for bacteria or occasionally break down, resulting in microscopic or macroscopic

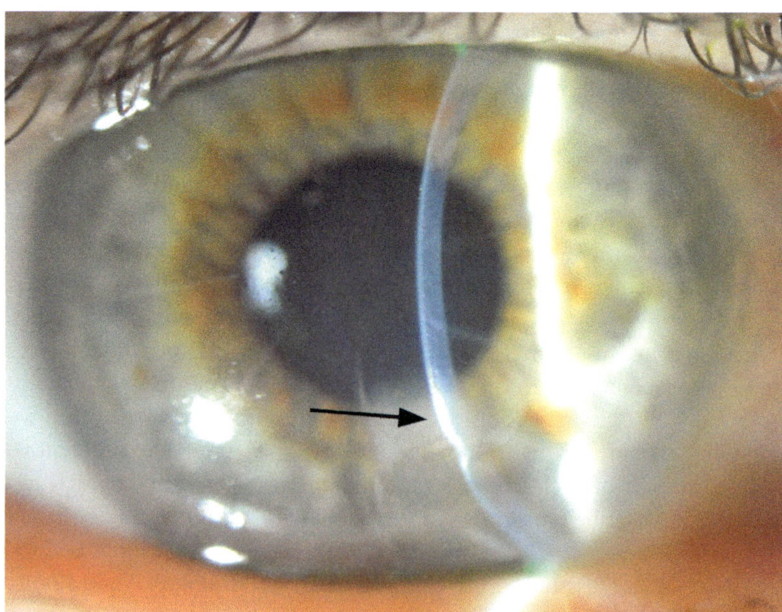

Fig. 4.3 Slit lamp photograph of infectious infiltrate along a radial keratotomy incision. Note the *black arrow* indicating the location of the infiltrate

erosions [21]. Incisional keratotomy infections can potentially lead to endophthalmitis.

Iatrogenic RK Incision Damage

Patients with previous RK can present a challenge when other ocular surgeries are necessary. Similar to blunt trauma, secondary surgical procedures can have an effect on RK wounds. There have been reports describing rupture of RK incisions during corneal transplant trephination, keratomileusis, phacoemulsification [18, 19, 22, 23], scleral buckling, and scleral depression [16].

Astigmatic Keratotomy

Introduction

Corneal astigmatism (mainly regular astigmatism) can be addressed by several astigmatic keratotomy techniques, often performed concurrently with cataract surgery. There are both incisional and ablative methods available to reduce or correct astigmatism. Astigmatic keratotomy incisional options (Fig. 4.4 a) include tangential (horizontal/linear) keratotomy, arcuate keratotomy (AK), and limbal relaxing incisions (LRI). All of these incisions are corneal relaxing incisions made parallel to the limbus that lead to flattening in the meridian of the incision and steeping in the meridian 90° away. With tangential and arcuate incisions, the incisions are placed closer to the visual axis compared to an LRI incision. Since AK incisions are closer to the visual axis, this may amplify any errors if there is misalignment between the planned and treated axes. In contrast, LRI incisions are more peripheral, mitigating the potential for error and preserving the central corneal optical clarity. There is less patient discomfort with the LRI incisions and fewer corneal irregularities leading to reduced glare. More recently, the femtosecond laser has become an additional platform that can create precise AK incisions (Fig. 4.4b).

LRI Procedure

For axis orientation, the cornea is marked at 12 and 6 o'clock in the upright position. After the patient has been positioned supine, the treatment axis and incision lengths can be marked based on

(a) (b)

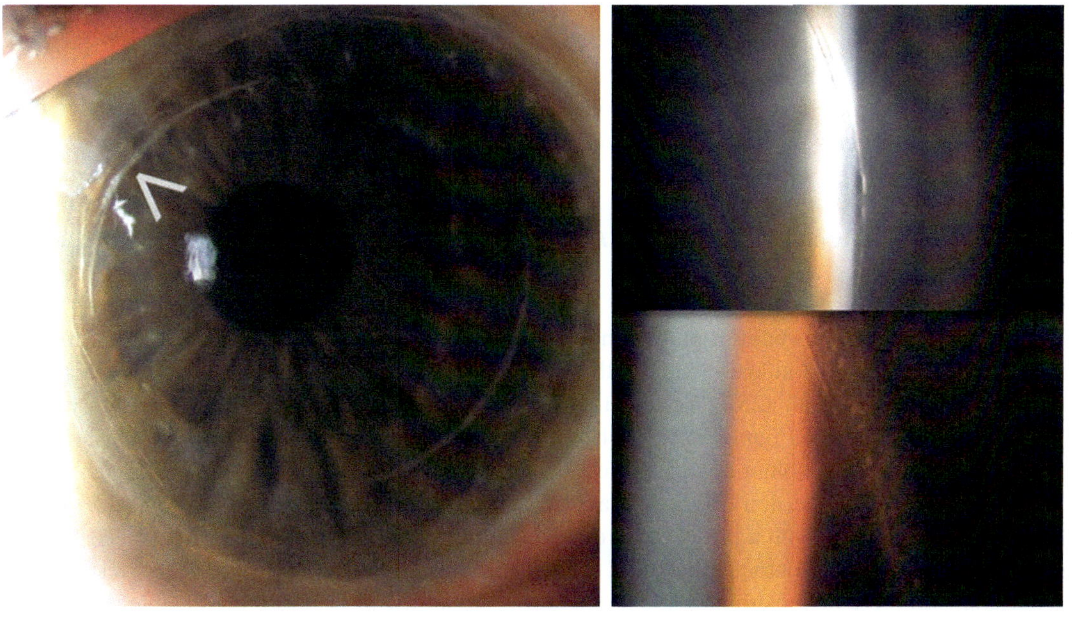

Fig. 4.4 **a** Slit lamp photograph of a normal astigmatic keratotomy. **b** Slit lamp photograph of femtosecond laser creation of limbal relaxing incision

the prior reference marks. Arcuate and tangential keratotomies can be performed either manually using a keratome or a diamond knife (often front-cutting), or by means of the femtosecond laser. These incisions are made approximately 95% depth in the steep meridian of the mid-peripheral cornea at the 7 mm optical zone. There are nomograms available, based on pre-operative degree of cylinder and patient age, to direct a surgeon as to the placement of incisions.

The LRI incision is commonly made using a diamond knife (often back-cutting), although disposable and reusable metal LRI knives are also available. Both types often have preset depths for surgeon convenience, and the usual depth is 600 microns (range 450–650 microns) or 50 microns less than the thinnest limbal corneal thickness.

Structural Effects of AK on the Cornea

Deg et al. [24] found that wound healing after astigmatic keratotomy appears similar to the healing process following standard radial keratotomy with the exception that AK incisions promoted faster wound healing. This was attributed to the better apposition of tangential incisions while semi-radial/radial incisions tend to gape as a result of the mechanical stress of intraocular pressure (IOP). Tangential incisions were also found to have a shallower depth which can both aid in better wound healing as well as corneal structural integrity.

Trauma-Associated Complications with AK

Wound Rupture/Dehiscence

There are reports of AK wound rupture although it has only been reported in association with RK wound rupture. Lee et al. [25] reported a case where 4 out of 8 RK and 1 out of 1 AK incisions dehisced following direct blunt trauma to the eye. The 45-degree arcuate incision had been made at a 7.00 mm optical zone with a preset blade depth of 105% of the central corneal thickness [25]. Eggleston [26] presented a similar patient where half of the RK incisions were completely or partially ruptured, and a single transverse incision (2–3 mm from the limbus) also ruptured following blunt trauma. The radial incision ruptures had intersected the transverse incision to combine both into one rupture wound.

Jammal et al. [3] reported traumatic wound dehiscence appearing only in RK scars but not in any of the four transverse incision scars. It is unclear whether the decreased likelihood of AK incision dehiscence is based on a difference in geometry, incision orientation, or location in thicker corneal tissue. Both RK and AK incisions are typically placed at a similar depth in the cornea; however, the amount of residual intact corneal tissue is larger with transverse incisions, possibly making them less vulnerable to rupture. To date, there are no reports of isolated rupture of astigmatic keratotomy incisions or LRIs.

Incisional Infectious Keratitis

Incisions from AK are at risk for late-onset infectious keratitis following trauma in a similar manner as RK incisions (See Infectious Keratitis section under RK).

Intrastromal Corneal Ring Segments (ICRS)

Introduction

The concept of an intrastromal corneal implant was introduced in 1978 by Reynolds [27]; however, it was not used until 1991 when the first complete polymethyl methacrylate (PMMA) ring was inserted into the stroma for the correction of myopia. The procedure subsequently evolved from complete ring insertion to the insertion of two C-shaped rings in order to avoid insertion-related complications. The initial indication for the ICRS procedure was low myopia (−1.00 D to −3.00 D) and emerged as a unique, potentially removable refractive surgical device that does not invade the central optical zone [28]. The procedure has since been replaced by photoablative corneal surgery as the results have been shown to be more predictable. ICRS have been adopted for the treatment of corneal ectasia

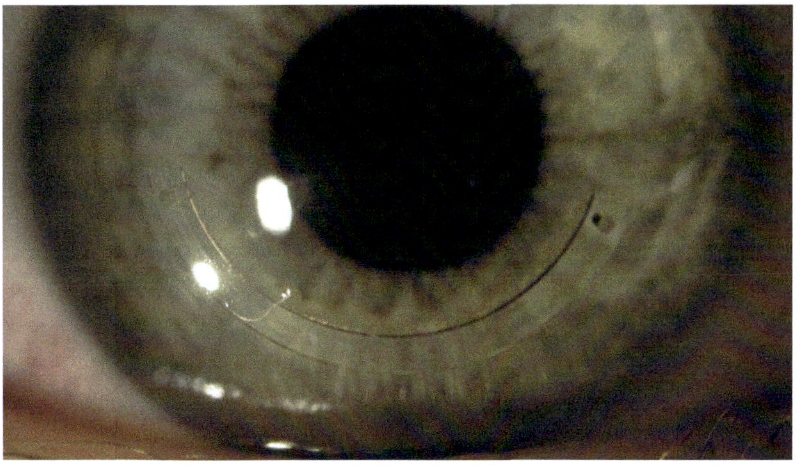

Fig. 4.5 Slit lamp photograph of a normal intrastromal ring placed inferiorly

following LASIK [29] as well as severe keratoconus for treatment of irregular astigmatism and corneal instability (Fig. 4.5) [30, 31].

Procedure

The surgeon marks the geometric center of the cornea with a Sinsky hook as a reference point. This procedure may be performed mechanically or with femtosecond laser-assisted technology. To complete the surgery mechanically, a 1 mm radial incision at 70–80% of the corneal thickness is created with a diamond blade knife along the steepest meridian. During the next step of the procedure, two continuous stromal tunnels are dissected by blunt separation of corneal lamellae for the insertion of the intrastromal ring segments. The dissected tunnels are created at 80% stromal depth with inner and outer diameters of 6.50 and 8.10 mm respectively. This step may be performed using a semi-automated suction ring and semicircular dissectors or using femtosecond laser technology. When using femtosecond laser technology, a single continuous circular tunnel is created rather than two tunnels. The ring segments are then manually inserted into the stromal tunnel. The radial incision may then be closed with glue or 10-0 Nylon suture.

Structural Effects of ICRS on the Cornea

The structural goal of refractive surgery for the correction of myopia is to flatten the cornea. The insertion of ICRS achieves this goal by the "arc shortening effect" in which the segment acts as a spacer between arching bundles of corneal lamellae therefore shortening the central corneal arc length. The stroma anterior to the ring segment is elevated while the posterior cornea is steepened resulting in central cornea flattening [32]. Without invading the central optical zone, this procedure induces morphologic change to reduce corneal steepening and astigmatism. Therefore, it does not depend on the healing properties of the cornea in order to have an effect.

There are four types of intrastromal ring segments that differ in various characteristics including the shape of the ring cross-section, arc length, radius, and thickness. These include INTACs, Ferrara rings, Bisantis segments, and the Myoring. The INTACs are the only intrastromal segment rings approved by the FDA in the United States. This segment has a hexagonal cross-section and is created with either a conical or oval longitudinal section. The ring thickness and proximity to the visual axis are two parameters that most directly induce the refractive changes created by ICRS insertion. In normal human corneal tissue, there is an almost linear relationship between the thickness of the segment and the degree of corneal flattening [33, 34].

Clinical and histologic studies of human corneas following ICRS show lamellar channel deposits of intracellular lipids around the segments that currently have unknown significance.

Histologic evaluation of corneal stroma in rabbits following ICRS by Twa et al. [35] demonstrated new keratocyte activation, intracellular lipid accumulation, and new collagen formation.

Trauma-Associated Complications with ICRS
There are reports of patients with ICRS and history of microtrauma who present with intermittent worsening of vision that improve with rubbing the eye. On slit lamp examination, it was noted that the intrastromal ring segments migrated, leading to superimposed distal segments. Surgical repositioning and ring segment fixation can be performed with 10-0 nylon suture to the cornea for stabilization of the intrastromal ring segments. In this case, a complete circular tunnel created by the femtosecond laser technique may have provided more opportunity for ring migration and override [36]. Other traumatic complications could include extruded segments and segments penetrating into the anterior chamber.

Incisional Refractive Surgery: Examination

Evaluation requires a complete general and ophthalmic examination. Similar to other types of eye-related trauma, when approaching a patient with a history of refractive surgery, it is important to differentiate a penetrating wound (passes into a structure) from a perforating wound (passes through a structure). Vigilant examination with a narrow slit beam can help determine the depth of the incision and/or injury. If not obvious, a Seidel test with fluorescein can confirm one's suspicion for a perforating corneal injury (Fig. 4.6). In addition, patients with ICRS should be examined for malposition including overriding segments, extruded segments, and segments penetrating into the anterior chamber.

Incisional Refractive Surgery: Treatment

For most wound ruptures, definitive treatment will require closure with sutures, typically 10-0 nylon (Fig. 4.7). At times, the rupture may be small and self-sealed. In these cases, a bandage contact lens (BCL) may be considered along with aqueous suppressants. A BCL may also be used to treat a partial thickness laceration/dehiscence.

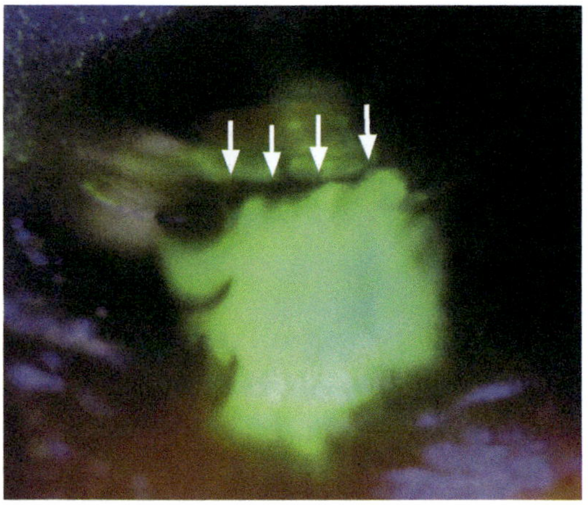

Fig. 4.6 Slit lamp photograph of Seidel positive wound. Note the *white arrows* indicating the wound. Photograph courtesy of David Heidemann, MD

As the cornea is the primary refracting component of the eye, wound repair can often induce decreased visual acuity secondary to scar formation and irregular astigmatism. Keratometry and corneal topography may help evaluate for irregular astigmatism. Rigid gas permeable (RGP) contact lenses can often provide improved visual acuity by correcting irregular astigmatism. This can be combined with a soft prosthetic contact lens for cosmesis (piggyback contact lens system).

Once the RK cornea has sustained injury and ruptured, some have advocated that suture removal should be avoided after the initial repair, especially if the sutures are not causing irregular astigmatism. Sony [37] reported a repeat dehiscence of 18-year-old RK incisions two days following suture removal 14 months after the initial wound repair.

As a broad spectrum of microorganisms have been found to cause incisional keratitis, management should include initial cultures and aggressive treatment with broad spectrum anti-microbials until the offending microorganism is identified.

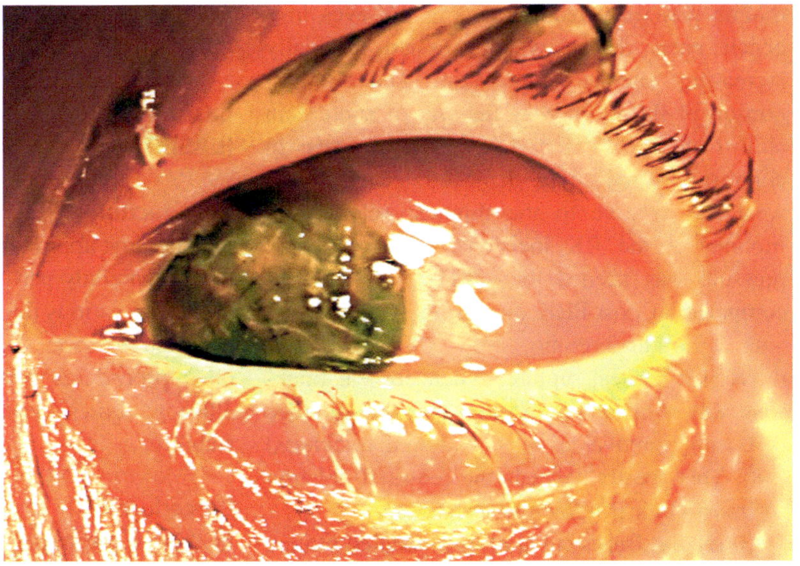

Fig. 4.7 External photograph of repaired radial keratotomy incisions with 10-0 nylon following rupture. Photograph courtesy of Lori Stec, MD

Laser Refractive Surgery

Laser Refractive Surgery: Procedures

Photorefractive Keratectomy (PRK)

Introduction

PRK utilizes the excimer laser to change the shape of the cornea similar to laser-assisted in situ keratomileusis (LASIK); however, in PRK, there is no flap creation. PRK emerged after RK as a new way to change the refractive state of the cornea without the disadvantages that can accompany RK incisions, including the potential susceptibility to trauma. While the final visual acuity results of PRK surgery are comparable to LASIK outcomes, PRK visual recovery is initially slower because it takes weeks for the epithelial layer to regenerate and form a stable refractive corneal surface. The entire thickness of the underlying stroma is available for treatment because a flap including epithelium and anterior stroma is not removed. Phototherapeutic keratectomy (PTK) is practically the same technique as PRK but typically refers to using the excimer laser for treatment of other corneal diseases (instead of refractive indications).

Procedure

Following topical anesthetic, the corneal epithelium in the ablation zone is first removed to allow for accurate ablation of the stromal tissue. This is often accomplished by placing a circular well over the ablation zone and filling it with 20% absolute alcohol for 20–45 s. Once the epithelium is loosened, it can be removed with a weck-cell sponge. Other debridement techniques include using a sharp blade, blunt spatula, rotary brush, or transepithelial ablation by the excimer laser. The excimer laser can then be applied to the exposed corneal stroma. Following the treatment, a BCL is then placed over the cornea. Topical antibiotic, NSAIDs, and corticosteroid are administered postoperatively. Visual acuity slowly improves after the epithelium heals and the refractive state stabilizes 3–6 months following surgery.

Structural Effects of PRK on the Cornea

Several studies have looked at whether PRK can potentially weaken the cornea structurally and increase the likelihood of damage with trauma. Campos et al. [38] tested a 10-diopter PRK treatment in porcine eyes with lateral compression blunt trauma and found that these post-PRK eyes behaved similarly to unoperated eyes. The trauma was delivered by placing the eyes in a bench press device which applied gradually increasing lateral compression. The thinnest portion of the sclera was the site of rupture in almost all post-PRK and nonoperated eyes. In contrast, post-RK eyes demonstrated structural weakness relative to the thinnest sclera with ruptures at the RK incisions. Lower average pressure was needed to rupture post-RK eyes compared to post-PRK eyes. Interestingly, porcine eyes undergoing deep PTK ablations developed corneal ruptures when corneal thickness was reduced to 0.45 mm from an average 0.90 mm (removal of >40% stromal thickness) [38]. This greatly exceeds the required ablation for most clinical refractive scenarios.

Similarly, Burnstein et al. [39] studied human eye-bank eyes and subjected them to PRK treatment ranging between 6 and 54 diopters. They demonstrated that PRK does not weaken the corneal integrity with ablation depths commonly used in the clinical setting. In their experiment, IOP was increased gradually using nitrogen gas in human eye-bank eyes until the globes ruptured. Rupture only occurred at the ablation site with ablations greater than 37% of corneal thickness and pressures greater than 65 psi [39]. Most clinical PRK protocols do not exceed 15% of corneal thickness. Using a similar pressurizing system, Alcaraz et al. [40] looked at wound integrity following excimer laser photoablation compared to RK. There was leakage at the incision only in the RK group and burst pressures were significantly lower in the RK group. Galler [41] found that PRK in porcine eyes does not affect ocular integrity after blunt trauma when subjected to a squash ball impacting the cornea axially.

Trauma-Associated Complications with PRK

There are no reported cases of isolated globe rupture after PRK treatment to date. Artola [42] reported a case of ruptured RK incisions following blunt trauma 6 years after combined RK/PRK. Four of the eight radial incisions ruptured with extrusion of intraocular tissues. They believed that PRK carried out on a thin cornea already weakened by RK may have compromised the structural integrity of the eye.

Laser-Assisted in Situ Keratomileusis (LASIK)

Introduction

LASIK, first approved in 1999, is now one of the most commonly performed refractive procedures to correct various degrees of myopia, hyperopia, and astigmatism. LASIK has replaced many other procedures because of its relative safety, efficacy, quick visual recovery, and visual stability.

Procedure

In this procedure, a corneal suction ring is first applied to the topically anesthetized eye. Traditionally, a microkeratome was used to create a 300° flap of corneal tissue by creating an incision along the corneal stromal lamellae to separate the epithelium, Bowman's layer, and the anterior stroma from the rest of the remaining posterior stroma. More recently, the femtosecond laser has been commonly used to create this flap (Fig. 4.8). The laser has allowed surgeons to optimize the flap dimensions and create a more precise flap. This flap is then reflected back at the hinge, the 60° that was not incised, to reveal the stroma.

Next, the excimer laser is used to reshape the residual corneal stromal bed using precisely guided pulses to disrupt the stromal carbon–carbon bonds. This ultraviolet laser energy can be titrated to an exact depth, which makes it ideal for manipulating the surface of the stroma. Once the stroma has been ablated to achieve the intended optical shift, the corneal flap is then refloated and repositioned on the stromal bed. Healing then takes place over the next several days to weeks.

Structural Effects of LASIK on the Cornea

The LASIK flaps created by the microkeratome and femtosecond laser have been studied histologically. After the first day following LASIK, the epithelial layer starts to regenerate at the flap

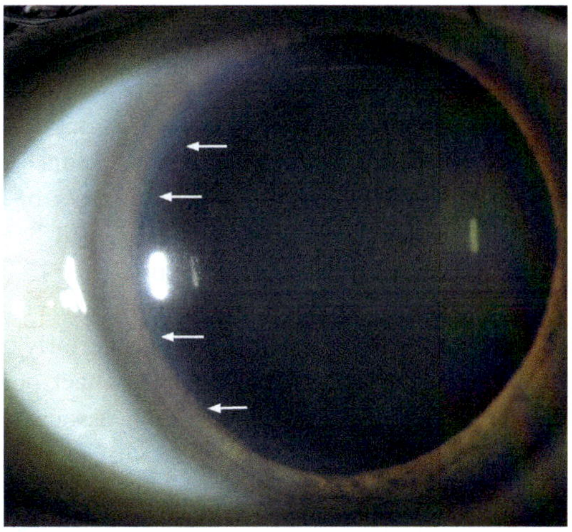

Fig. 4.8 Slit lamp photograph of a normal LASIK flap created by a femtosecond laser. Note *arrow* indicating the flap edge

margin. Over the next several weeks, a collagenous scar forms at the LASIK flap edge between the severed edges of Bowman's layer.

There are two types of reparative stromal wound healing responses associated with LASIK surgery: a hypercellular fibrotic scar at the flap-wound margin (this holds the corneal flap in place) and a weaker transparent, hypocellular primitive scar in central/paracentral areas of the lamellar wound [43]. The hypocellular primitive scar develops without reconnection of severed collagen lamellae, and the scar regains only 2.4% of normal stromal strength without evidence of remodeling even 6.5 years after LASIK surgery [44]. The LASIK flap-wound margin heals in a more complete manner, averaging 28.1% of normal corneal stromal strength [43–46].

Wound healing appears to only occur superficially (in the epithelial cell layers) as the collagen lamellae do not bond with each other in the area of the primitive scar. This can explain why the biomechanical properties of the post-LASIK cornea are primarily determined by the residual stromal bed with the LASIK flap only contributing minimally to the tectonic corneal strength and stability [47, 48]. Peacock et al. [49] studied the force needed to cause ocular rupture in RK, LASIK, automated lamellar keratoplasty (ALK), and PRK cadaver eyes. All operated eyes required less energy to rupture as compared with that of control eyes; however, unlike RK eyes, the level of energy required to rupture PRK and LASIK eyes were much greater [49].

Due to this wound healing, the interface between the flap and underlying stromal bed interface can be detected several years after its creation, with a clear absence of reconnection between adjacent severed lamellae despite close approximation of the flap-stromal interface. This lack of reconnection between the flap-stromal interface is what contributes to traumatic dislocations of the LASIK flap even many years following surgery. Two rabbit model studies have compared the force required to dislodge LASIK flaps at 1, 3 months, and at 75 days [50]. In both studies, femtosecond flaps were significantly stronger than their microkeratome counterparts. That being said, the flaps do take a substantial amount of force to create a dehiscence. This has been demonstrated by numerous authors; for example, the force from a cockpit ejection seat simulator was insufficient to dislodge microkeratome LASIK flaps 1 month after surgery in a rabbit model [51]. Additionally, subjecting rabbit eyes to high-speed wind trauma as early as 24 h after LASIK found microkeratome flaps to be stable, probably as a combined result of epithelial bridging across the flap edge and the osmotic gradient across the interface [52].

Mousavi et al. [53] simulated the effect of a blunt foreign body in PRK and LASIK eye models using finite element analysis. They showed that rupture occurs at higher velocities in the corneal stromal bed of the LASIK model than in the cornea of the PRK model [53]. In the clinical range of application of the excimer laser for PRK and LASIK (corneal thickness 500–350 μm), the required velocity for corneal rupture decreases nonlinearly with reduced corneal thickness. This reflects the reduction in impact force that occurs when the force is transferred from the upper separated corneal flap to the lower stromal bed in the LASIK model.

Trauma-Associated Complications with LASIK

Flap Dislocation/Displacement

While it is most vulnerable for spontaneous dislocation during the period immediately following surgery, the corneal flap created in LASIK is at a risk of dislocation at any time following ocular trauma secondary to the limited healing at the flap-stromal interface (Fig. 4.9). Following trauma with a substantial force, patients may present with either a dislocated corneal flap or a completely detached flap. Traumatic flap dislocation may occur in up to 1% of patients (and can predispose patients to a host of other subsequent complications, such as epithelial ingrowth, diffuse lamellar keratitis, infectious keratitis, and interface foreign bodies [54].

Dislocation or subluxation of the flap is possible, even many years after the procedure is performed. Cases of dislocation up to 14 years after the initial LASIK procedure have been reported. Because of the absence of reconnection between adjacent severed lamellae at the flap-stromal interface, a flap dislocation, theoretically, will always be a risk [55].

Flap Avulsion and Tears

Compared to flap dislocations, a flap avulsion is much less common [56]. Trauma to completely detach a flap likely requires substantial shearing force at a particular angle to sever the hinge. Because of the resultant irregular astigmatism, RGP lens fitting may be necessary to optimize visual acuity. Loss of the flap may induce a refractive error, reported up to 6 diopters of a myopic shift. PRK with Mitomycin C can be a potential option to treat this refractive error [57].

If not completely avulsed, a flap tear can result in the flap being flipped either anteriorly or posteriorly relative to the remaining intact portion of the flap [58]. This has been associated with epithelial ingrowth at the areas of exposed stroma (Fig. 4.10). The exposed stromal bed may also develop opacities that are visually significant. Even with slit lamp examination, there may be difficulty identifying the proper orientation of a flipped flap. Anterior segment optical coherence tomography (OCT) can be valuable in these situations. Its high magnification and resolution can identify the orientation of the flap and can reveal the location of epithelial ingrowth.

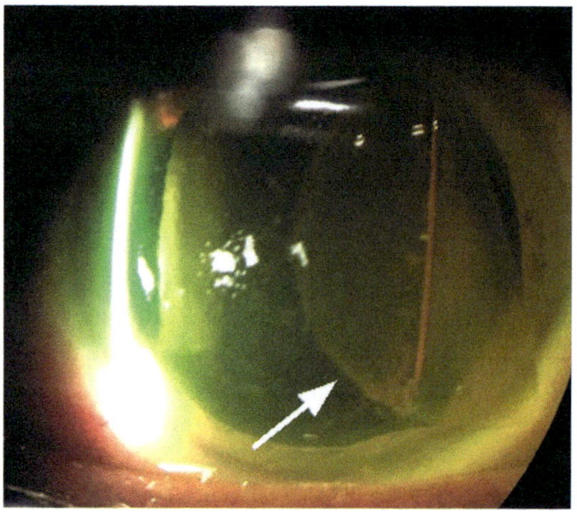

Fig. 4.9 Slit lamp photograph of a dislocated LASIK flap. Note the *arrow* indicating the dislocated flap edge. Photograph courtesy of Aparna Shah, MD

Corneal Penetrating/Perforating Injuries

When corneal injuries occur in patients with a history of LASIK, one must evaluate how both the flap and the stromal bed have been affected. Careful slit lamp examination can help determine partial and full-thickness injuries. The Seidel test may be falsely negative in a corneal perforation if the flap is slightly offset from the stromal bed because the aqueous fluid may accumulate in the interface and may not be apparent on the epithelial surface (see next section: Interface Fluid Syndrome).

Interface Fluid Syndrome (or Pressure-Induced Stromal Keratopathy [PISK])

Lamellar interface fluid accumulation is a well-described LASIK complication described by Lyle and Jin that is typically seen following corticosteroid-related IOP elevation [59]. Here, fluid collects in the interface potential space as aqueous humor diffuses into the corneal stroma in the setting of compromised endothelium. Interface fluid syndrome has also been reported following blunt, penetrating/perforating, and barotrauma [60–62]. The time from ocular trauma to development

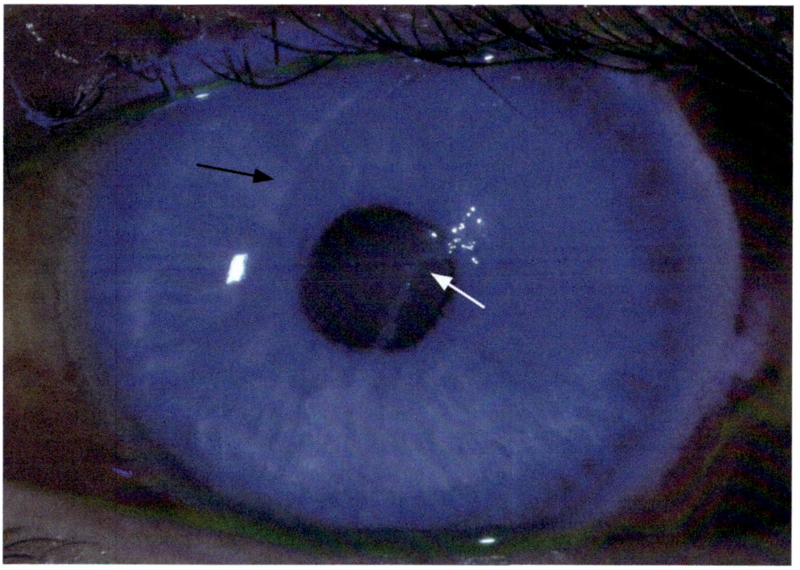

Fig. 4.10 Slit lamp photograph of a partially amputated LASIK flap with re-epithelialization over the bare stroma. Note the *black arrow* indicating the edge of the remaining flap. Note also the *white arrow* indicating the ridge of epithelium growing over the bare stroma. Photograph courtesy of Marius Miron

of interface fluid syndrome is much shorter (~2–3 days) than that associated with corticosteroids (typically after 10–21 days of use). Anterior segment OCT may prove valuable as the interface fluid may masquerade as interface hyperreflection (haze)/keratitis on slit lamp examination. Bushley et al. [62] reported a case of a paracentral full-thickness corneal laceration in an eye with prior LASIK that developed microcystic edema confined to the flap and fluid in the interface following initial laceration repair with 10-0 nylon. An additional 10-0 nylon suture was placed in the area of presumed posterior wound gape, and there was resolution of the microcystic edema and interface fluid within 24 h. In blunt trauma, as there is no direct pathway for fluid to sequester in the interface, it has been hypothesized that direct traumatic force to the flap and anterior chamber inflammation contribute to the formation of interface fluid (Fig. 4.11). For interface fluid syndrome associated with blunt trauma, treatment with anti-glaucoma medications and corticosteroids often leads to resolution.

Diffuse Lamellar Keratitis

Diffuse lamellar keratitis (DLK) is a well-known complication of LASIK, with overall incidence in most published series reported as less than 3% [63]. It was first described by Robert Maddox as "Sands of Sahara Syndrome," [64] and it was later termed "DLK" by Smith and Maloney [65]. DLK classically develops 2–6 days following LASIK (Fig. 4.12a, b) and typically resolves 5–8 days after the initiation of appropriate therapy

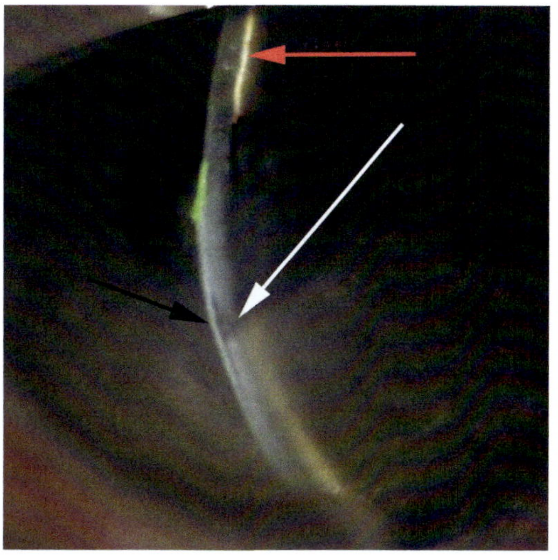

Fig. 4.11 Slit lamp photograph of an intact LASIK flap with an underlying stromal perforation. The *red arrow* indicates a flat anterior chamber. The *black arrow* indicates the intact LASIK flap. The *white arrow* indicates the perforation site. Between the *black* and *white arrows* demonstrates fluid within the interface. Photograph courtesy of David Heidemann, MD

(corticosteroids with or without lifting the flap) [65]. Although more rare, there have also been reported cases of late-onset DLK ranging from months to years after surgery with trauma being one of the more common triggering etiologies. This demonstrates the persistence of the potential space made upon flap creation.

Traumatic epithelial defects, blunt trauma [66], flap dislocation [67], metallic foreign body [68], and surgical trauma (including conductive keratoplasty [69], epithelial debridement [70], and cross-linking) [71] have all been associated with late-onset DLK. The etiology of late-onset DLK is not well understood. While early-onset DLK has been thought to be an inflammatory reaction to certain exogenous exposures, late-onset cases may illustrate how the interface continues to remain unhealed many years after lamellar surgery, resulting in a potential space for endogenous inflammatory debris/cells to collect in this space [72].

Epithelial Ingrowth

Epithelial ingrowth is a complication in which epithelial cells in the peripheral flap interface advance inwards along the lamellar interface (Fig. 4.13). It can be an early postoperative complication or can accompany trauma involving full or partial dehiscence of the corneal flap [73]. Epithelial ingrowth typically advances from the periphery where the flap was disrupted; however, any corneal penetrating/perforating injury along the flap can be associated with epithelial ingrowth in that area.

Flap Folds

Flap folds, otherwise known as striae, can appear within the first 24 h, but most occur within the first week following LASIK. They are classified as either macrostriae or microstriae. Macrostriae represent full-thickness folds and microstriae represent partial thickness folds. There have been cases of striae reported without corneal flap dislocation following trauma years after the initial photorefractive surgery [74]. It is important to consider the formation of striae when examining LASIK patients with ocular trauma even in the absence of flap slipping, subluxation, or dislocation. Flap striae tend to occur more frequently in cases of delayed presentations following trauma.

(a) (b)

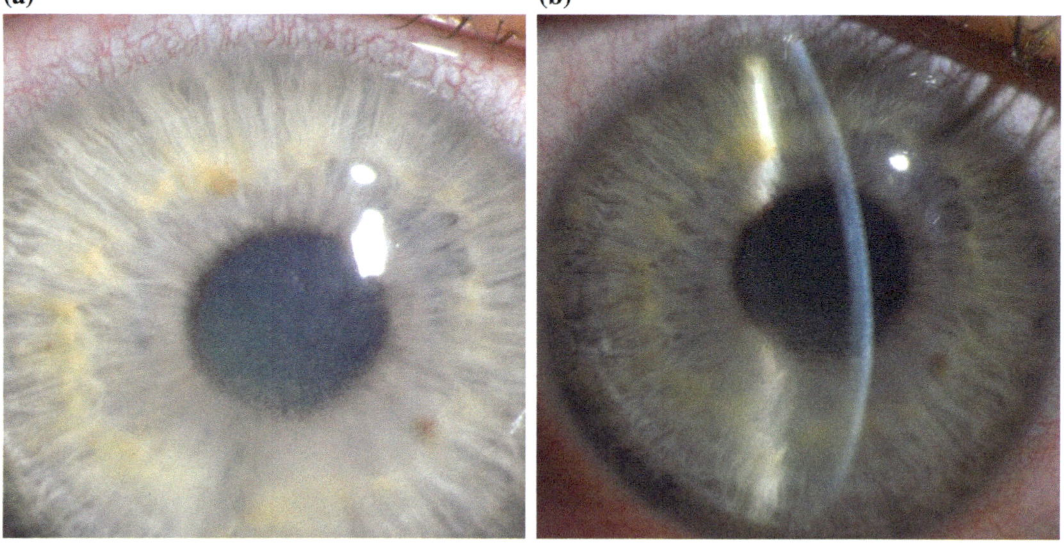

Fig. 4.12 Slit lamp photograph of a diffuse lamellar keratitis (DLK). There LASIK flap demonstrating a ground glass appearance consistent with inflammation confined to the flap. **a** Diffuse illumination redemonstrating the ground glass appearance. **b** Slit beam illumination inflammation confined to LASIK

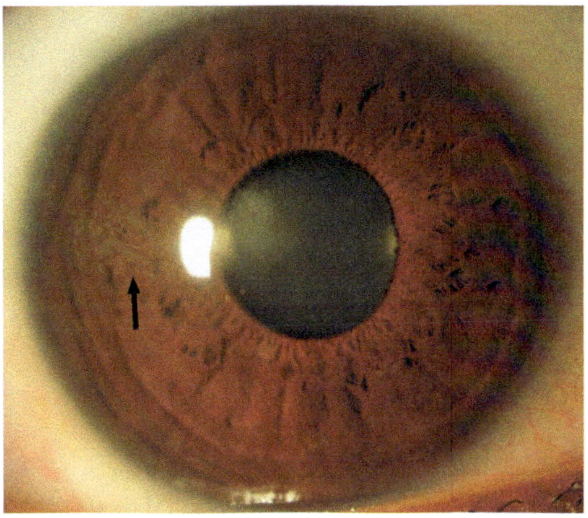

Fig. 4.13 Slit lamp photograph with direct illumination shows epithelial ingrowth at the edge of the LASIK flap between 9 and 10 o'clock growing towards the central cornea. Note the *black area* is denoting the area of epithelial ingrowth

Histological studies with rabbit corneas that have undergone LASIK and developed corneal flap folds have demonstrated that the formation of macrostriae leads to neutrophil infiltration around the incisional area, as well as irregular epithelial growth due to the disruption in the epithelial basement membrane [75]. This inflammatory reaction and asymmetrical hyperplasia fixes the folds into place, which leads to persistent visual deficits.

Folds can be visualized with a slit lamp under direct illumination or via fluorescein stain. If untreated, folds may cause a decrease in acuity. Smaller striae that are asymptomatic with no loss of BCVA may resolve spontaneously. Larger flap folds may not be responsive to flap massage, and may require sutures.

Infectious Keratitis (IK)

Trauma increases the risk of infectious keratitis in patients who have previously undergone LASIK. Infectious keratitis can have very severe complications, which include decreased visual acuity, pain, flap melting, astigmatism, and corneal scarring. Infectious keratitis may be differentiated from DLK in that the latter is usually confined to the plane of the flap creation, whereas infectious keratitis can extend above and below the interface and appear as an area of focal inflammation. The risk for infectious keratitis persists for years following a LASIK procedure. Vieira et al. described two cases developing 2 and 6 years after the initial procedure [76]. Counseling on these long term possible complications is vital to minimize the chance of infection throughout the patient's life.

Time between the procedure and onset of symptoms can be indicative of the etiology of the patient's symptoms. For cases occurring within 10 days of LASIK surgery, the responsible organisms are likely to be gram positive bacteria. Infections with later onset are more likely to be atypical mycobacteria or fungi (Fig. 4.14). Infections with nontuberculous mycobacteria may be confused with that caused by herpes simplex virus and may require surgical debridement [77]. Trauma can be a risk factor for late-onset infections, especially fungal keratitis [78, 79]. The clinical course of acute bacterial and fungal keratitis following trauma (especially with organic matter) in the post-LASIK patient may also be consistent with acanthamoeba. Although acanthamoeba keratitis is a rare cause of posttraumatic microbial keratitis, up to 25% of patients who develop acanthamoeba keratitis have an antecedent history of trauma [80]. Kaur et al. [81] demonstrated that acanthamoeba can divide and spread rapidly in the LASIK flap and deeper layers of the stroma.

Any infiltrate after LASIK should be considered infectious until proven otherwise. LASIK eyes are predisposed to infections compared to unoperated eyes. LASIK flaps may induce a permanent entry point in the peripheral cornea for microorganisms, allowing for delayed keratitis. Additionally, an epithelial break occurring any time after LASIK allows superficial microorganisms to penetrate the flap and reach the interface [82]. An infection may progress more rapidly as it can spread within the interface potential space. Interface infections can be more difficult to treat as the microorganisms are protected from the natural ocular surface defenses, and the antimicrobials do not penetrate well [78].

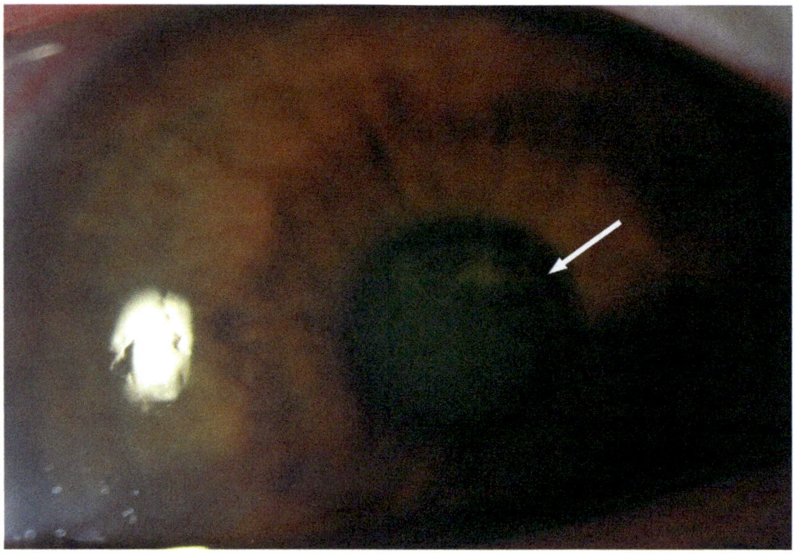

Fig. 4.14 Slit lamp photograph showing a focal area of opacification indicative of infectious keratitis secondary to atypical mycobacteria. Note the *white arrow* indicating the infiltrate

Interface Foreign Bodies

As described earlier, the flap-stromal interface is vulnerable given the limited healing that occurs. Foreign bodies and debris can be introduced into this potential space with or without an associated flap dislocation. While flap dislocation introduces a clear entrance to the interface for foreign body debris, Choi and Kim [83] described a case where crystalline material debris was introduced following trauma from a tree sprig. This caused a corneal abrasion without any flap dislocation. The presumed mechanism involved sharp ocular trauma with high velocity that may open the potential space and leave foreign body debris in the LASIK interface. The interface debris can also incite an inflammatory reaction.

Iatrogenic Flap Damage

Patients with previous LASIK can present a challenge when other ocular surgeries are necessary. Other ophthalmic surgical procedures can damage or alter the LASIK flap. Sakurai et al. [84] describe a case of a flap dehiscence during a scleral buckle procedure. Flap displacement has also been reported during epithelial debridement during vitrectomy surgery [85, 86]. In a technique to avoid flap displacement, Lopez-Guajardo et al. [87] advocate suturing a contact lens over the LASIK flap. Over this, a lens ring (OLV-1; Ocular instruments Inc., Bellevue, WA) is sutured to the sclera. Before suturing the lens ring, they place a drop of viscoelastic in the interface between contact lens and corneal surface.

Trauma to post-LASIK eyes may uncover an underlying subclinical ectasia process. Mearza et al. [88] described a patient who presented with bilateral reduced vision following a traffic accident where there was airbag deployment. Examination revealed intact LASIK flaps, bilateral inferior steepening on topography, and corneal pachymetry of 377 OD and 392 OS. They hypothesized that the airbag trauma created enough force to manifest an underlying subclinical ectasia.

While LASIK in itself does not appear to structurally weaken the globe in prior in vivo studies, post-LASIK ectasia may predispose to rupture following trauma secondary to increased thinning in the ectatic areas.

Small Incision Lenticule Extraction (SMILE)

Introduction

Small Incision Lenticule Extraction (SMILE) is a recently developed femtosecond laser-based refractive surgery procedure. In this procedure,

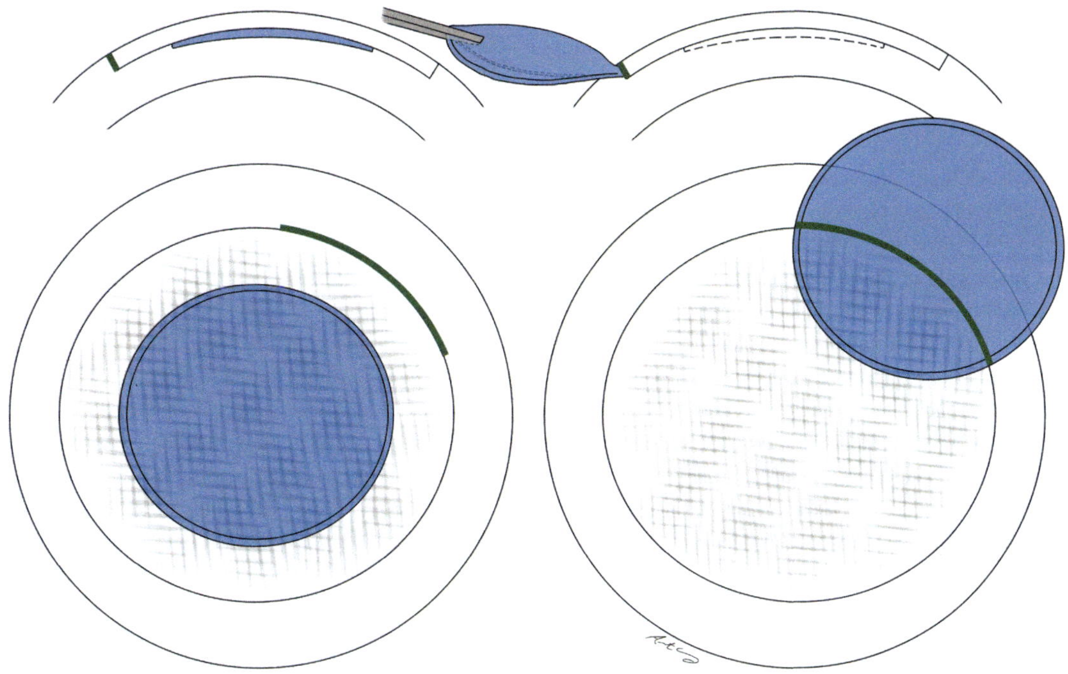

Fig. 4.15 This is an artist's rendition of the SMILE Procedure. The diagram shows the lenticule to be extracted (*blue*), the area of lamellar treatment (*gray* checkered pattern), and the corneal incision (*green*) through which the lenticule is removed with forceps. Diagram courtesy of Albert Cheung, MD

an intrastromal lenticule is dissected and extracted for the correction of myopia without the generation of a flap (Fig. 4.15). The SMILE procedure is a less invasive alternative that has evolved from the Femtosecond Lenticule Extraction technique that was introduced in 2007. A few small studies have shown that the visual and refractive outcomes of SMILE have been similar to those of LASIK [89]. Furthermore, following lenticule extraction, the anterior stroma remains intact offering increased biomechanical stability and faster recovery of corneal sensation when compared with LASIK [90]. It has also been suggested that the extracted lenticule may be stored for future donation or reimplantation. This technique is limited in use to patients with myopia ($\leq$ 10.00 D) with only mild to moderate cylindrical error ($\leq$ 6.00 D).

Procedure

The first stage of the procedure involves initial docking of the patient at the femtosecond laser using a curved contact glass and patient fixation on a target. The second stage requires the verification and maintenance of suction until all the femtosecond incisions have been made. The surgeon makes four intrastromal photoablative incisions to create the lenticule and one 2–3 mm corneal "cap opening" for the manual extraction of the lenticule. The corneal incision is typically made superiorly or superotemporally. In the third stage, the surgeon completes the manual lenticule extraction by inserting a dissector with a rounded end to separate any residual lenticular appendages and extracting the lenticule with microforceps. The lenticule diameter typically measures from 5.75 to 7.00 mm and the minimum lenticule thickness is 15 μm [91].

Structural Effects of SMILE on the Cornea

In the human cornea, the anterior stroma is known to have greater biomechanical strength than the posterior lamellae. The intrastromal incisions of SMILE are less invasive than alternative refractive surgical procedures, leaving the anterior stroma and Bowman layer intact. Therefore, a theoretical advantage to SMILE is increased corneal stability. Studies by Agca et al., Wu et al., and others have compared corneal hysteresis and corneal resistance factor as parameters of relative corneal biomechanical strength following SMILE and LASIK, however, the results have been inconclusive [90, 92].

The anatomy of the anterior stroma also includes the sub-basal nerve bundles that grow radially inward from the periphery toward the central cornea. Leaving the anterior stroma intact has been shown to cause less of a decrease in sub-basal nerve density and faster recovery of corneal sensation. Although studies have demonstrated the preserved nerve fiber density and corneal sensitivity following SMILE compared with LASIK, a significant difference in subjective symptoms of dry eye has not been established [93, 94].

Trauma-Associated Complications with SMILE

Given the recent development and novelty of SMILE, there are no current case reports of trauma related to this surgery to date. Theoretically, complications might include inflammation within the lenticule extraction site, epithelial ingrowth, or other complications of corneal incisional surgery.

Laser Refractive Surgery: Examination

While the flap edge can be difficult to visualize many years out from LASIK, broad beam illumination can help highlight this border. Although broad beam illumination often readily demonstrates a flap dislocation or displacement, fluorescein can help identify the gutter along the flap edge to visualize subtle displacements. As mentioned above, anterior segment OCT can be valuable in determining the orientation of flipped flaps as well as identify epithelial ingrowth. Careful examination with a thin slit beam can help determine partial and full-thickness injuries as well as identify fluid in the interface. The examiner should also proactively look for subsequent DLK, epithelial ingrowth, and flap folds following any trauma to the post-LASIK eye. When approaching a patient with history of SMILE, these same examination principles should be applied.

Surface Refractive Surgery: Treatment

Surgical repositioning for a flap dislocation or displacement should be performed as soon as possible. Under topical or subconjunctival anesthesia, the peripheral flap margin is approached with a Sinskey hook or spatula to free the edges of the LASIK flap. The flap is then irrigated, making sure to meticulously clean debris, inflammatory cells, and epithelial ingrowth. The flap is then repositioned. It could also be sutured into place with 10-0 nylon sutures or glued using fibrin glue. A BCL may be placed to decrease formation of striae and movement of the flap. Topical antibiotics and corticosteroids should then be prescribed.

If there is delayed presentation of a flap dislocation, the approach is different as epithelium has inevitably migrated over the stromal bed. Prior to repositioning, thorough epithelial debridement of the stroma bed and between each fold will give the best chance of repositioning a smooth flap. Flap sutures or glue can help minimize the potential for recurrent epithelial ingrowth.

Following a flap avulsion, the cornea should be treated with antibiotics with or without BCL, followed by subsequent corticosteroids. Mitomycin C may also be used early on to decrease the subsequent haze that can develop. One may consider restoring the original flap, if the amputated flap is found [95]. The free corneal cap should be carefully inspected to ensure it has not been excessively damaged or necrotic. If viable, the free cap should be cultured, irrigated, and replaced following careful removal of epithelium from both the free cap and stromal bed. One must be careful to orient the free cap properly and not place it epithelial side down. Misalignment can result in irregular astigmatism and predispose to epithelial ingrowth. Under high magnification, Bowman's layer surface will appear smooth and shiny while the stromal surface will appear dull and rough. A BCL should be placed over the eye following the repair. After the flap has been allowed to heal, resultant irregular astigmatism may necessitate RGP lens fitting to optimize visual acuity.

Management of corneal penetrating and perforating injuries in the post-LASIK patient should follow the basic tenets of open globe repair. Depending on the size of laceration, anterior chamber depth, and degree of aqueous leakage from the wound, treatment modalities include simple patching, contact lens, suture closure, and cyanoacrylate tissue adhesive [96]. If the leakage is too brisk for a contact lens and if proximity to the visual axis makes suture repair an unsatisfactory option, cyanoacrylate adhesive can seal small perforations without causing cornea flap striae and irregular astigmatism induced by a nylon suture [96].

Most cases of late-onset DLK will respond well to medical therapy, most often with a combination of topical corticosteroid and antibiotic (antibiotic indicated if the epithelium or flap has been disrupted). Oral corticosteroids, either initially or subsequently added to topical treatment, may help in cases not responding to topical corticosteroids [71, 97]. Other successful regimens have included topical NSAIDS (i.e., ketorolac) [98, 99], oral doxycycline [100, 101], and topical cyclosporine [102]; all of these were used in conjunction with corticosteroids. The authors recommend aggressive treatment with oral and topical corticosteroids before lifting the LASIK flap as long as an infection is not suspected or inciting debris is not seen in the flap as the vast majority resolve with such therapy.

Epithelial ingrowth does not need to be treated if it does not advance and does not disrupt the patient's vision. However, when it induces astigmatism or corneal melting, ingrowth should be removed mechanically with a microcurette. Following surface epithelial debridement, treatment most commonly involves lifting the flap from the periphery by first gaining access to the flap with an instrument such as a Sinskey hook or spatula. Next, the undersurface of the flap and the surface of the stromal bed are thoroughly scraped to remove any offending epithelium. Adjuvant treatments to remove epithelium include alcohol (30–100%), mitomycin C, and excimer laser PTK. Finally, the flap is replaced. Suturing the flap or use of fibrin glue (Tisseel tissue glue) at the corneal flap edge can reduce chances of recurrent epithelial ingrowth [103, 104]. An unconventional method in the setting of a penetrating or perforating corneal wound is to enter the flap interface through the wound track [105]. The surface epithelium is then debrided, and the flap interface is delineated by blunt dissection (e.g., tying forceps) through the wound. After the stromal bed and the undersurface of the flap is devoid of epithelium, the central portion of the flap overlying the laceration is then sutured with 10-0 nylon (without incorporating the underlying stromal bed).

Treatment for flap folds is most effective when initiated as soon as possible, before the folds become fixed in place. Treatment may include flap massage or stretching with forceps, alongside hydration and flap refloatation [106]. Donnenfeld et al. advocate the use of hyperthermic massage as a viable treatment for visually significant striae with no adverse flap consequences [107]. Smaller striae that are asymptomatic with no loss of BCVA may resolve spontaneously. Larger flap folds may not be responsive to flap massage, and may require sutures [108, 109]. Meticulous removal of all epithelium from the interface and between the fold will help relax the fold. Additionally, sterile water can be used to hydrate the flap, which creates local swelling of the flap. This can often aid in removing macrostriae and allow better reapproximation of the flap [55]. The use of a BCL has been reported to reduce the chance of postoperative flap wrinkling [110].

Regarding the management of infectious keratitis, any suspicious appearing infiltrate following LASIK should be cultured and managed aggressively. Superficial cultures can be attempted; however, if these are negative, the flap should be lifted for smears and cultures [78]. Karp et al. [78] recommend culture of the cornea with a 69 blade for the smears and plates after lifting the flap. Given the suspicion for atypical organisms and fungus, they recommended inoculation on blood, chocolate, Sabouraud, Lowenstein–Jensen agar, and blood heart infusion. They also routinely performed gram stain smears for Giemsa, Calcofluor white (fungus), and Ziehl–Neelsen stains (acid-fast bacteria). Treatment for bacterial pathogens includes tobramycin and vancomycin. Fourth generation fluoroquinolones have also been demonstrated to be effective against bacterial keratitis [111]. First-line fungal defense agents are Natamycin and Amphotericin B. Chang et al. [112] found that early flap lifting and repositioning performed within three days of the onset of symptoms was associated with better visual outcome in the treatment of infections following LASIK. At the time of flap lifting, immediate culture and smear should be performed, with subsequent irrigation of the bed and flap. Additionally, irrigation with a broad-spectrum antibiotic such as tobramycin and cefazolin can be considered. In cases that do not respond to antimicrobial therapy or when corneal melting has occurred, it may be necessary to amputate the corneal flap to improve antimicrobial penetration [78]. Penetrating keratoplasty may be considered in recalcitrant cases to remove the nidus of infection.

If foreign bodies are suspected to be the cause of an inflammatory reaction, early flap lifting with irrigation is imperative to prevent further complications, including the progression of infective keratitis, epithelial ingrowth, and diffuse lamellar keratitis.

Intraocular Refractive Surgery

Intraocular Refractive Surgery: Procedures

The stability and predictability of laser in situ keratomilieusis (LASIK) declines for higher levels of myopia and hyperopia given the limitations of corneal thickness, residual stromal bed, and keratometric measurements [113, 114]. In addition, side effects including dry eye syndrome, glare, halos, and irreversibility may favor alternative procedures including the placement of a phakic IOL (pIOL). pIOL implantation offers an alternative procedure for the correction of a wide range of myopia and hyperopia that are not limited by corneal thickness. Three anatomical placements for the pIOL include anterior chamber iris fixated (Artisan/Verisyse), anterior chamber angle supported (Kelman Duiet, Acrysof Cachet), or posterior chamber with no fixation (Implantable Collarmer Lenses).

Prior to surgery, the dioptric power of the pIOL is calculated using the Van der Heijde or similar post-refractive surgery formula, taking into account the patient's refraction (spherical equivalent), anterior chamber depth, and keratometric dioptric values. Ancillary preoperative testing may include ultrasonography and OCT examination for accurate angle to angle and sulcus to sulcus measurements and proper sizing of the pIOL.

Iris Fixated Intraocular Lens

Introduction

The iris-fixated lens was introduced for secondary lens implantation by Worst in 1978. It is now manufactured as Artisan or Verisyse lens as a convex/concave polymethyl methacrylate (PMMA) lens model with two low shoulders and connected haptics that secure the lens to the mid-peripheral iris stroma (Fig. 4.16) [114]. It is 8.5 mm in length. Variations of this lens model are used to treat high myopia, hyperopia and astigmatism in adults to correct from −23.5 to +12 Diopters of spherical equivalent [115–117]. Other indications include treatment of refractive errors following penetrating keratoplasty [117], treatment of anisometropic amblyopia in children, secondary implantation for aphakia correction, treatment of refractive errors in patients with keratoconus [114]. It requires an anterior chamber depth of greater than or equal to 2.7 mm. A more recent foldable model (Artiflex) is now available which allows for a smaller incision for insertion of the IOL. The artiflex lens is a three-piece lens with a silicone optic and

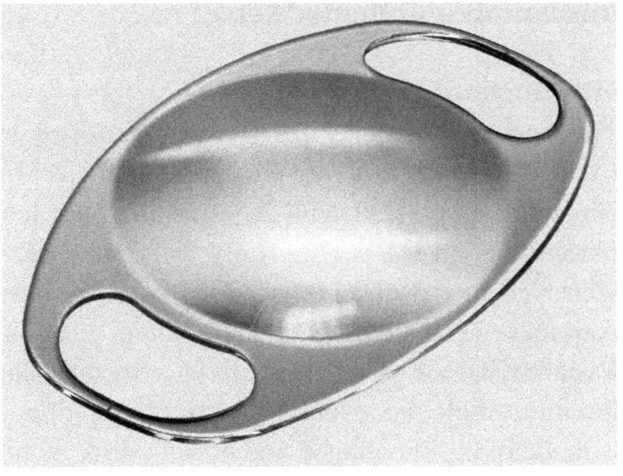

Fig. 4.16 Photograph of the Artisan lens. Permission obtained from Ophtec USA

PMMA claws that secure the lens to the mid-peripheral iris stroma.

Procedure

The limbus is marked at the horizontal and vertical axes as well as at the axis for the lens enclavation into the iris. A 2-Plane 5.2–6.2 mm corneoscleral incision is then made, centered at 12 o'clock along with 2 stab incisions placed at locations that would most easily facilitate enclavation with orientation toward the enclavation sites. The surgeon then administers an intracameral injection of acetylcholine prior to introducing the lens with Budo forceps under ophthalmic viscosurgical device (OVD). The lens is then fixated with a disposable enclavation needle which buries the diametrically opposed claws of the haptics beneath a layer of iris tissue in the mid-peripheral iris. A slit iridotomy is performed to decrease risk of pupillary block and the wound is closed with 3–5 interrupted 10-0 nylon sutures. Postoperatively, the patient is treated with topical antibiotic/steroid combination, such as tobramycin/dexamethasone as well as an NSAID, such as ketorolac-trometamol in a tapered fashion over 3 weeks. Selective suture removal is performed as needed given subjective refraction [115–117].

Trauma-Associated Complications of Iris Fixated Intraocular Lens

Traumatic dislocation of the Artisan IOL is rare, with seven cases reported in literature [118–124]. A patient may present years after lens implantation with complaint of decreased vision or monocular diplopia following blunt trauma. Examination at the slit lamp more commonly will reveal a pair of iris haptic claws that have released free from the iris stroma with one side of the lens resting in the angle.

One case report describes the possibility of blunt trauma causing complete aniridia, with expulsion of the crystalline lens and vitreous through the 6 mm incision wound 6 months following Artisan lens implantation [123]. The Artisan lens was not found on examination in this case. It was hypothesized that the trauma caused the enclavated lens to shear the iris from its root thereby creating a complete iridodialysis resulting in aniridia.

A case has also been reported of a patient with bilateral Artiflex lenses who suffered severe blunt trauma causing partial aniridia [124]. In this report, the optic haptic junction was stuck in the incision wound. The smaller incision wound required for insertion the foldable iris-fixated lens may decrease risk of complete aniridia and expulsion of the Artisan lens following blunt trauma. This patient was treated with iris repositioning and excision resulting in partial aniridia.

Angle Supported Phakic Intraocular Lens

Introduction

AcrySof Cachet is a single-piece foldable hydrophobic acrylic phakic IOL (pIOL) with a vaulted 6 mm optic with haptics designed to allow compression of the angle to maintain IOL stability without creating excessive force. It is available for the correction of −6.00 to −16.50 D [125, 126].

A less common, second variant, the Kelmen Duet, is a PMMA tripod haptic that allows for compression of the angle for IOL stability. This tripod haptic is connected to a silicone optic by optic eyelets, which fit over haptics tabs, securing the optic in place [127].

The sizing of the angle supported pIOL may present a challenge and requires accurate measurement of the angle-to-angle distance. Correct sizing is crucial for successful visual outcomes and reduce the risk of pupil ovalization, IOL decentration, endothelial touch, inflammation, and secondary glaucoma. The lens length may range from 11.5 to 14 mm [114].

Procedure

AcrySof Cachet: The pupil is constricted with 2% pilocarpine, as well as intracameral acetylcholine (1%). The surgeon creates 2 limbal paracentesis ports, then makes a 3–3.5 mm clear corneal incision along the steepest meridian or at a location based on surgeon preference. Cohesive viscoelastic is injected into the angle to inflate and maintain the anterior chamber. The pIOL is then folded and inserted with a delivery system. IOL placement is confirmed by visualization of the IOL loops and on gonioscopic examination. Diamox is given postoperatively to prevent IOP spikes and postoperative examination is performed on the same day. The patient is treated with antibiotic and corticosteroid for at least 1 week following the procedure [128, 129].

Kelman Duet: The surgeon creates a 2.5 mm incision and then inserts the tripod haptic first using an injector system. The optic is then placed in the anterior chamber and attached by the optic eyelets and haptic tabs using a Sinskey hook [127].

Trauma-Associated Complications with Angle Supported Phakic Intraocular Lens

There were no specific case reports found in the literature of trauma related to pIOLs. Alio et al. [130] reviewed 240 cases of pIOL explantation. They found that cataract was the main cause of explantation for all pIOL locations (angle-fixated, iris-fixated, and posterior chamber) with nearly 100% of cataracts being nuclear. pIOL decentration/dislocation was another common indication for explantation. While they did not specifically attribute trauma as the cause, decentration/dislocation was noted in all types of pIOLs and affected 6.67% of cases overall. The angle-supported group had the highest incidence of decentration/dislocation (7.64%) leading to explantation [130]. It is reasonable to envision trauma as a potential cause of dislocation.

Implantable Collamer Lens

Introduction

The posterior chamber pIOL was developed by Fyodorov in 1986 to avoid endothelial decompensation associated with anterior chamber lens placement [131]. The only current FDA approved model on the market is an implantable collamer lens (ICL) manufactured as the Visian ICL V4 (Fig. 4.17). It is a rectangular, flexible, single piece lens with central vaulting. It is made of 0.2% collagen and 60% hydroxylethyl methacrylate copolymer. This hydrophilic material enables permeability of gas and metabolites for normal metabolism of the lens, decreasing the risk of cataract formation [132]. It requires an anterior chamber depth of >2.8 mm for myopia and greater than or equal to 3.0 mm for hyperopia with endothelial cell density parameters based on the age [114].

Procedure

The pupil is dilated with topical mydriatic prior to surgery. The surgeon creates a 3.0 mm clear corneal incision temporally. Cohesive viscoelastic is placed into the anterior chamber and the posterior IOL is inserted into the ciliary sulcus with an injector. The orientation of the lens is established by the placement of the footplates beneath the iris using a flat manipulator. Following lens placement, an intraoperative iridectomy is performed. The patient is treated with corticosteroid and antibiotic drops postoperatively.

Trauma-Associated Complications of an Implantable Collamer Lens

Dislocation of the pIOL is rare with five reported cases in literature [133]. There is one report of spontaneous dislocation with hypothesized zonular dehiscence with posterior movement into the vitreous. There are four reported cases of traumatic dislocation of the pIOL secondary to blunt ocular and occipital injury. In these cases, there was no pattern of footplate dislocation and the lens was repositioned within one week with good visual outcomes. Risk of endothelial cell damage and resulting corneal decompensation

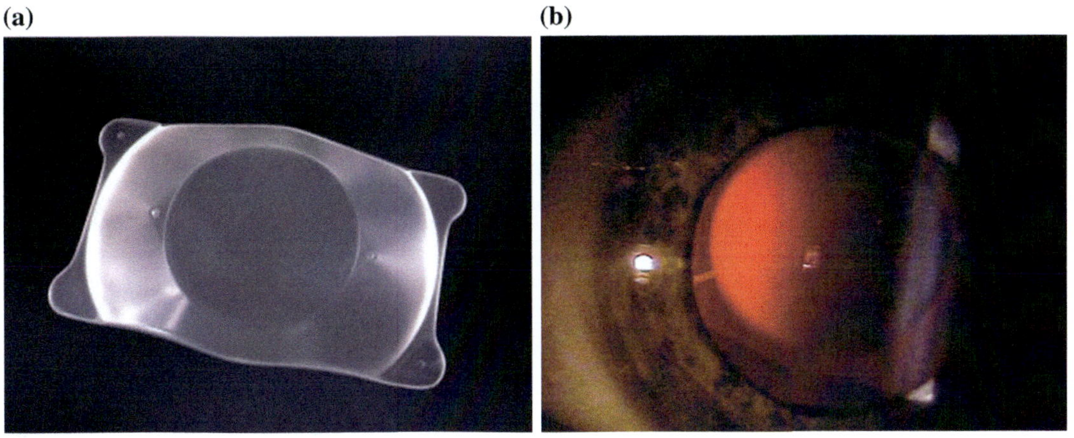

Fig. 4.17 **a** Photograph of Visian ICL (Implantable Collamer Lens). Permission obtained from Staar Surgical USA. **b** Slit lamp photograph of implanted ICL. Photograph courtesy of William Goldstein, MD

was the most serious injury associated with dislocations.

Theoretically, patients with chronic eye rubbing, improperly sized pIOL, or zonular pathology could be at risk for dislocation of the pIOL (Fig. 4.18) [133]. Otherwise, the ICL has been noted to be resistant to dislocation during trauma with reported stability even during grenade explosion [134].

Intraocular Refractive Surgery: Examination

Slit lamp examination in patients with a history of pIOL implantation must be performed with special attention to the haptic enclavation sites on the mid-peripheral iris for iris-fixated pIOLs and to the haptic position for the other pIOL types. The cornea should be examined for edema, which may be suggestive of endothelial cell damage or loss. IOP must be measured, and a gonioscopic examination should be performed if possible given the patient's risk of PAS (2–18% following lens implantation) and potential iridodialysis or cyclodialysis [130]. Pupil irregularity, iris atrophy, and iris tears should be noted and may be associated with pupillary ovalization. Pupillary ovalization is a complication that may present in 7–22% of patients with an angle supported IOL caused by compression of the angle structure due to an oversized lens, inflammation in the angle, PAS formation, and iris sectoral hypoperfusion/ischemia [135]. The irregular pupil can be indicative of a dislocated IOL and/or a partially extruded IOL (Fig. 4.19). The slit beam must also be directed toward the pIOL and natural lens to verify the distance between the posterior surface of the IOL and the lens. IOL/lens touch following trauma may also be associated with increased risk of cataract formation. The anterior chamber should also be evaluated for hyphema as well as cell and flare.

Intraocular Refractive Surgery: Treatment

Management of displacement/dislocation often involves explantation or repositioning of the pIOL. This can be performed in conjunction with cataract extraction if a cataract develops from the trauma of the adjacent pIOL. Repositioning of the lens should be done promptly as endothelial cell injury represents a potentially serious problem. If the haptic claws of the iris-fixated pIOL are malpositioned, these cases can be treated by re-enclavation of the haptic claws into the mid-peripheral iris stroma with a good visual prognosis [136].

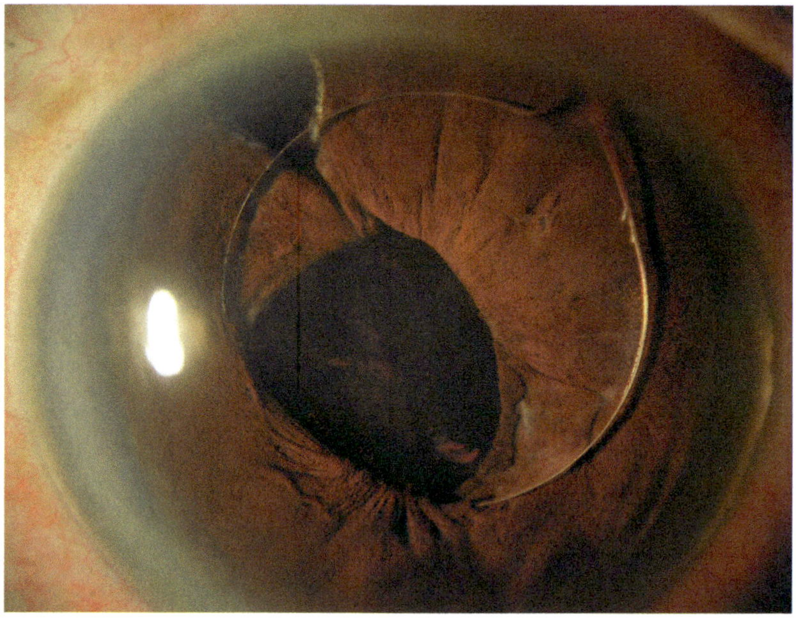

Fig. 4.18 Slit lamp photograph of a dislocated intraocular lens. Although it is not an implantable collamer lens, however, it is representative of traumatic dislocation of an intraocular lens

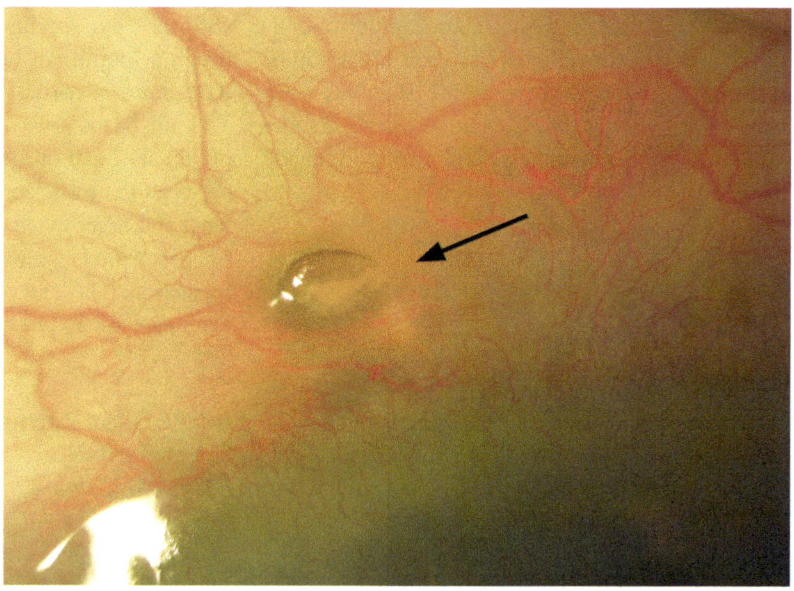

Fig. 4.19 Slit lamp photograph of a partially extruded IOL. Note the *black arrow* indicating the extruded footplate

Cases

Case 1

A 46-year-old male with a history of bilateral LASIK 17 years prior presented with blurred vision 3 weeks after sustaining an injury involving a finger to his right eye. Prior treatment included topical antibiotics and BCL for a corneal ulcer followed by topical prednisolone acetate 1% QID. Initial visual acuity in the right eye was 20/80 (pinhole 20/30). Examination revealed a focal mid-peripheral corneal scar

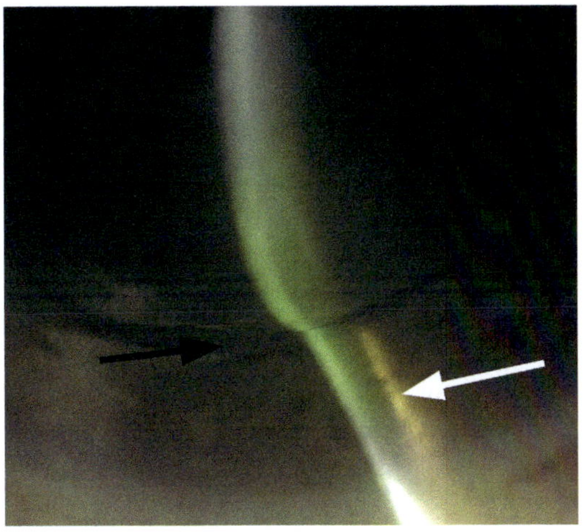

Fig. 4.20 Slit lamp photograph demonstrating a perforated LASIK flap noted by the *black arrow* at the flap edge. Note also the *white arrow* indicating the flat anterior chamber. Photograph courtesy of David Heidemann, MD

accompanied by stage II DLK (Fig. 4.12a, b). Topical prednisolone acetate was increased to every 2 h. The DLK resolved, topical corticosteroids were tapered, and vision improved to 20/40 2 weeks later. Six weeks following presentation, the stromal haze resolved with only trace scarring after being off corticosteroids for 1 month, and visual acuity returned to 20/30.

Case 2

A 42-year-old male with a history of bilateral LASIK 9 years prior that had developed bilateral post-LASIK keratectasia presented with decreased vision after sustaining trauma secondary to a fist to his left eye. He had been wearing gas-permeable contact lenses (GPCL) for best corrected visual acuity.

On initial physical examination, his visual acuity was 20/40 (with a GPCL) in the right eye and count fingers in the left eye. Slit lamp examination of the left eye revealed a posterior rupture of the inferior paracentral posterior stroma with an intact overlying LASIK flap. The inferior edge of LASIK flap was Seidel positive, and the anterior chamber was flat (Fig. 4.20). There was fluid noted in the interface that had tracked through the posterior rupture and was leaking around the inferior periphery of the LASIK flap. The right eye was remarkable for an intact LASIK flap with anterior thinning/protrusion consistent with post-LASIK keratectasia.

A large area of cyanoacrylate glue was applied around the flap periphery, followed by a BCL (9.1 base curve). The anterior chamber quickly reformed, and 40 min later it appeared

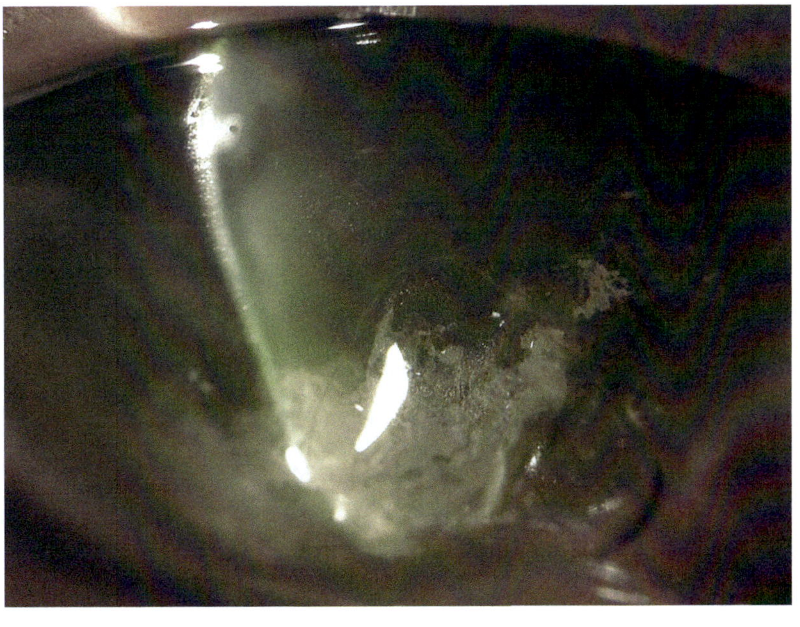

Fig. 4.21 Slit lamp photograph showing cyanoacrylate glue at the flap periphery covering a flap perforation. Note also the bandage contact lens overlying glue as well as the deep anterior chamber. Photograph courtesy of David Heidemann, MD

moderate in depth (Fig. 4.21). Lumigan and Istalol were both given once in the office. A fox shield was applied, and the patient was treated with topical gatifloxacin 0.5% QID and oral moxifloxacin 400 mg daily.

The following morning the anterior chamber was flat again although the glue and BCL appeared intact. The decision was made to proceed with tectonic penetrating keratoplasty that same day. The postoperative course was unremarkable, and over 1 year later, the visual acuity OS was 20/25 with −7.50 + 2.00 × 050 [137].

References

1. Fyodorov SN, Durnev VV. Operation of dosage dissection of corneal circular ligament in cases of myopia of a mild degree. Ann Ophthalmol. 1979;11:1885–90.
2. Binder PS, Stainer GA, Zavala EY, et al. Acute morphologic features of radial keratotomy. Arch Ophthalmol. 1983;101:1113–6.
3. Jammal HM, Dolat WM. Ruptured globe 20 years after radial and transverse keratotomy. Int Ophthalmol. 2012;32:51–3.
4. Glasgow BJ, Brown HH, Aizuss DH, et al. Traumatic dehiscence of incisions seven years after radial keratotomy. Am J Ophthalmol. 1988;106:703–7.
5. Bryant MR, Szerenyi K, Schmotzer H, McDonnell PJ. Corneal tensile strength in fully healed radial keratotomy wounds. Invest Ophthalmol Vis Sci. 1994;35:3022–31.
6. Luttrull JK, Jester JV, Smith RE. The effect of radial keratotomy on ocular integrity in an animal model. Arch Ophthalmol. 1982;100:319–20.
7. Larson BC, Kremer FB, Eller AW, Bernardino VB Jr. Quantitated trauma following radial keratotomy in rabbits. Ophthalmology. 1983;90:660–7.
8. Alvi NP, Donohue EK, Curnyn K, Sugar J. Rupture of radial keratotomy sites after presumed blunt trauma. Ophthalmic Surg Lasers. 1995;26:574–5.
9. Bloom HR, Sands J, Schneider D. Corneal rupture from blunt trauma 22 months after radial keratotomy. Refract Corneal Surg. 1989;6:197–9.
10. Pinheiro MN Jr, Bryant MR, Tayyanipour R, et al. Corneal integrity after refractive surgery. Effects of radial keratotomy and mini-radial keratotomy. Ophthalmology. 1995;102:297–301.
11. Steinemann TL, Baltz TC, Lam BL, et al. Mini radial keratotomy reduces ocular integrity. Axial compression in a postmortem porcine eye model. Ophthalmology. 1998;105:1739–44.
12. McDonnell PJ. Sight-threatening complications after radial keratotomy. Arch Ophthalmol. 1996;114:211–2.
13. Rylander HG, Welch AJ, Fremming B. The effect of radial keratotomy in the rupture strength of pig eyes. Ophthalmic Surg. 1983;14:744–9.
14. Vinger PF, Mieler WF, Oestreicher JH, Easterbrook M. Ruptured globes following radial and hexagonal keratotomy surgery. Arch Ophthalmol. 1996;114:129–34.
15. McKnight SJ, Fitz J, Giangiacomo J. Corneal rupture following radial keratotomy in cats subjected to BB gun injury. Ophthalmic Surg. 1988;19:165–7.
16. Binder PS, Waring GO, Arrowsmith PN, Wang C. Histopathology of traumatic corneal rupture after radial keratotomy. Arch Ophthalmol. 1988;106:1584–90.
17. Casebeer JC, Shapiro DR, Phillips S. Severe ocular trauma without corneal rupture after radial keratotomy: case reports. J Refract Corneal Surg. 1994;10(1):31–3.
18. Bouchard CS, Vaziri B. Dehiscence of radial keratotomy wounds without globe rupture following explosion injury. J Refract Surg. 2001;17:561–3.
19. Nemi A, Bahadur RP, Randleman JB. Traumatic epithelial downgrowth after radial keratotomy. J Cataract Refract Surg. 2008;34:327–9.
20. Forstot SL, Damiano RE. Trauma after radial keratotomy. Ophthalmology. 1988;95:833–5.
21. Heidemann DG, Dunn SP, Chow CY. Early-versus late-onset infectious keratitis after radial and astigmatic keratotomy: clinical spectrum in a referral practice. J Cataract Refract Surg. 1999;25:1615–9.
22. Behl S, Kothari K. Rupture of a radial keratotomy incision after 11 years during clear corneal phacoemulsification. J Cataract Refract Surg. 2001;27:1132–4.
23. Freeman M, Kumar V, Ramanathan US, O'Neill E. Dehiscence of radial keratotomy incision during phacoemulsification. Eye. 2004;18:101–3.
24. Deg JK, Binder PS. Wound healing after astigmatic keratotomy in human eyes. Ophthalmology. 1987;94:1290–8.
25. Lee BL, Manche EE, Glasgow BJ. Rupture of radial and arcuate keratotomy scars by blunt trauma 91 months after incisional keratotomy. Am J Ophthalmol. 1995;120:108–10.
26. Eggleston RJ. Surgical repair of multiple ruptures of radial and transverse incisions under topical anesthesia. J Cataract Refract Surg. 1996;22:1394.
27. Burris TE. Intrastromal corneal ring technology: results and indications. Curr Opin Ophthalmol. 1998;9:9–14.
28. Schanzlin DJ, Asbell PA, Burris TE, Durrie DS. The intrastromal corneal ring segments. Phase II results for the correction of myopia. Ophthalmology. 1997;104:1067–78.

29. Park J, Gritz DC. Evolution in the use of intrastromal corneal ring segments for corneal ectasia. Curr Opin Ophthalmol. 2013;24(4):296–301.
30. Rabinowitz YS. Intacs for keratoconus. Curr Opin Ophthalmol. 2007;18:279–83.
31. Carrasquillo KG, Rand J, Talamo JH. Intacs for keratoconus and post-LASIK ectasia: mechanical versus femtosecond laser-assisted channel creation. Cornea. 2007;26(8):956–62.
32. Pinero DP, Alio JL, Barraquer RI, Michael R. Corneal biomechanical changes after intracorneal ring segment implantation in keratoconus. Cornea. 2012;31:491–9.
33. Burris TE, Ayer CT, Evensen DA, Davenport JM. Effects of intrastromal corneal ring size and thickness on corneal flattening in human eyes. Refract Corneal Surg. 1991;7:46–50.
34. Burris TE, Baker PC, Ayer CT, et al. Flattening of central corneal curvature with intrastromal corneal rings of increasing thickness: an eye-bank eye study. J Cataract Refract Surg. 1993;19 (Suppl):182–7.
35. Twa MD, Ruckhofer J, Kash RL, et al. Histologic evaluation of corneal stroma in rabbits after intrastromal corneal ring implantation. Cornea. 2003;22:146–52.
36. Colin J, Buestel C, Touboul D. Unusual secondary displacement of intacts segments—superimposition of distal ends. J Refract Surg. 2010;26:924–5.
37. Sony P, Panda A, Pushker N. Traumatic corneal rupture 18 years after radial keratotomy. J Refract Surg. 2004;20:283–4.
38. Campos M, Lee M, McDonnell PJ. Ocular integrity after refractive surgery: effects of photorefractive keratectomy, phototherapeutic keratectomy, and radial keratotomy. Ophthalmic Surg. 1992;23:598–602.
39. Burnstein Y, Klapper D, Hersh PS. Experimental globe rupture after excimer laser photorefractive keratectomy. Arch Ophthalmol. 1995;113:1056–9.
40. Alcaraz LG, Banez MA, Height DH, et al. Comparative study of wound integrity after excimer laser photoablation and radial keratotomy. Invest Ophthalmol Vis Sci. 1992;33(Suppl):999.
41. Galler EI, Umlas JW, Vinger PF, Wu HK. Ocular integrity after quantitated trauma following photorefractive keratectomy and automated lamellar keratectomy. Abstract presented at: Association for Research in Vision and Ophthalmology, May 16, 1995; Ft. Lauderdale, FL. Abstracts in: Invest Ophthalmol Vis Sci 1995;36(Suppl):580.
42. Artola A, Ayala MJ, Ruiz-Moreno JM, et al. Rupture of radial keratotomy incisions by blunt trauma 6 years after combined photorefractive keratectomy/radial keratotomy. J Refract Surg. 2003;19:460–2.
43. Dawson DG, Kramer TR, Grossniklaus HE, et al. Histologic, ultrastructural, and immunofluorescent evaluation of human laser assisted in situ keratomileusis corneal wounds. Arch Ophthalmol. 2005;123:741–56.
44. Schmack I, Dawson DG, McCarey BE, et al. Cohesive tensile strength of human LASIK wounds with histologic, ultrastructural, and clinical correlations. J Refract Surg. 2005;21:433–45.
45. Davies JB, Randleman JB. Successful delayed surgical revision of a dislocated LASIK flap. Ophthalmic Surg Lasers Imaging. 2008;39:221–4.
46. Kramer TR, Chuckpaiwong V, Dawson DG, et al. Pathologic findings in postmortem corneas after successful laser in situ keratomileusis. Cornea. 2005;24:92–102.
47. Roberts C. The cornea is not a piece of plastic. J Refract Surg. 2000;16:407–13.
48. Chan C, Wachler BB. Corneal ectasia and refractive surgery. Int Ophthalmol Clin. 2006;46(3):13–25.
49. Peacock LW, Slade SG, Martiz J, et al. Ocular integrity after refractive procedures. Ophthalmology. 1997;104:1079–83.
50. Knorz MC, Vossmerbaeumer U. Comparison of flap adhesion strength using the Amadeus microkeratome and the IntraLase iFS femtosecond laser in rabbits. J Refract Surg. 2008;24:875–8.
51. Goodman RL, Johnson DA, Dillon H, et al. Laser in situ keratomileusis flap stability during simulated aircraft ejection in a rabbit model. Cornea. 2003;22:142–5.
52. Laurent JM, Schallhorn SC, Spigelmire JR, Tanzer DJ. Stability of the laser in situ keratomileusis corneal flap in rabbit eyes. J Cataract Refract Surg. 2006;32:1046–51.
53. Mousavi SJ, Nassiri N, Masoumi N, et al. Finite element analysis of blunt foreign body impact on the cornea after PRK and LASIK. J Refract Surg. 2012;28:59–64.
54. Stulting RD, Carr JD, Thompson KP, et al. Complications of laser in situ keratomileusis for the correction of myopia. Ophthalmology. 1999;106:13–20.
55. Holt DG, Sikder S, Mifflin MD. Surgical management of traumatic LASIK flap dislocation with macrostriae and epithelial ingrowth 14 years postoperatively. J Cataract Refract Surg. 2012;38:357–61.
56. Tetz M, Werner L, Müller M, Dietze U. Late traumatic LASIK flap loss during contact sport. J Cataract Refract Surg. 2007;33:1332–5.
57. Motwani M, Lizano GJ, Yam K, English C. Photorefractive keratectomy after late traumatic LASIK flap loss. J Refract Surg. 2011;27:542–4.
58. Kim JS, Chung B, Lee T, et al. Management of long-standing partially torn and flipped laser in situ keratomileusis flaps. J Cataract Refract Surg. 2015;41:464–7.
59. Lyle WA, Jin GJ. Interface fluid associated with diffuse lamellar keratitis and epithelial ingrowth after laser in situ keratomileusis. J Cataract Refract Surg. 1999;25:1009–12.

60. Kumar S. Traumatic interface oedema two years after LASIK. Clin Exp Optom. 2009;92:395–6.
61. Liu X, Ling S, Gao X, et al. Pressure-induced stromal keratopathy as a result of ocular trauma after laser in situ keratomileusis. JAMA Ophthalmol. 2013;131:1070–2.
62. Bushley DM, Holzinger KA, Winkle RK, et al. Lamellar interface fluid accumulation following traumatic corneal perforation and laser in situ keratomileusis. J Cataract Refract Surg. 2005;31:1249–51.
63. Gritz DC. LASIK interface keratitis: epidemiology, diagnosis and care. Curr Opin Ophthalmol. 2011;22:251–5.
64. Maddox R, Hatsis AP. Sands of Sahara syndrome interface inflammation with flap melt following LASIK. Ocular Surgery news. Thorofare, NJ: SLACK, Inc; 1998. p. 41–2.
65. Smith RJ, Maloney RK. Diffuse lamellar keratitis. A new syndrome in lamellar refractive surgery. Ophthalmology. 1998;105:1721–6.
66. Bouveret B, Orucoglu F. Late-onset diffuse lamellar keratitis after blunt trauma without epithelial or flap damage. JCRS Online Case Rep. 2015;3:32–4.
67. Melki SA, Talamo JH, Demetriades AM, et al. Late traumatic dislocation of laser in situ keratomileusis corneal flaps. Ophthalmology. 2000;107:2136–9.
68. Weisenthal RW. Diffuse lamellar keratitis induced by trauma 6 months after laser in situ keratomileusis. J Refract Surg. 2000;16:749–51.
69. Davis EA, Fahmy AM. Stage III diffuse lamellar keratitis following conductive keratoplasty over a LASIK flap. J Cataract Refract Surg. 2009;35:1141–3.
70. Steinert RF, McColgin AZ, White A, Horsburgh GM. Diffuse interface keratitis after laser in situ keratomileusis (LASIK): a nonspecific syndrome. Am J Ophthalmol. 2000;129:380–1.
71. Kymionis GD, Bouzoukis DI, Diakonis VF, et al. Diffuse lamellar keratitis after corneal crosslinking in a patient with post-laser in situ keratomileusis corneal ectasia. J Cataract Refract Surg. 2007;33:2135–7.
72. Cheng AC, Rao SK, Leung GY, et al. Late traumatic flap dislocations after LASIK. J Refract Surg. 2006;22:500–4.
73. Kim JS, Chung B, Lee T, et al. Management of long-standing partially torn and flipped laser in situ keratomileusis flaps. J Cataract Refract Surg. 2015;41:464–7.
74. Ursea R, Feng MT. Traumatic Flap Striae 6 years after LASIK: case report and literature review. J Refract Surg. 2010;26:899–905.
75. Liu L, Song FZ, Bao LY. Histopathological study of corneal flap striae following laser in situ keratomileusis in rabbits. Exp Ther Med. 2015;9:895–900.
76. Vieira AC1, Pereira T, de Freitas D. Late-onset infections after LASIK. J Refract Surg. 2008;24:411–3.
77. Moorthy RS, Valluri S, Rao NA. Nontuberculous mycobacterial ocular and adnexal infections. Surv Ophthalmol. 2012;57:202–35.
78. Karp CL, Tuli SS, Yoo SH, et al. Infectious keratitis after LASIK. Ophthalmology. 2003;110:503–10.
79. Read RW, Chuck RS, Rao NA, Smith RE. Traumatic Acremonium atrogriseum keratitis following laser-assisted in situ keratomileusis. Arch Ophthalmol. 2000;118:418–21.
80. Lee GA, Gray TB, Dart JK, et al. Acanthamoeba sclerokeratitis: treatment with systemic immunosuppression. Ophthalmology. 2002;109:1178–82.
81. Kaur H, Maguire LJ, Salomao DR, Cameron JD. Rapid progression of amebic keratitis 1 week after corneal trauma and 1 year after LASIK. Cornea. 2007;26:212–4.
82. Karp KO, Hersh PS, Epstein RJ. Delayed keratitis after laser in situ keratomileusis. J Cataract Refract Surg. 2000;26:925–8.
83. Choi JA, Kim MS. LASIK interface-captured foreign bodies after mild traumatic corneal scratch without flap displacement. Korean J Ophthalmol. 2012;26:222–5.
84. Sakurai E, Okuda M, Nozaki M, Ogura Y. Late-onset laser in situ keratomileusis (LASIK) flap dehiscence during retinal detachment surgery. Am J Ophthalmol. 2002;134:265–6.
85. Jonas JB. Displacement of a laser in situ keratomileusis flap during retinal detachment surgery. Acta Ophthalmol Scand. 2004;82:314–5.
86. Chaudhry NA, Smiddy WE. Displacement of corneal cap during vitrectomy in a post-LASIK eye. Retina. 1998;18:554–5.
87. López-Guajardo L, Drake-Rodríguez P, Paz-Moreno J, et al. Possibility of flap displacement during retinal surgery. Retina 2007;27:393–4; author reply 394.
88. Mearza AA, Koufaki FN, Aslanides IM. Airbag induced corneal ectasia. Cont Lens Anterior Eye. 2008;31:38–40.
89. Reinstein DZ, Archer TJ, Gobbe M. Small incision lenticule extraction history, fundamentals of a new refractive surgery technique and clinical outcomes. Eye Vis (Lond). 2014;1:3.
90. Wu W, Wang, Y. The correlation analysis between corneal biomechanical properties and the surgically induced corneal high order aberrations after small incision lenticular extraction and femtosecond laser in situ keratomileusis. J Ophthalmol. 2015. Epub Sep 21.
91. Moshirfar M, McCaughey MV, Reinstein DZ, et al. Small-incision lenticule extraction. J Cataract Refract Surg. 2015;41:652–65.
92. Agca A, Demirok A, Cankaya K, et al. Comparison of visual acuity and higher-order aberrations after femtosecond lenticule extraction and small-incision lenticule extraction. Cont Lens Anterior Eye. 2014;37:292–6.

93. He J, Bazan NG, Bazan HE. Mapping the entire human corneal nerve architecture. Exp Eye Res. 2010;91:513–23.
94. Reinstein DZ, Archer T, Gobbe M, Bartoli E. Corneal sensitivity after small incision lenticule extraction and laser in situ keratomileusis. J Cataract Refract Surg. 2015;41:1580–7.
95. Haw WW, Manche EE. Successful corneal flap replacement following complete traumatic flap amputation after laser-assisted in situ keratomileusis. Arch Ophthalmol. 2004;122:275–6.
96. Korn BS, Korn TS. Cyanoacrylate repair of laser in situ keratomileusis corneal flap perforation by a snake bite. J Cataract Refract Surg. 2005;31:2224–6.
97. Asano-Kato N, Toda I, Tsubota K. Severe late-onset recurrent epithelial erosion with diffuse lamellar keratitis after laser in situ keratomileusis. J Cataract Refract Surg. 2003;29:2019–21.
98. da Reitz Pereira C, Narvaez J, King JA, et al. Late-onset traumatic dislocation with central tissue loss of laser in situ keratomileusis flap. Cornea 2006;25:1107–10.
99. Yeoh J, Moshegov CN. Delayed diffuse lamellar keratitis after laser in situ keratomileusis. Clin Exp Ophthalmol. 2001;29:435–7.
100. Díaz-Valle D, Arriola-Villalobos P, Sánchez JM, et al. Late-onset severe diffuse lamellar keratitis associated with uveitis after LASIK in a patient with ankylosing spondylitis. J Refract Surg. 2009;25:623–5.
101. Symes RJ, Catt CJ, Males JJ. Diffuse lamellar keratitis associated with gonococcal keratoconjunctivitis 3 years after laser in situ keratomileusis. J Cataract Refract Surg. 2007;33:323–5.
102. Chung MS, Pepose JS, El-Agha MS, Cavanagh HD. Confocal microscopic findings in a case of delayed-onset bilateral diffuse lamellar keratitis after laser in situ keratomileusis. J Cataract Refract Surg. 2002;28:1467–70.
103. Anderson NJ, Hardten DR. Fibrin glue for the prevention of epithelial ingrowth after laser in situ keratomileusis. J Cataract Refract Surg. 2003;29:1425–9.
104. Yeh DL, Bushley DM, Kim T. Treatment of traumatic LASIK flap dislocation and epithelial ingrowth with fibrin glue. Am J Ophthalmol. 2006;141:960–2.
105. Meskin SW, Seedor JA, Ritterband DC, Koplin RS. Removal of epithelial ingrowth via central perforating wound tract 6 years post LASIK. Eye Contact Lens. 2012;38:266–7.
106. Sinha R, Shekhar H, Tinwala S, et al. Late post-traumatic flap dislocation and macrostriae after laser in situ keratomileusis. Oman J Ophthalmol. 2014;7:25–7.
107. Donnenfeld ED, Perry HD, Doshi SJ, et al. Hyperthermic treatment of post-LASIK corneal striae. J Cataract Refract Surg. 2004;30:620–5.
108. Biser SA, Bloom AH, Donnenfeld ED, et al. Flap folds after femtosecond LASIK. Eye Contact Lens. 2003;29:252–4.
109. Jackson DW, Hamill MB, Koch DD. Laser in situ keratomileusis flap suturing to treat recalcitrant flap striae. J Cataract Refract Surg. 2003;29:264–9.
110. Pannu JS. Incidence and treatment of wrinkled corneal flap following LASIK. J Cataract Refract Surg. 1997;23:695–6.
111. Solanki S, Rathi M, Khanduja S, et al. Recent trends: medical management of infectious keratitis. Oman J Ophthalmol. 2015;8:83–5.
112. Chang MA, Jain S, Azar DT. Infections following laser in situ keratomileusis: an integration of the published literature. Surv Ophthalmol. 2004;49:269–80.
113. Knorq MC, Wiesinger B, Liewnann A, et al. Laser in situ keratomileusis for moderate and high myopia and myopic astigmatism. Ophthalmology. 1998;105:932–40.
114. Ghanem RC, Allemann N, Azar DT. Phakic intraocular lenses. In: Yanoff M, editor. Ophthalmology. 4th ed. Philadelphia, PA: Elsevier Saunders Inc; 2014. p. 127–40.
115. Güell JL, Vázquez M, Malecaze F, et al. Artisan torik phakic intraocular lens for the correction of high astigmatism. Ophthalmology. 2003;136: 442–7.
116. Nuijts RM, Abhilakh Missier KA, Nabar VA, Japing WJ. Artisan toric lens implantation for correction of postkeratoplasty astigmatism. Ophthalmology. 2004;111:1086–94.
117. Tahzib NG, Cheng YY, Nuijts RM. Three-year follow up analysis of artisan toric lens implantation for correction of postkeratoplasty ametropia in phakic and pseudophakic eyes. Ophthalmology. 2006;113:976–84.
118. Ioannidis A, Nartley I, Little BC. Traumatic dislocation and successful re-enclavation of an artisan phakic IOL with analysis of the endothelium. J Refract Surg. 2006;22:102–3.
119. Day AC, Ramkissoon Y, George S, Corbett MC. Traumatic dislocation of an iris-fixated phakic intraocular lens. Eye (Lond). 2007;2:121–2.
120. Mertens E, Tassignon MJ. Detachment of iris claw haptic after implantation of phakic worst anterior chamber lens: case report. Bull Soc Belge Ophtalmol. 1998;268:19–22.
121. Yoon H, Macaluso DC, Moshirfar M, Lundergan M. Traumatic dislocation of an Ophtec Artisan phakic intraocular lens. J Refract Surg. 2002;18:482–3.
122. Harsum S, Tossounis C, Tappin MJ. Spontaneous dislocation of an Artisan phakic IOL causing corneal decompensation requiring an endothelial graft. Eye (Lond). 2010;24:1292.
123. Lee SJ. Traumatic aniridia and aphakia after Artisan intraocular lens implantation. J Cataract Refract Surg. 2007;33:1341–2.

124. Hyun J, Chung JK, Lee SJ. Traumatic partial aniridia and cataract after iris-fixated foldable phakic intraocular lens implantation. Case Rep Ophthalmol. 2013;4:210–5.
125. Knorz MC, Lane SS, Holland SP. Angle-supported phakic intraocular lens for correction of moderate to high myopia: three-year interim results in international multicenter studies. J Cataract Refract Surg. 2011;37:469–80.
126. Kohnen T, Klaproth OK. Three-year stability of an angle-supported foldable hydrophobic acrylic phakic intraocular lens evaluated by Scheimpflug photography. J Cataract Refract Surg. 2010;36: 1120–6.
127. Alio JL, Pinero D, Bernabeu G, et al. The Kelman Duet phakic intraocular lens: 1-year results. J Refract Surg. 2007;23:868–79.
128. Himbel H, Norton NR, Amritandand A. Angle-supported phakic intraocular lenses for the correction of myopia: three year follow up. J Cataract Refract Surg. 2015;41:2179–89.
129. Menezo JL, Peris-Martinez C, Cisneros AL, Martinez-Costa R. Phakic intraocular lenses to correct high myopia: Adatomed, Staar, and Artisan. J Cataract Refract Surg. 2004;30:33–44.
130. Alió JL, Toffaha BT, Peña-Garcia P, et al. Phakic intraocular lens explantation: causes in 240 cases. J Refract Surg. 2015;31:30–5.
131. Fellner P, Vidic B, Ramkissoon Y, et al. Pupil ovalization after phakic intraocular lens implantation is associated with sectorial iris hypoperfusion. Arch Ophthalmol. 2005;123:1061–5.
132. Fyodorov SN, Zuyev VK, Tumanyan ER. Modern approach to the stagewise complex surgical therapy of the high myopia. [Russian] Transactions of International Symposium of IOL Implantation and Refractive Surgery. Moscow, RSFSP Ministry of health; 1987. p. 274–79.
133. Jiménez-Alfaro I, Benítez del Castilo JM, Gàrcia-Feijoó J, et al. Safety of posterior chamber phakic Intraocular lenses for the correction of high myopia: anterior segment changes after posterior chamber phakic intraocular lens implantation. Ophthalmology. 2001;108:90–9.
134. Moshirfar M, Stagg BC, Muthappan V, Vasavada SA. Traumatic dislocation of implanted Collamer Phakic Lens: a case report and review of the literature. Open Ophthalmol J. 2014;8:24–6.
135. Alio JL, de la Hoz F, Perez-Santonja JJ, et al. Phakic anterior chamber lenses for the correction of myopia: a 7 year cumulative analysis of complications in 263 cases. Ophthalmology. 1989;106:458–66.
136. Moran S, Kirwan C, O'Keefe M, et al. Incidence of dislocated and subluxed iris-fixated phakic intraocular lens and outcomes following re-enclavation. Clin Exp Ophthalmol. 2014;42:623–8.
137. Cheung AY, Heidemann DG. Globe Rupture of a post-LASIK keratectasia eye from blunt trauma. Cornea 2016 Jul 27 [Epub ahead of print].

5 Glaucoma Considerations

Ilan Epstein, Prachi Dua, Edward Chay and Inci Dersu

Posttrauma Glaucoma

The posttraumatic patient, whether following accidental or postsurgical trauma, may develop secondary glaucoma by a variety of pathophysiologic mechanisms including open angle glaucoma, angle closure glaucoma with pupillary block, angle closure without pupillary block, or a mixed mechanism (Table 5.1). Intraocular pressure may rise subacutely or transiently, acutely to severe levels, or progressively with glaucomatous nerve damage occurring months to years following the original inciting trauma.

Chemical Injury

Monitoring intraocular pressure is critical in the early stages of chemical injury, especially with alkali burns. Acute secondary glaucoma may occur as a result of inflammation, shrinkage of scleral collagen, release of chemical mediators such as prostaglandins, direct injury to the angle, or compromise of the anterior uveal circulation.

The original version of this chapter was revised: Figure captions have been interchanged. The erratum to this chapter is available at https://doi.org/10.1007/978-3-319-47633-9_16

I. Epstein · P. Dua · E. Chay · I. Dersu (✉)
Department of Ophthalmology, The State University of New York (SUNY) Downstate Medical Center, Brooklyn, NY, USA
e-mail: Inci.dersu@downstate.edu

Oral carbonic anhydrase inhibitors may be used to lower intraocular pressure until the corneal epithelium adequately heals to allow for the introduction of topical intraocular pressure lowering agents. Chronic secondary open angle glaucoma may also occur months to years following chemical injury due to trabecular damage. (A more detailed discussion of chemical injury can be found in chapter Corneal Trauma on section Chemical Injury.)

Hyphema

Traumatic hyphema, following blunt or penetrating ocular trauma or intraocular surgery may cause acute rises in intraocular pressure. Typically, increased intraocular pressure leading to glaucomatous nerve damage occurs following a recurrent hemorrhage or in patients with sickle cell hemoglobinopathies. Elevated intraocular pressure may occur acutely following obstruction of the trabecular meshwork, pupillary block by a "buttonhole clot" involving both the anterior and posterior chambers, trauma to the trabecular meshwork, angle recession, or chronically by the formation of peripheral anterior synechiae.

Iridodialysis and Cyclodialysis

The three most common anterior chamber angle injuries found in a sample of posttraumatic glaucoma patients were angle recession, iridodialysis, and cyclodialysis [1]. Iridodialysis

S.C. Kaufman and D.R. Lazzaro (eds.), *Textbook of Ocular Trauma*,
DOI 10.1007/978-3-319-47633-9_5

Table 5.1 Mechanisms of post-traumatic glaucoma

Open angle glaucoma
Inflammatory (alkali burn, siderosis, postsurgical, hyphema, UGH)
Pigment dispersion (postsurgical, iridotomy)
Angle recession (angle recession glaucoma, hyphema)
Trabecular outflow obstruction (hemolytic/ghost cell glaucoma, hyphema, retained viscoelastic)
Angle closure glaucoma
Ectopia lentis
Postsurgical (aphakic, posterior chamber IOL, anterior chamber IOL, capsular)
Peripheral anterior synechia (inflammatory, post-hyphema, post-iridodialysis)
Aqueous misdirection
Postsurgical (scleral buckles, vitreous oil/gas)
Choroidal swelling (serous or hemorrhagic choroidal detachments or effusions)

refers to a separation of the iris root from the ciliary body. Secondary glaucoma may develop acutely if associated with significant hyphema or chronically by the formation of peripheral anterior synechiae if untreated. Cyclodialysis refers to a separation of the ciliary body from its attachment at the scleral spur, resulting in a cleft. Cyclodialysis typically causes hypotony that may result in visual damage; however, delayed closure of a cleft may result in an acute rise in intraocular pressure with a formed anterior chamber and open angle.

Angle Recession Glaucoma

Recession of the anterior angle may occur following blunt ocular trauma by tears in the ciliary body, usually between the longitudinal and circular fibers. Angle recession is often associated with injury to the trabecular meshwork as well. Glaucoma associated with angle recession, referred to as angle recession glaucoma or traumatic glaucoma, presents as chronic secondary open angle glaucoma with an insidious rise in intraocular pressure leading to glaucomatous nerve damage and visual field loss months to years following the trauma.

A population-based study conducted on inhabitants in Mamre, South Africa revealed a prevalence of angle recession at 14.6% of 987 inhabitants screened with gonioscopy, over half of which having bilateral angle recession. The prevalence of glaucoma in those with angle recession was 5.5 to 8.0% in eyes identified as having 360° angle recession [2]. Possible risk factors for the development of glaucoma with angle recession include increased pigmentation of the angle, elevated baseline intraocular pressure, hyphema, lens displacement, and angle recession of more than 180° [3].

All individuals sustaining blunt ocular trauma should undergo gonioscopic evaluation of the angle for recession, typically 6–8 weeks following the trauma. Gonioscopic findings may include a broad angle recess, absent or torn iris processes, a white glistening scleral spur, depression in the overlying trabecular meshwork, and peripheral anterior synechiae in the border of the recession (Fig. 5.1). Patients identified with recessed angles should be monitored routinely with intraocular pressure checks and adjunctive glaucoma testing.

Treatment of angle recession glaucoma is often initiated with topical medications such as aqueous suppressants, prostaglandin analogs, and alpha-2 adrenergic agonists. Laser trabeculoplasty has little utility [4]. Surgical intervention may be undertaken to lower the intraocular pressure. Angle recession glaucoma had been associated with a high rate of bleb failure in trabeculectomy; however, trabeculectomy with adjunctive mitomycin C has been shown to be effective [5, 6]. Glaucoma drainage devices are

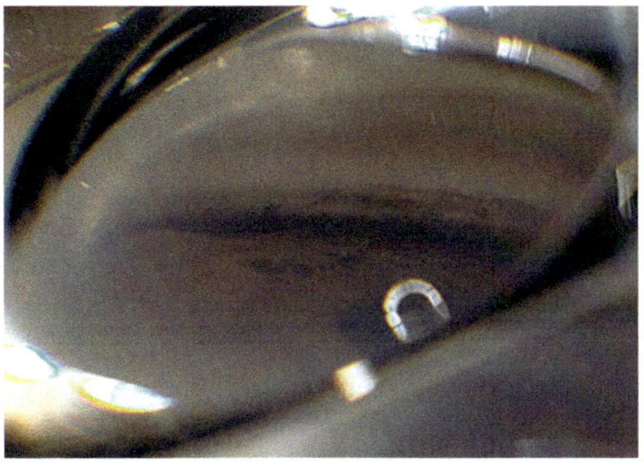

Fig. 5.1 Anterior chamber angle showing angle recession with widening of the ciliary body band and increased pigmentation

also gaining popularity for the treatment of this condition.

Ghost Cell and Hemolytic Glaucoma

Ghost cell glaucoma and hemolytic glaucoma are related forms of secondary open angle glaucoma that develop following a traumatic vitreous hemorrhage with a disrupted anterior hyaloid face that provides a communication between the posterior and anterior chambers. In ghost cell glaucoma, de-hemoglobinized red blood cells or "ghost cells" migrate to the anterior chamber to block trabecular outflow channels leading to elevated intraocular pressure; while in hemolytic glaucoma, hemoglobin-laden macrophages are the source of the obstruction. Theoretically, patients with a disruption of the anterior hyaloid face from previous ocular trauma or surgery are at risk for the development of hemolytic or ghost cell glaucoma following vitreous hemorrhage of any cause.

On examination, khaki-color cells are visualized in the anterior chamber out of proportion to aqueous flare and can be seen layering over the inferior trabecular meshwork on gonioscopy in ghost cell glaucoma. In hemolytic glaucoma, red-tinged cells are seen in the anterior chamber and a reddish-brown pigment is seen covering the trabecular meshwork on gonioscopy. Given the time course for the natural degradation of red blood cells, elevation in intraocular pressure tends to occur a few weeks to three months following the vitreous hemorrhage [7].

The incidence of hemolytic and ghost cell glaucoma following traumatic vitreous hemorrhage is not known. Regardless, intraocular pressure should be monitored closely in the posttraumatic vitreous hemorrhage patient for the development of secondary open angle glaucoma. Following clearance of the hemorrhage, which removes the source hemoglobin and red blood cells, the secondary open angle glaucoma typically resolves. Intraocular pressure may be managed with traditional topical aqueous suppressants although some patients may require anterior chamber washout or glaucoma filtration surgery. Pars plana vitrectomy may be indicated to clear the vitreous hemorrhage for visual improvement and for control of intraocular pressure.

Siderosis

Retained intraocular foreign body from previous penetrating ocular trauma composed of iron causes siderosis. If untreated, iron deposited in neuroepithelial tissue oxidizes to form powerful free radicals that promote chronic intraocular inflammation, where secondary chronic open angle glaucoma may develop. Also known as siderotic glaucoma, the retained iron-containing foreign bodies may also be associated with heterochromia, mydriasis, and rustlike discoloration of the anterior capsular and posterior corneal surfaces.

Postsurgical Glaucoma

Postsurgical Glaucoma Following Anterior Segment Surgery or Procedures

Secondary glaucoma may follow anterior segment surgery or various ophthalmic laser procedures. Peripheral iridotomy with neodymium: yttrium–aluminum–garnet (Nd:YAG) laser may cause an immediate spike in intraocular pressure that is usually transient but may occasionally be clinically significant. The photodisruptive properties of Nd:YAG laser on pigment-containing iris epithelial tissue can cause bleeding and secondary pigment dispersion that can obstruct aqueous outflow at the trabecular meshwork. A series of 734 Chinese patients reported intraocular pressure rises of >8 mmHg in 9.8 and 0.8% of treated patients at one hour and two weeks post-procedure, respectively [8]. The series also revealed an association between the incidence of intraocular pressure spikes with higher amounts of laser energy used for the procedure. Similarly, patients undergoing posterior capsulotomy with Nd:YAG laser can have long-term elevations in intraocular pressure when higher amounts of energy are used, as reported in one series comparing groups receiving <80 and >80 mJ treatments [9].

Patients undergoing Nd:YAG laser iridotomy typically are pretreated with intraocular pressure lowering agents such as brimonidine 0.15% and pilocarpine 2%. Previous series have shown higher incidences of intraocular pressure spikes, including clinically significant rises, in patients not receiving intraocular pressure lowering pretreatment [10]. Following the procedures with Nd:YAG laser, patients are typically given a short course of topical nonsteroidal or corticosteroids to reduce inflammation and associated intraocular pressure rises.

Intraocular pressure rise is relatively common following cataract surgery that may occur by a variety of mechanisms with either an open or closed anterior chamber angle (Table 5.2). Frequently, intraocular pressure can acutely rise in the immediate postoperative period due to retention of high viscosity dispersive viscoelastic material (sodium hyaluronate, sodium chondroitin sulfate-sodium hyaluronate), commonly utilized in the modern era of phacoemulsification for intraoperative endothelial cell protection [11]. In this scenario, the peak of intraocular pressure rise occurs about 4–6 hours following surgery usually due to an obstruction in aqueous outflow through the trabecular meshwork. Patients may present with acute pain and corneal haze with an

Table 5.2 Mechanisms of intraocular pressure rise following cataract surgery

Open angle
Retained viscoelastic material
Hyphema
Toxic Anterior Segment Syndrome
Endophthalmitis
Retained lens material (lens particle, phacolytic, phacoanaphylactic)
Uveitis
Pigmentary dispersion
Previous glaucoma
Steroid response
Vitreous in the anterior chamber
Ghost cell glaucoma
α-chymotrypsin
Closed angle
Pupillary block
Ciliary block
Epithelial ingrowth
Neovascular glaucoma
Peripheral anterior synechiae

open anterior chamber angle due to significantly elevated pressure. In addition to medical management, the surgeon may also provide gentle pressure on the posterior lip of the surgical paracentesis wound to release a small amount of aqueous humor to provide immediate pressure lowering. Over the course of a few days, intraocular pressure tends to normalize as the retained material resorbs.

Secondary glaucoma is also a common complication following penetrating keratoplasty. The glaucoma typically progresses in a chronic insidious nature due to wound distortion of the trabecular meshwork and progressive angle closure. Aphakic and pseudophakic patients and those with a second graft are more frequently affected. Various treatment options may be utilized. Glaucoma drainage implants and trabeculectomy combined with antimetabolite (mitomycin C) have shown similar efficacy [12].

Postsurgical Glaucoma

Uveitis-Glaucoma-Hyphema Syndrome

Inflammation, hyphema, and increased intraocular pressure can occur as a result of contact between the iris or ciliary body and a malpositioned intraocular lens implant. This entity, known as uveitis-glaucoma-hyphema syndrome, was first recognized in 1978 with the creation of poorly developed anterior chamber lens implants that resulted in iris chafing. This syndrome can lead to chronic inflammation, cystoid macular edema, hemorrhage, and glaucomatous optic neuropathy. Although the number of cases has been reduced with the advent of posterior chamber intraocular lenses, it can still occur because of posterior iris chafing. Treatment usually involves intraocular lens removal, repositioning, or exchange. Medical management involves the use of intraocular pressure lowering drops for glaucoma and topical steroids for uveitis [13].

Postsurgical Glaucoma Following Posterior Segment Surgery or Procedures

Secondary open or angle closure glaucoma can occur after retinal surgery including retinal detachment and macular hole repair. Scleral buckling may lead to anterior rotation of ciliary body, elevation in intraocular pressure, and acute angle closure. Use of expansile gases such as sulfur hexafluoride (SF6) and perfluoropropene (C3F8) can produce secondary angle closure with or without pupillary block (Fig. 5.2).

In these cases, aspiration of intraocular gas may be needed with a laser iridotomy.

Silicone oil is used for repair of complex retinal detachments. Emulsified oil can reach the anterior chamber and lead to endothelial damage and band keratopathy. In some cases, pupillary block glaucoma can also occur. In these cases, it is best to perform prophylactic inferior iridectomy at time of surgery to prevent pupillary block [14].

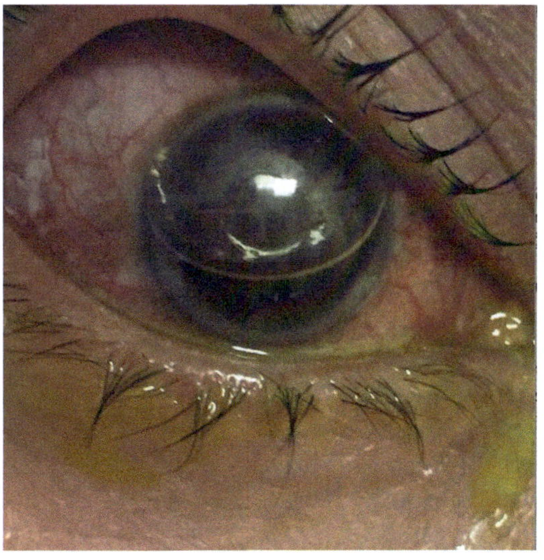

Fig. 5.2 C3F8 gas within anterior chamber leading to pupillary block glaucoma

Acute Angle Closure

Ectopia Lentis

Dislocation or subluxation of the crystalline lens can occur due to blunt trauma or head injuries. This leads to a force in the antero-posterior direction leading to equatorial expansion. When this occurs, zonules are disrupted and lens dislocation or subluxation can occur leading to pupillary block glaucoma. Some patients with the following conditions are at increased risk for lens dislocation or subluxation. These include Marfan syndrome, Weill–Marchesani syndrome, homocystinuria, or Ehlers–Danlos Syndrome.

Phacomorphic Glaucoma

Narrowing of the anterior chamber in conjunction with previous trauma and zonular weakening may occur with cataract formation. With aging, the lens increases in thickness. The iris is pushed forward with subsequent apposition of the iris root to the trabecular meshwork leading to obstruction of aqueous outflow. Acute angle closure glaucoma can then occur with significant increase in intraocular pressure, corneal edema, ocular pain, nausea, and vomiting. Treatment should focus on lowering intraocular pressure and preventing this phenomenon in the fellow eye. Medical management includes intraocular pressure lowering drops, cycloplegics, and patent iridotomy. Definitive management is surgical, however, with removal of the lens [15].

Lens Particle Glaucoma

With disruption of the anterior lens capsule during trauma, capsulotomy, or surgery, lens cortex material can migrate to the anterior chamber itself or obstruct the trabecular meshwork. This can lead to elevation in intraocular pressure, a persistent inflammatory anterior chamber reaction, and microcystic corneal edema. This event can occur weeks to years following the initial inciting event. Medical therapy should include intraocular pressure lowering drops, cycloplegics, and topical steroids to decrease inflammation. If intraocular pressure cannot be controlled with medical management, one must proceed with surgery to remove the lens material [15].

Aphakia

Aphakia can lead to pupillary block when the pupillary aperture becomes obstructed by the anterior hyaloid surface. In addition, postoperative inflammation can lead to the development of complete posterior synechiae between the iris and intact anterior hyaloid membrane. Medical management is comprised of cycloplegia, aqueous suppressants. Surgical care involves multiple iridotomies to relieve pupillary block or incision of the anterior hyaloid.

Pupillary block can also occur following anterior segment procedures. Viscoelastic substances are used during cataract surgery to maintain anterior chamber depth and prevent endothelial damage during surgery. Use of these substances can lead to increased intraocular pressures postoperatively if they block the trabecular meshwork. Dispersive substances are more likely to cause such a phenomenon because of its lower viscosity property and difficulty with removing the substance in its entirety.

Aqueous Misdirection

Aqueous misdirection is also known as malignant glaucoma, ciliary block glaucoma, and posterior aqueous diversion syndrome. Patients usually present with a shallow or flat anterior chamber and elevated intraocular pressures. Initially, on clinical exam, it may be difficult to distinguish this entity from choroidal effusion, pupillary block, or suprachoroidal hemorrhage. The underlying mechanism for aqueous misdirection is anterior rotation of the ciliary body with concomitant posterior misdirection of vitreous. Other proposed mechanisms include reduced vitreous conductivity and a propensity for choroidal expansion. This type of glaucoma usually presents in patients who have undergone intraocular surgery including cataract surgery, laser procedures, and retinal detachment repair. Medical management includes cycloplegics and aqueous suppression with IOP lowering drops. Parasympathomimetics should be discontinued if there is suspicion of aqueous misdirection. If patients do not respond to medical treatment, surgical options include disruption of anterior hyaloid face through Nd: Yag laser or vitrectomy [16, 17].

Ocular Hypotony

Intraocular pressure 5 mmHg or lower is considered as ocular hypotony. Normal pressure is measured between 10 and 20 mmHg in most individuals. Some glaucoma patients will have chronic hypotony after glaucoma surgery as a result of successful filtering surgery and this would not cause any vision problem and to be left untreated. Or eyes which are blind or near blind from old trauma or inflammation can have chronic hypotony that do not cause any symptoms. Therefore, history is very important to understand the cause and onset of hypotony. Gathering of medical history including chronic inflammatory diseases such as tuberculosis, syphilis, and sarcoidosis, as well as rheumatologic diseases is important (Table 5.3). Any history of trauma, even remote, is important and may explain chronic retinal detachment and reduced ocular volume (pre-phthisis or phthisis).

Examining the Trauma Patient

Diagnosing hypotony in the trauma patient could be challenging. Checking the eye pressure consists of applying small controlled amount of pressure of the eye, which could be deleterious and should be left to judgement of an eye specialist. When there is obvious destruction of eye and prolapse of its contents, it is recommended not to manipulate the eye as this could cause discomfort, subsequent squeezing of the eyes by the patient and make prolapse worse. In addition, a blood clot tamponing the wound could be released and more prolapsing and bleeding could occur. When the globe looks intact but chemosis and sub-conjunctival hemorrhage is evident, it is crucial to check the eye pressure in the injured eye and compare it to the contralateral eye. More than a 3–4 mmHg difference between the eyes would be suspicious. If the injured eye has a significantly lower pressure than the fellow eye, this could supportive evidence that there might be scleral perforation on the scleral portion of the eye hidden underneath subconjunctival hemorrhage, and this requires surgical exploration of the eye. During this process, the conjunctiva is excised and sclera exposed to identify and close any perforation. On the other side of the spectrum in the trauma patient, eye pressure could be

Table 5.3 Ocular conditions associated with hypotony

Entity	Other findings
Ruptured globe	Sub-conjunctival hemorrhage, uveal prolapse through cornea or conjunctiva, hyphema
Blunt trauma with no major perforation	Cyclodialysis cleft on gonioscopy hyphema
Following trabeculectomy	White cystic lesion at superior conjunctiva, wound leak
Following cataract surgery	Shallow anterior chamber, wound leak
Retinal detachment	Confrontational visual field defect
Inflammation	Keratic precipitates, posterior synechia
Pre/phthisical eye	Smaller globe, white cornea, ptosis

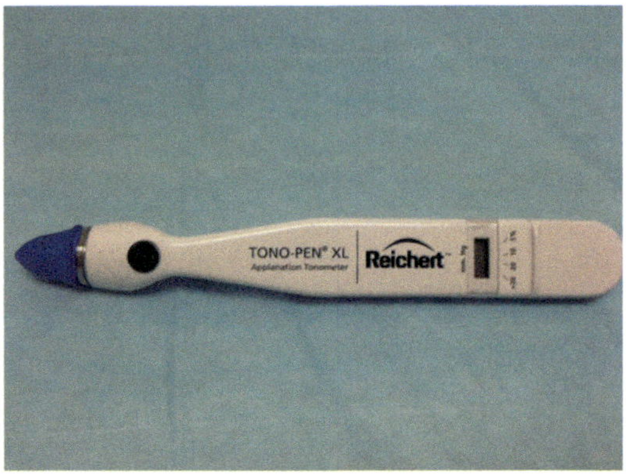

Fig. 5.3 Handheld applanation tonometer with 1 mm tip

found to be high due to various reasons including intraorbital hemorrhage.

To check intraocular pressure, applanation by a small tip, such as the Tonopen® (Reichert™ Technologies, Depew, New York), is preferred and easily applied when the patient is lying in supine position. (Fig. 5.3) A Hand held slit lamp could be utilized at the bedside to magnify the tissue and check for wound integrity. (Fig. 5.4) Existence of a leak from the ocular surface could be checked with fluorescent strip (Seidel test). Of note, the Fluorescein strip should be soaked with saline prior to use to avoid causing an abrasion in the eye. Gonioscopic exam is essential to examine the angle to look for cyclodialysis cleft, which could be associated with hypotony. In the hyphema patient, gonioscopy should be postponed until no re-bleeding is ensured as pressure from goniolens could restart the bleeding.

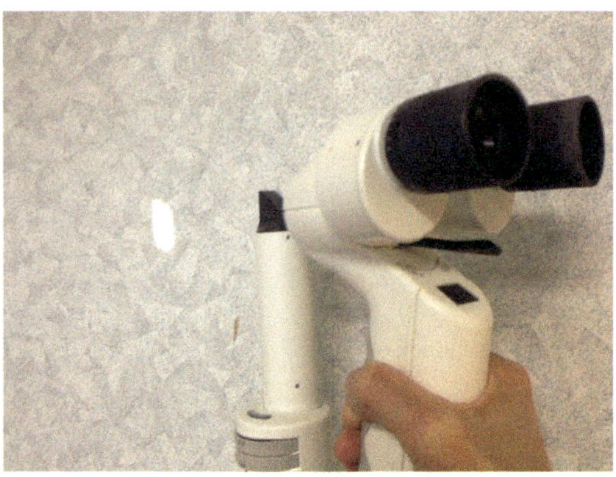

Fig. 5.4 Handheld slit lamp biomicroscopy

Postsurgical Patient

In the early period following major eye surgery, the ciliary body, which is responsible from producing fluid (aqueous) in the eye, may be ischemic and unable to generate enough aqueous fluid, leading to hypotony. Wound dehiscence leading to a leak should be kept in mind as well. Suprachoroidal effusion and cyclodialysis are other entities when patient present with hypotony in the early postoperative period. Ultrasound and ultrasound biomicroscopy are helpful tools to make this diagnosis. Even years after the glaucoma procedure, the surgical wound can leak and cause severe hypotony and infection, ranging from mild to severe. Even minor trauma such as vigourous eye-rubbing can cause this adverse event. The Eye pressure should be checked in every patient who is known to have had a glaucoma procedure. The Eye pressure could be so low that it may not be able to be measured with handheld applanation tonometer as the cutoff is 5 mmHg pressure. Severe hypotony affects the vision by causing hypotony maculopathy and refractive changes.

Management

Acute hypotony associated with ruptured globe should be treated urgently. Risk of infection, corneal decompensation, cataract development, and subsequent visual impairment among other problems increase significantly if the eye does not get immediate attention and anterior chamber stays flat considerable amount of time. The Patient should not eat or drink anything until assessed and cleared by the eye doctor or an appopriate consultant. Indicated imaging studies should be done and the injury should be repaired as soon as possible. Peri-operatively, the eye should be protected with an eye shield. The patient should be instructed not to touch the eye, and if the patient is agitated or unable to comply, adequate medical and physical measures should be taken to restrain the patient.

Glaucoma patients who are post-operative may also have special trauma considerations. Traumatic bleb leak related hypotony requires treatment with bandage contact lenses, antibiotic and topical aqueous suppressants. It is important to rule out blebitis or bleb related endophthalmitis in this setting. Chronic bleb leaks should be repaired surgically.

Small traumatic cylodialysis clefts (less than 1.5 clock hours) could be managed using cycloplegics such as atropine, larger ones will need surgical repair. Atropine relaxes the ciliary body muscles and facilitates reapposition of the ciliary longitudinal muscle to the scleral spur, thereby allowing re-establishment of its vascular supply and reversl of hypotony. Atropine also improves coexisting conditions such as inflammation by strengthening the blood-aqueous barrier. Trauma-related inflammation additionally requires topical steroids and cycloplegics [18].

Case 6.1

A 79-year-old man with history of heart disease on Coumadin and pseudoexfoliation glaucoma had Ahmed Valve placed in the right eye 5 days ago prior to Emergency Room visit. He had 2 days of severe pain and decreased vision in the right eye. There was associated tearing and redness. There was no fluctuation or improvement in symptoms since onset, and the patient complained of being unable to sleep because of the intense pain. Of note, on postoperative day 1, he was doing well with pressure at 10 mmHg; the tube was verified to be in position with a healthy conjunctival bleb overlaying the support plate; the anterior chamber was formed and without hyphema. He had a log in a notebook showing compliance with all postoperative drops including prednisolone acetate, atropine, and moxifloxacin.

On exam of the involved right eye (left eye was essentially normal), the patient's best-corrected vision was 20/100. The pressure was 64 mm Hg. Despite administration of dorzolamide, brimonidine, latanaprost, and timolol, pressure did not improve below 50 mm Hg. Acetazolamide tablets were added. The bleb, located superotemporally, was intact, diffusely elevated and had no purulent drainage. There was microcystic edema of the cornea limiting posterior visibility, and shallowing of the anterior chamber temporally and superotemporally with mild anterior displacement of the iris (Fig. 5.5). Though was no frank anterior chamber reaction, hyphema or hypopyon. B-scan showed dome shaped elevation of choroid consistent with suprachoroidal hemorrhage.

Initial differential diagnosis included poorly functioning glaucoma drainage device secondary to suboptimal positioning, suprachoroidal hemorrhage, pseudoexfoliation plugging trabecular meshwork or tube, postsurgical inflammation, and endophthalmitis. B-scan was performed and revealed a large suprachoroidal hyperintensity, most prominent near the glaucoma drainage device, with anterior rotation of the ciliary body—iris complex (Fig. 5.6). This finding, along with the pain and elevated intraocular pressure, was most consistent with delayed-onset suprachoroidal hemorrhage.

Two common entities with these findings must be recognized, characterized and promptly

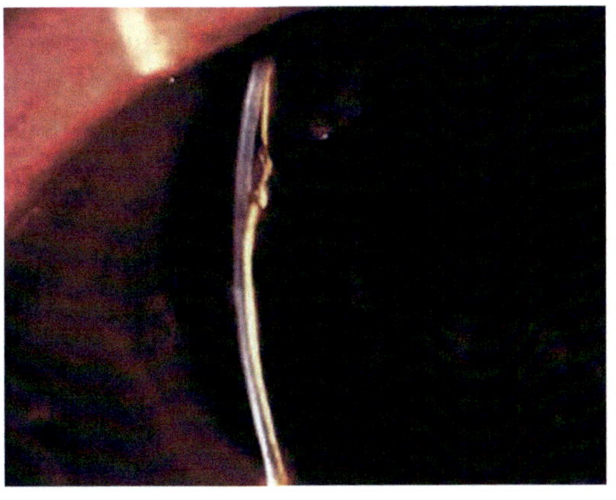

Fig. 5.5 Slit beam demonstrating shallowing of the temporal anterior chamber after delayed-onset suprachoroidal hemorrhage

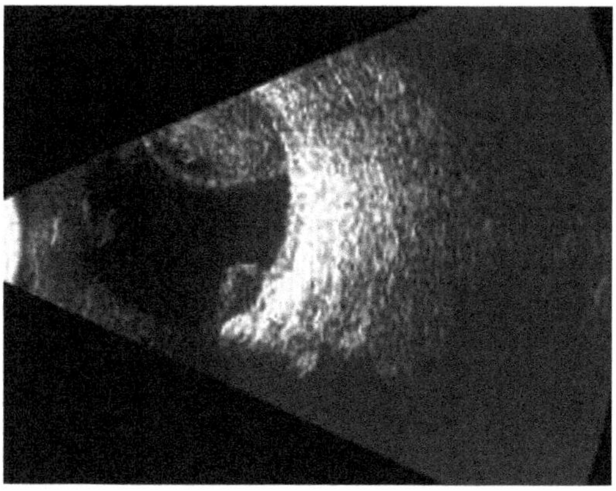

Fig. 5.6 B-Scan demonstrating large temporal suprachoroidal hemorrhage

dealt with: posttraumatic and perioperative suprachoroidal hemorrhages. In each, there is an accumulation of blood between the choroid and sclera, and the likely mechanism is hemorrhage after rupture of a short or long posterior ciliary artery secondary to hypotony. It is linked to poor visual prognosis, with only 34% of eyes achieving final visual acuity better than 20/200 [19].

One author discusses a case of traumatic ruptured globe and subsequent management. In this case, the ruptured globe was suffered while the patient was chopping wood. The vision was instantly reduced to light perception. Upon taking the patient to the operating room, a large Y-shaped laceration was found between the lateral rectus and superior rectus muscles 5 mm behind the limbus; though successfully closed, the patient suffered massive suprachoroidal hemorrhage. There was associated retinal detachment, found during the course of treatment which involved scleral parecentesis, vitrectomy, and silicone oil tamponade.

Suprachoroidal hemorrhage can also occur intraoperatively (termed expulsive) or after surgery (delayed-onset) as in our case. Delayed-onset suprachoroidal hemorrhages have an incidence of 0.7–6.1%, and more commonly after tube shunt than after trabeculectomy at a 2:1 ratio [20]. Postsurgical risk factors include high preoperative intraocular pressure (often higher in patients selected for tube shunts), severe postoperative hypotony, aphakia, pseudophakia, anticoagulation, white race, and prior intraocular surgery. Another risk factor is systemic anticoagulation, likely a complicating factor seen in our patient.

In both traumatic and surgical cases, early surgical intervention is rarely done and usually limited to cases of kissing choroidals or intraoperative expulsive suprachoroidal hemorrhage. Surgical techniques include choroidal tap and pars plana vitrectomy. Delayed-onset suprachoroidal hemorrhages, however, are usually managed nonsurgically; there are few published studies proving increased efficacy over conservative management with medications. Our patient was managed conservatively, intraocular pressure was controlled medically and suprachoridal hemorrhage dissolved on its own. He returned to clinic several weeks later with vision improved to 20/70 and intraocular pressure was 8 mmHg with no glaucoma drops.

Case 6.2

A 54-year-old African American gentleman presented with a complaint of one week of unilateral blurry vision in the right eye. He did not endorse pain, haze/glare, halos, or nausea or vomiting. He did not endorse noticing any constriction to his peripheral visual field. Previous ophthalmic history was significant for only myopic refractive error and remote blunt trauma to the right eye from being struck with a baseball bat at least 15 years prior.

On exam, his best-corrected visual acuity was 20/80 on the right and 20/25 on the left. There was a reverse afferent pupillary defect on the right. Color vision tested by Ishihara plates gave zero correct plates on the right, compared with 11 out of 11 on the left. Intraocular pressure by applanation tonometry was 48 mmHg on the

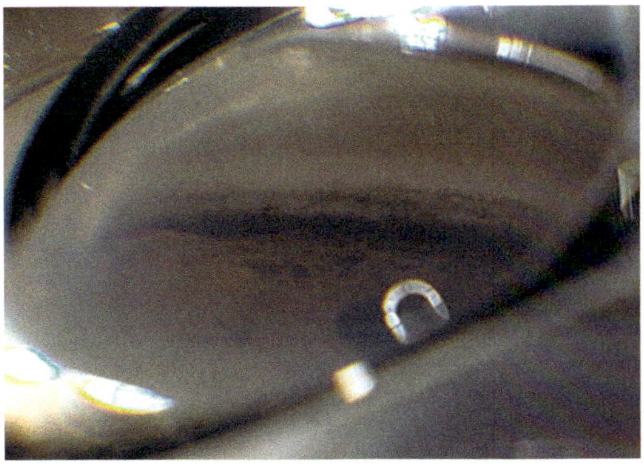

Fig. 5.7 Widened ciliary body band with heavy trabecular pigmentation in all quadrants on the *right*, compared to a normal appearing open angle with moderate pigmentation on the *left*, confirming the suspected diagnosis of angle recession glaucoma

right and 21 mmHg on the left. Corneal pachymetry revealed central corneal thicknesses of 531 and 541 μm for the right and left corneas, respectively. Slit lamp exam was significant for 2+ flare in the right anterior chamber. Gonioscopy revealed a widened ciliary body band with heavy trabecular pigmentation in all quadrants on the right (Fig. 5.7), compared to a normal appearing open angle with moderate pigmentation on the left, confirming the suspected diagnosis of angle recession glaucoma. Fundus exam revealed optic nerves with 0.9 and 0.5 symmetric cups, respectively (Fig. 5.8). Ocular coherence tomography confirmed retinal nerve fiber layer thinning of the vertical quadrants on the right, compared to normal thickness in all quadrants on the left (Fig. 5.9). Automated perimetry with Humphrey visual field 24-2 sita standard testing revealed diffuse constriction of the visual field of the right eye, compared to a full field on the left, (Fig. 5.10), confirming the advanced nature of the disease on presentation.

The patient was initially treated with 500 mg intravenous acetazolamide and two rounds of topical brimonidine tartrate/timolol maleate 0.2%/0.5%, and dorzolamide 2%, which brought the intraocular pressure down to 33 mmHg, and was continued on topical medications only. The following day, intraocular pressure was 13 mmHg. A short course of topical predisolone acetate 1% was also used, as concomitant inflammatory or glaucomatocyclic crisis to angle recession was considered in the differential diagnosis, to treat the aqueous flare that resolved in one week. At that time, intraocular pressure had risen to 24 mmHg. Topical corticosteroid was discontinued and latanoprost 0.005% was added. The patient was asked to return in one week but returned five weeks later and reporting non-compliance with eye drops. Vision fell to 20/200 and intraocular pressure was back up to 50 mmHg. Glaucoma drainage implant surgery was offered, which the patient refused, preferring to remain on eye drops.

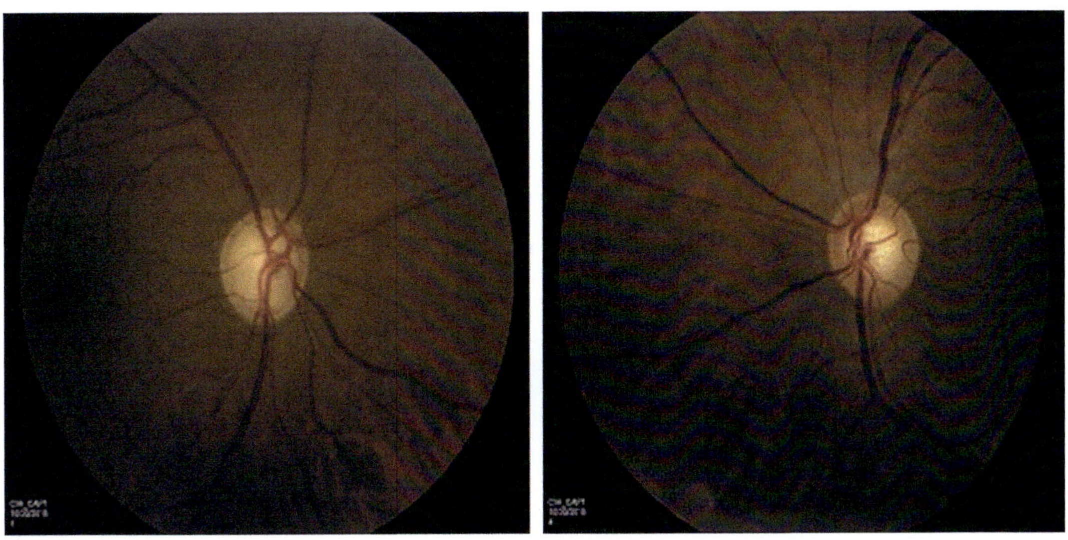

Fig. 5.8 Color fundus photos of the optic discs of the right and left eyes

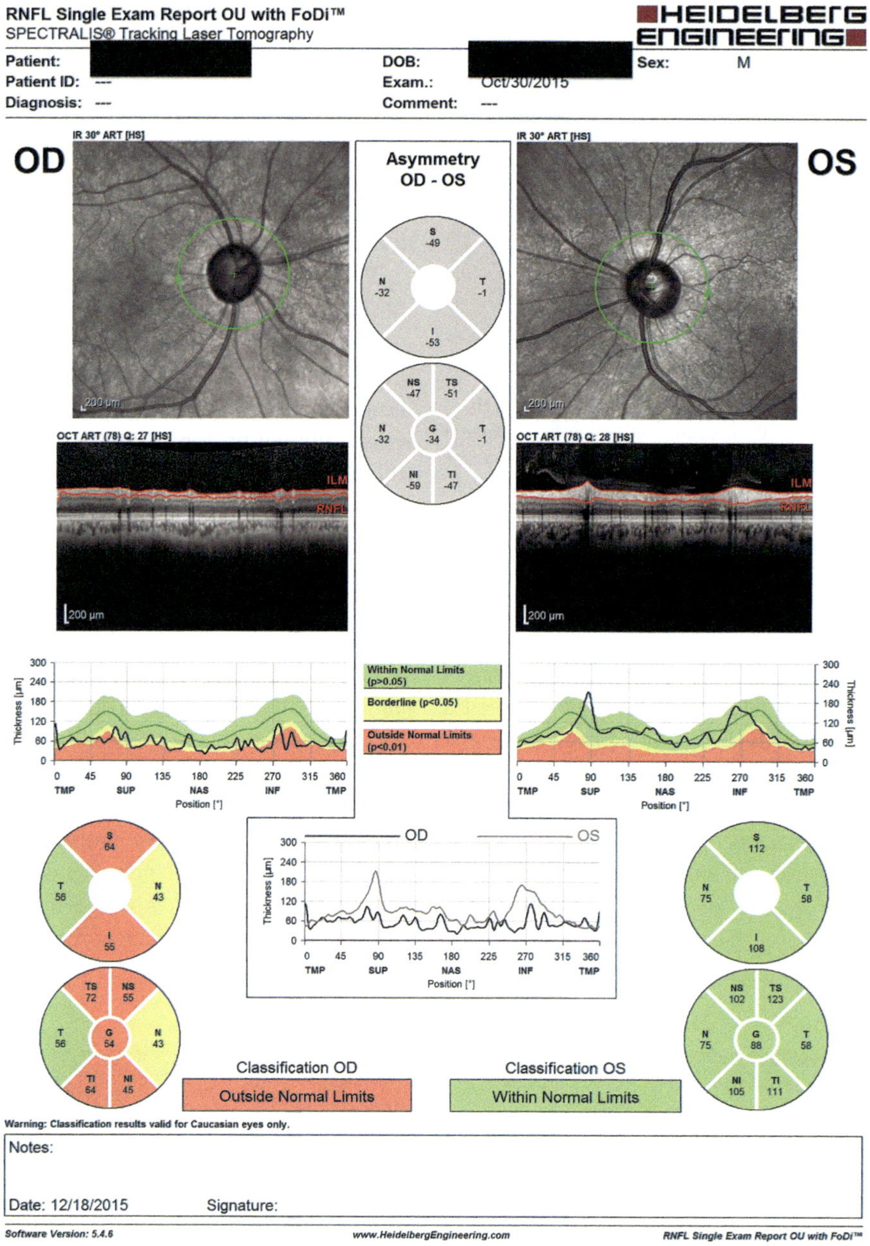

Fig. 5.9 Optical coherence tomography report on retinal nerve fiber layer thickness for the right and left eyes

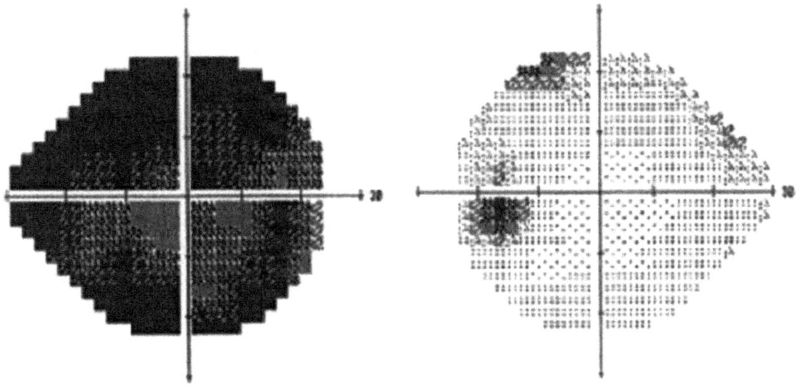

Fig. 5.10 Automated perimetry with Humphrey visual field 24-2 sita standard testing revealing diffuse constriction of the visual field of the right eye, compared to a full field on the left, confirming the advanced nature of the disease on presentation

References

1. Ellong A, Ebana Mogo C, et al. Post-traumatic glaucoma with irido-corneal angle injuries in Cameroon. Bull Soc Belge Ophtalmol. 2005;298:21–8.
2. Salmon JF, Mermoud A, et al. The detection of post-traumatic angle recession by gonioscopy in a population-based glaucoma survey. Ophthalmology. 1994;101(11):1844–50.
3. Sihota R, Kumar S, et al. Early predictors of traumatic glaucoma after closed globe injury. Arch Ophthalmol. 2008;126(7):921–6.
4. Fukuchi T, Iwata K, et al. Nd:YAG laser trabeculopuncture (YLT) for glaucoma with traumatic angle recession. Graefes Arch Ophthalmol. 1993;231:571–6.
5. Mermoud A, Salmon JF, Straker C, et al. Post-traumatic angle recession glaucoma: a risk factor for bleb failure after trabeculectomy. Br J Ophthalmol. 1993;77:631–4.
6. Manners T, Salmon JF, et al. Trabeculectomy with mitomycin C in the treatment of post-traumatic angle recession glaucoma. Br J Ophthalmol. 2001;85:159–63.
7. Campbell DG. Ghost cell glaucoma following trauma. Ophthalmology. 1981;88(11):1151–8.
8. Jiang Y, Chang DS, et al. Immediate changes in intraocular pressure after laser peripheral iridotomy in primary angle-closure suspects. Ophthalmology. 2012;119:283–8.
9. Ari S, Cingu AK, et al. The effects of Nd:YAG laser posterior capsulotomy on macular thickness, intraocular pressure, and visual acuity. Ophthalmic Surg Lasers Imaging. 2012;43(5):395–400.
10. Shani L, David R, et al. Intraocular pressure after neodymium:YAG laser treatments in the anterior segment. J Cataract Refract Surg. 1994;20:455–8.
11. Rainer G, Menapace R, et al. Intraocular pressure after small incision cataract surgery with Healon5 and Viscoat. J Cataract Refract Surg. 2000;26:271–6.
12. Ayyala RS, Pieroth L, Vinals AF, et al. Comparison of mitomycin C trabeculectomy, glaucoma drainage device implantation, and laser neodymium:YAG cyclophotocoagulation in the management of intractable glaucoma after penetrating keratoplasty. Ophthalmology. 1998;105:1550–6.
13. Piette, et al. Ultrasound biomicroscopy in uveitis-glaucoma-hyphema syndrome. Am J Ophthalmol. 2002;133(6):839–41.
14. Gedde SJ. Management of glaucoma after retinal detachment surgery. Curr Opin Ophthalmol. 2002;13(2):103–9.
15. Papconstantinou D, et al. Lens-induced glaucoma in the elderly. Clin Interv Aging. 2009;4:331–6.
16. Lundy DC. Ciliary block glaucoma. *Focal Points: Clinical Modules for Ophthalmologists*. 1999. San Francisco: American Academy of Ophthalmology (module 3).
17. Quigley HA, Friedman DS, Congdon NG. Possible mechanisms of primary angle-closure and malignant glaucoma. J Glaucoma. 2003;12:167–80.
18. Ioannidis AS, Barton K. Cyclodialysis cleft: causes and repair. Curr Opin Ophthalmol. 2010;21:150–4.
19. Jin W, Xing Y, Xu Y, Wang W, Yang A. Management of delayed suprachoroidal hemorrhage after intraocular surgery and trauma. Graefes Arch Clin Exp Ophthalmol. 2014;252:1189–93.
20. Chu TG, Green RL. Suprachoroidal haemorrhage. Surv Ophthalmol. 1999;43:471–86.

6 Eyelids

Jenny Temnogorod and Roman Shinder

Anatomy

Knowledge of eyelid anatomy is essential for proper evaluation, diagnosis, and treatment of periocular injuries. The eyelids play an important role in the maintenance of ocular health by protecting and lubricating the ocular surface. The goal of management of eyelid trauma is to restore the anatomy and maximize the appearance and the function of the eyelids.

Eyebrow

The eyebrow is the area in the superficial muscle plane where the frontalis and the orbicularis oculi muscles meet. The skin and the subcutaneous tissue layer are thicker in this region than in the eyelid. The skin contains large hair follicles that are arranged in a particular fashion which should be taken into account when reconstructing defects in this area. The cilia in the medial eyebrow are angled superotemporally. The remainder of the eyebrow cilia is divided into upper and lower portions, where it is angled inferotemporally and superotemporally, respectively [1].

J. Temnogorod · R. Shinder (✉)
Department of Ophthalmology, The State University of New York (SUNY) Downstate Medical Center, 541 Clarkson Ave, E Bldg, 8th Floor, Suite C, Brooklyn, NY 11203, USA
e-mail: shinder.roman@gmail.com

Eyelid

It is important to remember the superficial structural relationships of the eyelid when evaluating and managing trauma. In children the upper eyelid normally rests at the upper border of the cornea (the limbus), and in adults it falls about 2 mm below the limbus [1]. The angles formed at the junctions of the upper and lower eyelids are called medial and lateral canthi. Normally, the lateral canthal angle is about 2 mm higher than the medial canthal angle (Fig. 6.1) [1].

The eyelid margin is divided into the anterior and posterior lamella by the gray line, the terminal extension of the orbicularis oculi muscle. The anterior lamella consists of the skin, orbicularis oculi muscle and the eyelashes. The posterior lamella includes the tarsus and the conjunctiva (Fig. 6.2). The canaliculi of the lacrimal drainage system are found in the medial portion of the upper and lower eyelids, and the puncta are located in the medial eyelid margins.

The eyelid skin is the thinnest skin of the body. Careful repair of an eyelid skin laceration usually produces minimal scarring and cosmetically favorable results. There is loose subcutaneous tissue with minimal subcutaneous fat in this region.

The orbicularis oculi muscle is a superficial muscle covering the orbit and is found just posterior to the eyelid. It is innervated by the facial nerve and its main actions are involuntary blink and forced eyelid closure. Portions of the muscle surrounding the canaliculi participate in the

S.C. Kaufman and D.R. Lazzaro (eds.), *Textbook of Ocular Trauma*,
DOI 10.1007/978-3-319-47633-9_6

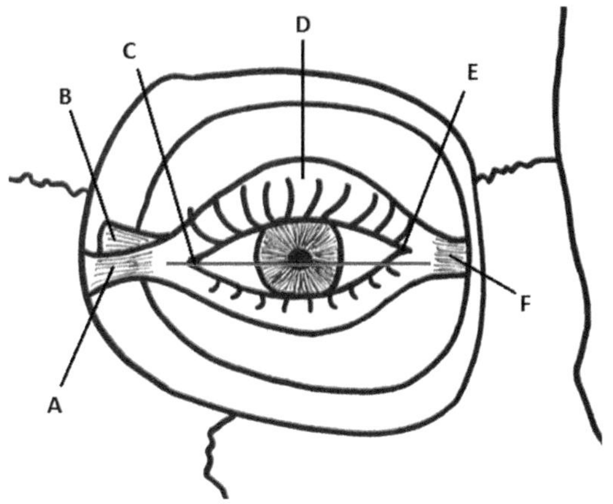

Fig. 6.1 Frontal view of the left periocular area with the superficial layers (eyelid skin and orbicularis oculi) removed. The medial and lateral canthal ligaments attach the eyelids to the orbital walls. The lateral canthal angle is about 2 mm higher than the medial canthal angle. The upper eyelid covers the superior limbus by about 2 mm in adults. *A* Superficial limb of the medial canthal ligament. *B* Deep limb of the medial canthal ligament. *C* Medial canthal angle. *D* Superior tarsus. *E* Lateral canthal angle; *F* Lateral canthal ligament

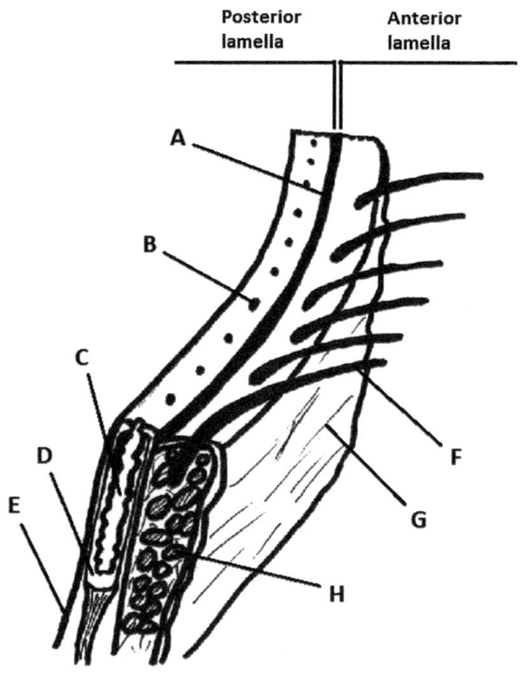

Fig. 6.2 Anterior and posterior lamella of the eyelid margin separated by the *gray line*. Anterior lamella includes the eyelid skin, orbicularis oculi muscle and the cilia. Posterior lamella includes the tarsus and the palpebral conjunctiva. *A Gray line*. *B* Meibomian gland orifice. *C* Meibomian gland. *D* Tarsus. *E* Palpebral conjunctiva. *F* Cilia. *G* Eyelid skin. *H* Orbicularis oculi muscle

lacrimal pump mechanism allowing egress of tears through the lacrimal outflow system.

Posterior to the orbicularis oculi muscle is the orbital septum, a thin membrane that arises from the periosteum of the orbital rim and marks the anterior border of the orbit. In the upper eyelid it fuses with the underlying levator aponeurosis 2–5 mm above the superior border of the tarsus. In the lower eyelid it inserts on the inferior border of the tarsus along with the lower eyelid retractors [1]. The septum is an important barrier protecting the vital orbital compartment and its structures from spread of infection or blood in cases of preseptal cellulitis or hemorrhage. Orbital fat, including the preaponeurotic and the lower eyelid fat pads, are found directly posterior to the septum.

The muscles that elevate the upper eyelid and depress the lower eyelid are called the eyelid retractors (Fig. 6.3). They are found deep to the orbital fat and include the levator palpebrae superioris and Müller's muscle in the upper eyelid and the lower eyelid retractors in the lower eyelid. The retractors of the upper eyelid are more developed than their counterparts in the lower eyelid because the upper eyelid requires greater range of motion.

The levator palpebrae superioris is innervated by the oculomotor nerve and is the main elevator of the upper eyelid. It arises in the posterior orbit in the orbital apex and travels anteriorly through the superior orbit. Near the superior orbital rim a fibrous condensation, Whitnall's ligament, is attached to the levator muscle sheath transversely and redirects the course of the muscle inferiorly. At Whitnall's ligament, the muscular body of the levator changes to the fibrous levator aponeurosis. The levator aponeurosis inserts at the anterior surface of the tarsus, with other distal attachments to the overlying orbicularis oculi muscle and skin forming the upper eyelid crease. Medially and laterally the levator aponeurosis attaches to the bony orbit. The lateral horn of the aponeurosis divides the lacrimal gland into the

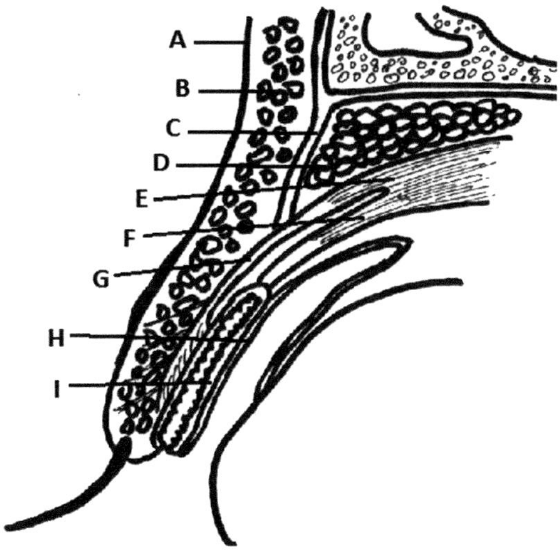

Fig. 6.3 Cross-section of the upper eyelid. *A* Eyelid skin. *B* Orbicularis oculi muscle. *C* Orbital septum. *D* Preaponeurotic orbital fat. *E* Levator palpebrae superioris muscle. *F* Müller's muscle. *G* Levator aponeurosis. *H* Palpebral conjunctiva. *I* Tarsus

orbital and palpebral lobes as it passes toward the lateral orbital wall.

Müller's muscle is sympathetically innervated and contributes 2 mm of elevation to the upper eyelid. It arises from the underside of the levator muscle in the superior orbit and inserts at the superior border of the tarsus. The lower eyelid retractors arise from the capsulopalpebral fascia and insert into the inferior border of the lower lid tarsus. Just posterior to Müller's muscle in the upper lid, and the lower eyelid retractors in the lower lid, is the palpebral conjunctiva.

The tarsal plates and the palpebral conjunctiva comprise the posterior lamella of the eyelid. The tarsal plates contribute to the form and support of the eyelids. Centrally, the upper tarsus is 10 mm in height, while the lower tarsus is 3–5 mm [1]. It is composed of dense connective tissue and contains sebaceous meibomian glands. The glands secrete the oily component of the tear film with their orifices located at the eyelid margin. The palpebral conjunctiva is adherent to the posterior tarsal surface and extends over the eyelid margin to the mucocutaneous junction, just posterior to the meibomian gland orifices. This conjunctiva represents a smooth mucous membrane important for comfortable contact between the lid and globe during the blink cycle and eye movements.

The tarsal plates are attached to the bony orbit by fibrous connections called the medial and lateral canthal ligaments (Fig. 6.1). The medial canthal ligament consists of a superficial and deep limb, which attach to the anterior and posterior lacrimal crest, respectively. The posterior attachment is important in maintaining the apposition of the eyelids against the convex globe and allowing normal tear drainage. Disruption of this anatomic relationship by trauma can result in chronic tearing (epiphora). Laterally, the fibrous strands from the tarsal plates form a common lateral canthal ligament, which attaches just inside the lateral orbital rim at the lateral orbital tubercle. It is important to recreate this posterior insertion during reconstruction after lateral canthal avulsion injuries.

The eyelids have a rich vascular supply that promotes healing. This includes an extensive network of anastomoses between branches from the external and internal carotid arteries. The angular and the superficial temporal arteries from the external carotid and the ophthalmic artery and its terminal branches from the internal carotid participate in this vascular network. They form the marginal and the peripheral arcades in the upper eyelid. The marginal arcade is found 2–4 mm superior to the eyelid margin, while the peripheral arcade is located at the superior tarsal border between the levator aponeurosis and Müller's muscle [1]. The lower eyelid often has one arcade.

The eyelids are supplied by two sensory nerves, the ophthalmic and maxillary divisions of the trigeminal nerve. Sensory input travels from the upper eyelid via the ophthalmic division and from the lower eyelid via the maxillary division of the trigeminal nerve.

Eyelid Trauma

Evaluation

It is important to elicit a detailed history of the trauma when possible. The mechanism and timing of injury can provide clues as to whether deeper ocular or orbital damage has occurred or when the presence of a foreign body should be suspected. A penetrating injury with a long, sharp object can appear as a small puncture wound on the surface, but may extend deep into the orbit or globe causing significant damage. Lacerations due to bites have a higher prevalence of canalicular involvement than those due to other causes [2–4]. An orbital fracture should be considered in cases of blunt injury to the periorbital area.

A careful and systemic ocular and adnexal examination should be performed with the goal of determining the extent of injury. The examination of the eye should be performed first to exclude the presence of a serious ocular injury, such as a ruptured globe, that can be exacerbated by manipulation of the surrounding soft tissues. Often eyelid injuries coexist with severe ocular injuries that need to be addressed first to decrease the risk of potential vision loss [5]. Next, the eyelid should be examined. Careful cleaning of the traumatic area with saline and gauze will often uncover a more complex injury than was suspected during initial gross inspection as recent lacerations may splay apart disclosing their true extent. Careful inspection of the eyelid margin is critical in assessing margin involving full thickness lacerations. Special attention should be directed at the eyelid margins medial to the puncta to determine whether the canaliculi have been injured. If there is any suspicion, a lacrimal probe should be used to inspect for a canalicular laceration. The presence of orbital fat in a wound confirms that the orbital septum has been violated and trauma extends to orbital structures. Careful inspection of any deep wounds should be carried out using cotton tipped applicators to assess for presence of foreign bodies. Movement of the upper eyelid should be evaluated in a vertical direction to assess levator function. Based on the history and physical examination, orbital imaging may be warranted.

Management

Intravenous antibiotics should be administered if the injury is extensive or the wound appears contaminated. A history of tetanus immunization should be obtained. Human tetanus immunoglobulin 250 units should be administered unless the patient is up to date with this vaccination. If the patient's immunization was more than 5 years ago, 0.5 mL of tetanus toxoid prophylaxis should be given [2].

Primary repair of eyelid wounds produces the best functional and cosmetic results. It is recommended that eyelid lacerations be repaired within 12–24 h of trauma; however, life and vision-threatening conditions should be addressed first. If a delay occurs, all attempts should be made to perform delayed primary closure rather than allowing the wounds to heal by secondary intention. Eyelid lacerations can be repaired after 24–72 h without significant negative outcomes, though the wound margins may have to be freshened during repair [2]. While awaiting repair, tissues should be repositioned into their anatomic locations and a robust supply of ophthalmic antibiotic ointment placed over the wounds. Systemic antibiotics should also be considered.

Repair can be performed using local anesthesia at bedside or in a minor procedure room for most minor injuries. More extensive injuries can be repaired in the operating room under sedation or general anesthesia. Local anesthesia can be achieved by injecting 1% lidocaine with 1:100,000 epinephrine. The authors prefer to combine lidocaine in a 50:50 mixture with 0.5% bupivacaine with epinephrine for a longer lasting effect and postoperative pain control. Betadine should be used to prep the surgical area. As always, consider medication allergies.

The first step in surgical repair is thorough cleaning and exploration of the wounds. To avoid chronic infection and abscess formation, removal of foreign bodies is essential. Avoid excising any tissue unless clearly devitalized. Decontamination of wounds using high-pressure sterile saline irrigation reduces the rate of wound infection by 90% [2]. If the wounds are visibly contaminated, irrigation with an antibiotic solution should also be performed.

When planning surgical repair, any injuries to the lacrimal apparatus, canthal ligaments, or the levator aponeurosis should be addressed first, and repair of eyelid margin and skin should follow. It may seem as if tissue is missing from a wound but this is uncommon in eyelid lacerations, and the appearance may actually be due to swelling and retraction of the wound edges. Care should be taken to carefully reapproximate the wound margins, unfolding any rolled tissue edges. Identifying landmarks such as the eyebrow hairline can help in proper realignment of the tissue. It is important not to mistakenly capture the septum during wound closure, to avoid secondary lid retraction and lagophthalmos.

Blunt Trauma

Blunt trauma is often caused by impact during motor vehicle accidents, assaults and accidental trauma. It can result in periocular contusion or hematoma (Fig. 6.4), skin abrasion, irregularly shaped lacerations or avulsions. Periocular contusions and skin abrasions do not require surgical intervention and can be treated with thorough cleaning, antibiotic ointment to prevent infection and ice packs to decrease swelling. Repair of irregularly shaped lacerations follows the same principles as that for simple lacerations but requires patience to carefully identify and close the opposing edges of the wound with carefully placed interrupted sutures.

Avulsion of Medial and Lateral Canthal Ligaments

Avulsions are caused by tearing of tissue, which often occurs with injuries on pavement. The wound edges often separate, which may appear as if there is loss of tissue. However, tissue loss is very rare so careful examination with reapposition of wound edges is essential in determining the extent of injury [6].

Avulsion of the medial canthal tendon is suspected when there is lateral displacement of the punctum upon lateral traction on the eyelid. Medial canthal injuries are often associated with canalicular lacerations, which should be addressed first. During evaluation of a medial canthal injury, it is important to establish whether the posterior limb of the medial canthal ligament has avulsed from its bony attachment. Proper repositioning of the posterior limb is a key to reestablishing adequate lid apposition to the globe and maintaining normal lacrimal pump function. Failure to perform this critical step can result in chronic tearing, telecanthus, and facial asymmetry.

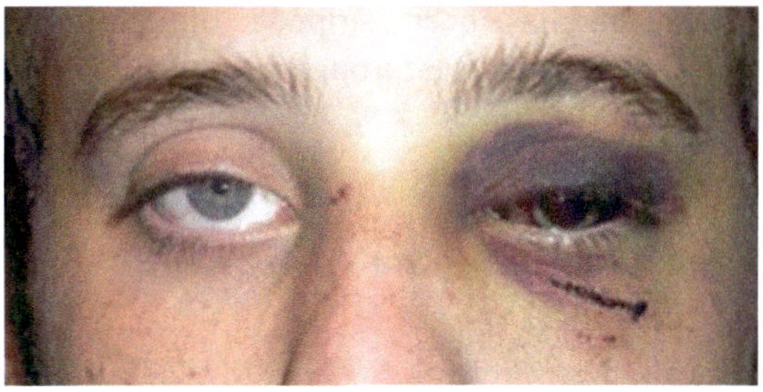

Fig. 6.4 16-year-old male with a left periocular contusion after assault with a closed fist

Fixation of the avulsed medial canthal ligament to the periosteum of the posterior lacrimal crest can be performed with a nonabsorbable suture such as polypropylene. In cases where the periosteum is completely stripped from the bone, a titanium microplate and drill holes can be used to anchor the medial canthal ligament [7]. If there is a medial orbital wall fracture that cannot be stabilized, transnasal wiring may be required to reposition the medical canthal ligament [7].

Repair of an avulsed lateral canthal ligament also requires posterior fixation to maintain the proper lid-globe apposition and avoid rounding of the lateral canthal angle and lateral canthal dystopia [8]. This can be achieved by using polypropylene suture and attaching the distal severed end of the ligament or the lateral edge of the lower lid tarsus to the periosteum on the inner aspect of the lateral orbital rim. The suture should be passed slightly above the normal anatomic position of the lateral canthal ligament at the lateral orbital tubercle to avoid the angle being pulled inferiorly by wound contracture [2]. This will help retain the correct anatomic orientation of the lateral canthal angle, which is 2 mm higher than the medial canthal angle. If the periosteum has been stripped off the bone, sutures can be passed through holes drilled in the lateral orbital rim.

Penetrating Trauma

Penetrating trauma is caused by sharp objects and results in simple and complex lacerations and puncture wounds, depending on the object and mechanism of injury.

A long, sharp object can create a small entrance wound through the skin but may extend deep into the orbit. Simple lacerations are linear, involve the skin and the underlying orbicularis oculi muscle and have minimal tissue loss. Complex lacerations can be stellate, with damage to deeper eyelid structures and have significant tissue loss. It is important to differentiate lacerations involving the eyelid margin from those that do not, as marginal laceration repair involves specific surgical techniques to restore proper eyelid anatomy.

Simple Extramarginal Lacerations

Repair of simple extramarginal lacerations (Fig. 6.5) can be performed at bedside in the emergency room or in a minor procedure room in the office. After injection of a local anesthetic, a thorough examination should be performed to confirm that the injury is superficial. The key to wound closure is to eliminate tension on the skin. If the skin edges are not well apposed, which often occurs with vertical lacerations through the orbicularis, the muscle should be reapproximated with deep long-lasting absorbable sutures such as 5-0 or 6-0 polyglactin to remove tension from the skin. Then the skin should be closed with either absorbable (6-0 plain or fast absorbing gut) or nonabsorbable (6-0 polypropylene, silk or nylon) suture. If the laceration involves the thicker eyebrow skin, a larger 5-0 suture can be used. Nonabsorbable sutures can be removed in 5–7 days. In cases of trauma where patient follow up is questionable, absorbable sutures may be prudent.

To maximize cosmetic results, wound margins should be everted during suturing. This will minimize the risk of a depressed scar, which occurs due to tissue contraction during healing. Linear wounds can be closed with a running suture, but interrupted sutures should be used for any nonlinear wounds.

Topical skin adhesives or glues are options for repair of small superficial lacerations where little to no tension exists at the laceration site. They are especially useful for management of lacerations in the pediatric population, avoiding the need for sedation or repair in the operating room [9–11]. However, glue should not be used for gaping wounds that require suture for proper reconstruction. It is also not adequate for repair of marginal lacerations.

Application of the glue is quick and simple and the cosmetic results are similar to a wound closed with suture [9–11]. In addition, skin adhesives prevent infectious organisms from reaching the wound, thereby eliminating the need for antibiotic ointment [9]. Tissue glue should be applied to the skin and not inside the wound as it can delay healing. Care should be taken to prevent glue from coming into contact with the globe as it can cause the lashes to stick together, interfering with vision and leading to irritation of the ocular surface [12].

Complex Extramarginal Lacerations

Complex eyelid lacerations include irregularly shaped lacerations (Fig. 6.6) and those with injuries deep to the orbicularis or with significant tissue loss. If tissue loss is present, the size and location of the defect are important considerations when planning surgical repair. Options for surgical repair include direct closure if wound tension allows or local flaps may be necessary. Skin grafting is usually avoided during initial closure in a trauma situation [2].

Direct closure of smaller defects is an option as long as this does not distort the eyelid margin. Vertical tension should be minimized during repair to avoid risk of eyelid retraction, ectropion and lagophthalmos. Wide undermining of tissue is helpful in minimizing skin tension [2]. In general, older patients have more skin laxity and simple stretching can aid in closing a wound that might be more difficult to

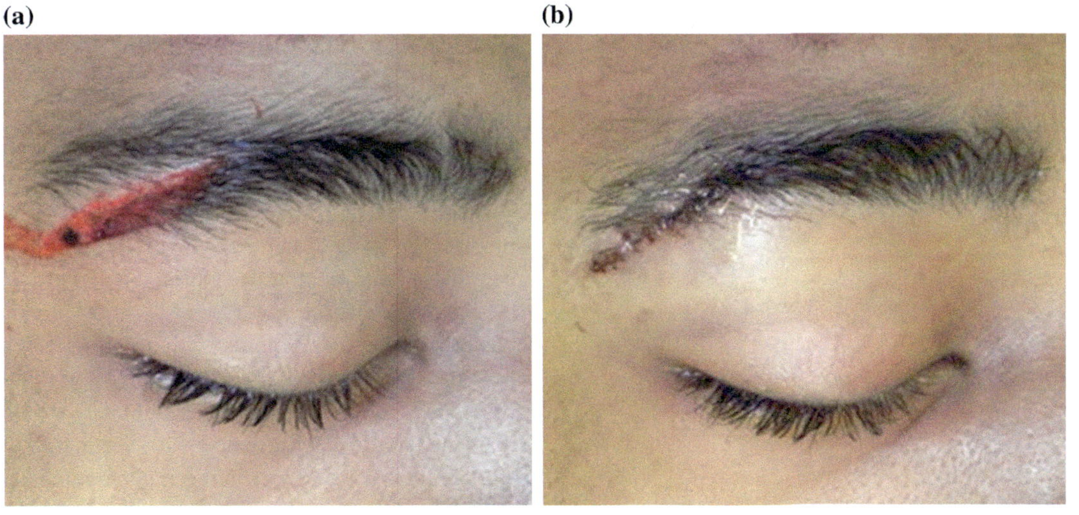

Fig. 6.5 **a** 10-year-old male with a superficial linear laceration of the right eyebrow and lateral upper lid. **b** Laceration immediately after repair using a running absorbable suture

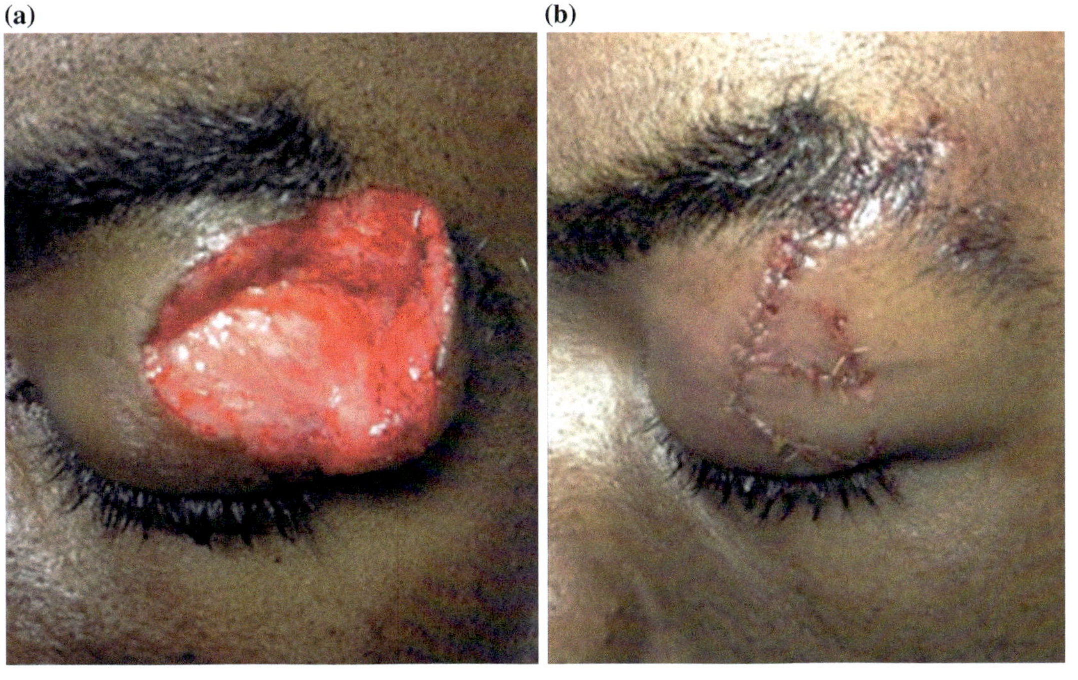

Fig. 6.6 **a** 19-year-old male with an irregularly shaped laceration of the left upper eyelid and temporal brow after trauma with barbed wire. The laceration extended deep into the orbicularis muscle without injury to deeper structures or the eyelid margin. **b** Laceration immediately after repair with deep absorbable suture and superficial interrupted and running absorbable suture

close in a younger patient. Larger defects may be repaired using myocutaneous flaps. Sometimes skin grafts are required to close the wound when there is significant loss of tissue and lack of good local tissue for flap repair (Fig. 6.7).

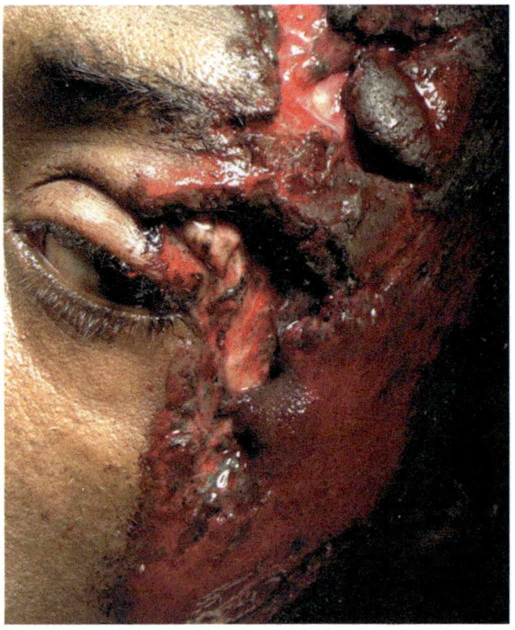

Fig. 6.7 34-year-old male with lateral left upper eyelid, lateral canthus and brow wound with loss of tissue after being struck by a car. A retroauricular full thickness skin graft was used to close the eyelid wound due to significant amount of tissue loss and lack of adequate local tissue for flap repair

Simple Marginal Lacerations

Proper repair of lacerations involving the eyelid margin (Fig. 6.8) is essential in restoring the normal eyelid anatomy and preventing complications, including irregular eyelid contour, notching at the margin, lagophthalmos with corneal exposure, and corneal irritation from incorrectly placed sutures. It is important to carefully examine the laceration and evert the eyelid to determine the extent of injury to the posterior lamella. Wounds with minimal tissue loss can be repaired at bedside or in a minor procedure room. Irregular or angulated wound margins should be freshened with vertical excision of tarsus, usually creating a pentagonal full thickness wound, to avoid wound dehiscence and notching [2].

Many techniques have been described to repair marginal lacerations, the authors will describe their current preferred technique. First the cut tarsal edges are aligned with multiple interrupted 6-0 polyglactin sutures. This is the most important step in providing structural integrity to the eyelid. The sutures should be passed partial-thickness through the tarsus with

(a) (b)

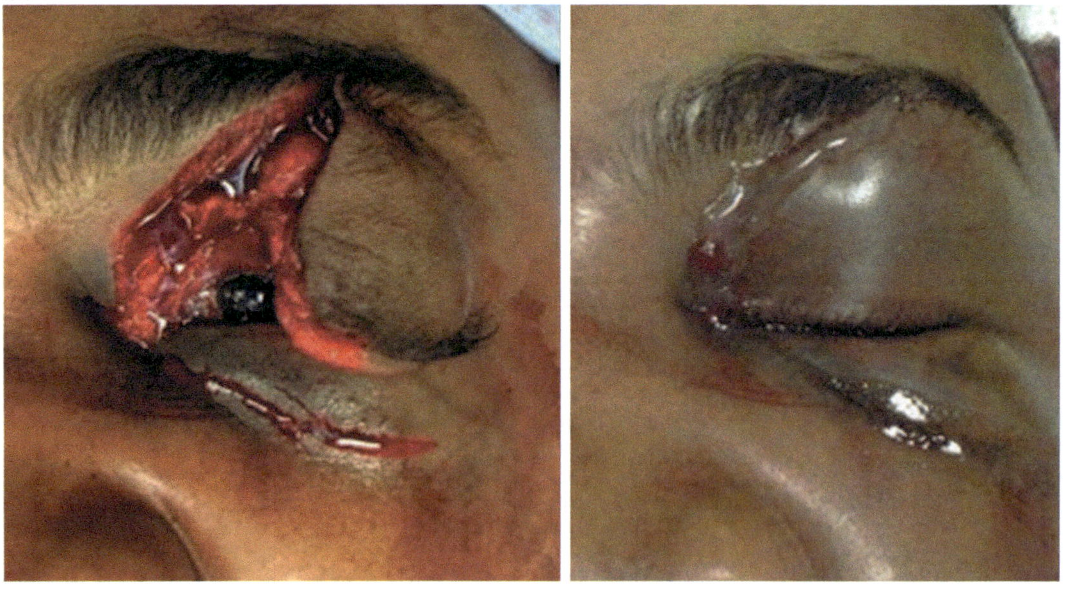

Fig. 6.8 **a** 31-year-old male with a *left upper* eyelid full thickness margin involving laceration and a *left lower* eyelid superficial laceration. **b** Lacerations immediately after repair

the knots placed anteriorly, avoiding the palpebral conjunctiva and protecting the corneal surface from potential irritation by the suture. Tarsal closure can be achieved with three sutures for upper lid lacerations and two for lower lid lacerations. To realign the margins, a 6-0 silk suture is first passed through the gray line on each side of the laceration and left long. An additional 6-0 silk marginal suture is used to realign the lash line. A third marginal silk suture through the tarsus should then be considered, but typically is not needed in the authors' experience.

The lid skin can then be closed with 6-0 silk suture. The long marginal silk tails are secured taught within the last skin suture which prevents them from irritating the ocular surface. The authors prefer to remove the marginal silk sutures 10 days after repair to allow adequate time for the marginal tissues to heal. In young children and patients with questionable compliance with follow up, absorbable 6-0 polyglactin suture can be used to realign the margin [2].

Complex Marginal Lacerations

Primary closure is an option for eyelid margin lacerations when tissue loss is less than 25–33% of the margin, depending on the patient's age and skin laxity. When the defect is too large for primary closure, horizontal tissue recruitment via a canthotomy and cantholysis can enable closure without significant tension. When defects involve 33–50% of the eyelid margin, use of advancement flaps such as a Tenzel semicircular flap from the adjacent lateral eyelid is recommended. For large defects involving more than 50% of the eyelid margin, lid sharing tarsoconjunctival flap procedures or large rotating cheek flaps for the lower lid are usually required [2, 8].

Traumatic Levator Dehiscence

The levator aponeurosis can dehisce from its attachment to the tarsus secondary to blunt and penetrating trauma. Initially after trauma, swelling of the eyelid can produce mechanical blepharoptosis that can make it appear that the levator has been damaged. In cases of penetrating trauma, the presence of fat in the wound suggests disruption of the septum and increased likelihood of potential levator injury. In such cases, the wound and the levator aponeurosis should be thoroughly explored with good tissue retraction. Levator dehiscence should be repaired during initial closure by reattaching the levator aponeurosis to the tarsus with a nonabsorbable suture such as 6-0 silk. A levator laceration that does not disrupt its attachment to the tarsus can be sutured using 6-0 polyglactin to restore normal anatomy. Patients whose levator lacerations are not repaired initially or those who develop ptosis after trauma should be observed for at least 6 months prior to surgical consideration because spontaneous improvement is possible [2]. When surgery is considered, levator function should be measured and documented. If there is adequate levator function, reattachment of the aponeurosis to the tarsus can be performed. Poor levator function requires the use of a frontalis sling procedure for ptosis repair [13].

Animal and Human Bites

Evaluation of patients with wounds secondary to animal or human bites is similar to that of other traumatic injuries with several special considerations. It is important to note any history of immunosuppression since the most common complication of bites is infection, which tends to be more severe in immunocompromised patients. The status of the animal's rabies immunization should be determined and rabies immunization for the patient, both passive and active, should be considered as indicated. Primary repair of facial lacerations is recommended due to improved cosmetic results. Infection is less common in this area likely secondary to the abundant facial blood supply [2]. To further decrease the risk of infection, treatment with oral antibiotics is recommended to cover for the polymicrobial flora commonly encountered in such injuries. Amoxicillin-clavulanate is a good first line antibiotic and can be substituted with a combination of clindamycin and a fluoroquinolone for those with a penicillin allergy [2]. Immunocompromised patients might require admission for IV antibiotics as they are at risk for life-threatening infection. In cases of human bites, HIV and hepatitis B status of the biter and the victim should be obtained. HIV prophylaxis is generally not recommended, while hepatitis B vaccination and immunoglobulin should be administered to those without antibodies [2].

Burns

Ocular adnexal burns can be secondary to thermal, chemical or electric current injury. Of these, thermal burns, which can be due to flame or explosions, are the most common [14]. These burns are usually more superficial than the others and the ocular surface is usually protected. Chemical burns tend to result in more ocular surface injury. Alkali burns cause tissue necrosis and cause deep injury to the eye, as well as the adnexa. Electric burns are well demarcated and may appear localized on the surface while causing significant deep tissue damage [15].

As with any trauma, initial goal in management is to stabilize the patient. Burns to the face have a higher likelihood of airway obstruction which should be addressed first [14]. The globe should be examined before the eyelids. Immediate treatment of thermal adnexal burns includes gentle cleaning and removal of all debris and

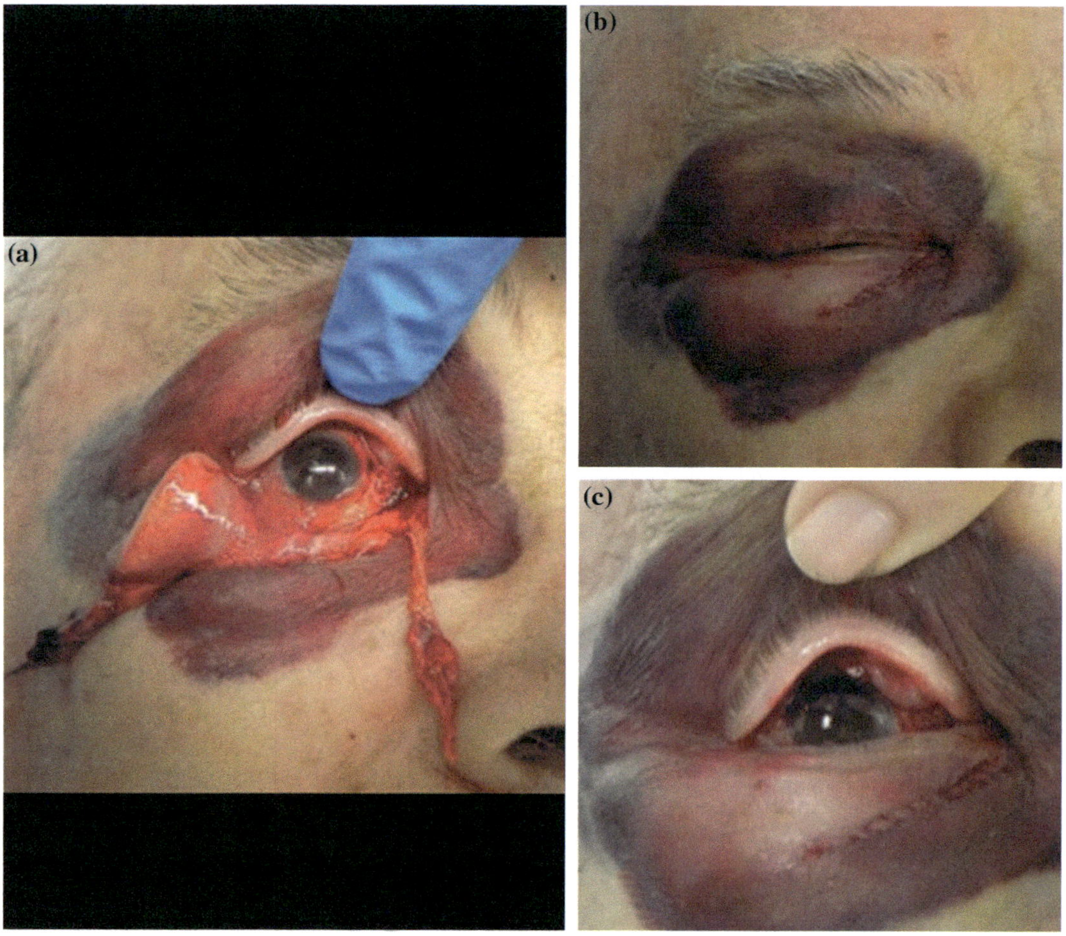

Fig. 6.9 **a** Avulsed full thickness right lower lid laceration. **b**, **c** Postoperative day 1 after reconstruction

application of cool, moist compresses. For chemical burns, the most important first step is irrigation and removal of the chemical, to prevent further damage. pH strips should be used after the initial irrigation to make certain that a physiologic neutral pH has been attained. Broad-spectrum topical antibiotic should then be applied to all wounds. Wound contracture associated with healing may result in lagophthalmos, requiring frequent lubrication of the ocular surface.

Over time, scarring of the anterior lamella pulls the eyelid margin away from the globe resulting in a cicatricial ectropion and corneal exposure. The risk of this occurring depends on the depth of penetration of the initial injury [14]. Acid burns usually cause superficial injuries and rarely lead to scarring, whereas alkali burns tend to penetrate deeper into the tissue and cause significant cicatrization [6]. The treatment for this often requires scar lysis and skin grafting, which should be delayed 3–12 months [6].

Case: Eyelid Trauma

An 87-year-old male presented to the emergency room after trauma to the right eye and periocular region with a metal hook. Examination of the adnexa was significant for a periocular hematoma and a full thickness lower eyelid laceration extending from the medial canthal region laterally, creating an avulsed flap of the lower lid without compromise of the medial canthal ligament (Fig. 6.9a). The patient was given systemic antibiotics and tetanus prophylaxis in the emergency room. The patient was taken to the operating room for repair under general anesthesia. The orbicularis muscle was reapproximated with deep 5-0 vicryl interrupted suture. The skin was then closed with a running 6-0 plain gut suture. The wound appeared well apposed with normal lower eyelid position after repair (Fig. 6.9b, c).

References

1. Lemke BN, Lucarelli MJ. Anatomy of the ocular adnexa, orbit, and related facial structures. In: Black EH, Nesi FA, Calvano CJ, et al., editors. Smith and Nesi's ophthalmic plastic and reconstructive surgery. 3rd ed. New York: Springer; 2012. p. 3–58.
2. Rattan GH, et al. Management of ocular adnexal trauma. In: Black EH, Nesi FA, Calvano CJ, et al., editors. Smith and Nesi's ophthalmic plastic and reconstructive surgery. 3rd ed. New York: Springer; 2012. p. 207–27.
3. Sadiq MA, Corkin F, Mantagos IS. Eyelid lacerations due to dog bite in children. J Pediatr Ophthalmol Strabismus. 2015;52(6):360–3.
4. Wladis EJ, Dewan MA. Periorbital trauma from pit bull terrier attacks. Orbit. 2012;31(3):200–2.
5. Mishra A, Baranwal VK, Parihar JKS, Verma AK. Simple laceration wound of the eyelid? Always remember to look under the lids! Med J Armed Forces India. 2013;69(3):301–4.
6. Pargament JM, Armenia J, Nerad JA. Physical and chemical injuries to eyes and eyelids. Clin Dermatol. 2015;33(2):234–7.
7. Howard GR, Nerad JA, Kersten RC. Medial canthoplasty with microplate fixation. Arch Ophthalmol. 1992;110(12):1793–7.
8. Mathijssen IM, van der Meulen JC. Guidelines for reconstruction of the eyelids and canthal regions. J Plast Reconstr Aesthet Surg. 2010;63(9):1420–33.
9. Devrukhkar VN, Hedge RJ, Khare SS, et al. Evaluation of isoamyl 2-cyanoacrylate tissue adhesive in management of pediatric lacerations: an alternative to suturing. Ann Maxillofac Surg. 2015;5(1):49–54.
10. Farion KJ, Osmond MH, Hartling L, et al. Tissue adhesives for traumatic lacerations: a systematic review of randomized controlled trials. Acad Emerg Med. 2003;10(2):110–8.
11. Ong TK, Dudley M. Craniofacial trauma presenting at an adult accident and emergency department with an emphasis on soft tissue injuries. Injury. 1999;30(5):357–63.
12. Coutts SJ, Sandhu R, Geh VS. Tissue glue and iatrogenic eyelid gluing in children. Pediatr Emerg Care. 2012;28(8):810–1.
13. Srinath N, Balaji R, Basha MS. Ptosis correction: a challenge following complex orbital injuries. J Maxillofac Oral Surg. 2012;11(2):195–9.
14. Cabalag MS, Wasiak J, Syed Q, et al. Early and late complications of ocular burn injuries. J Plast Reconstr Aesthet Surg. 2015;68(3):356–61.
15. Ratnarajan G, Calladine D, Bird KJ. Delayed presentation of severe ocular injury from a button battery. BMJ Case Rep. 2013;2013.

The Lacrimal System

7

Nora Silverman and Roman Shinder

Lacrimal System—Secretory and Excretory System: Anatomy and Function

The lacrimal system is composed of a secretory portion (the main and accessory lacrimal glands) and an excretory portion (the puncta, canaliculi, lacrimal sac, and nasolacrimal duct). The maintenance of this system allows for lubrication of the globe and drainage of excess tears. The lacrimal gland, which is located superotemporally to the globe within the lacrimal fossa of the frontal bone, secretes tears that are spread over the surface of the cornea. Accessory lacrimal glands, which are located within the palpebral conjunctival stroma, also provide lubrication by supplying tear fluid onto the surface of the globe via small ducts [1]. Tears accumulate as a tear lake along the margin of each eyelid. The puncta, which are 0.3 mm concavities located at the medial aspect of both the superior and inferior lid margins, sit somewhat posteriorly so as to better receive tears from the tear lake. The puncta connect to the superior and inferior ampullae, which are 2 mm in length and oriented vertically to each punctum. The ampullae then lead medially into superior and inferior canaliculi, which have a length of 8 mm and come together as a common canaliculus. The common canaliculus opens into the lacrimal sac, which has a length of 10–12 mm and is located within the lacrimal sac fossa, a concavity, which is composed anteriorly by the frontal process of the maxillary bone and posteriorly by the lacrimal bone. The sac is continuous with the nasolacrimal duct, which has a length of 12–18 mm and empties into the nasal cavity just inferior to the inferior nasal meatus (Fig. 7.1).

The mechanism of tear drainage is facilitated by a combination of capillary action and a negative pressure suction within the drainage apparatus and positive pressure created by blinking. At the beginning of a blink, the lacrimal system contains tears from the previous blink—as the lids close, the pretarsal orbicularis oculi muscle compresses the canaliculi and moves the puncta medially. Co-contraction of the lacrimal portion of the orbicularis muscle forces tears down the nasolacrimal duct into the nasal cavity [1]. Once the blink is complete, the components of the lacrimal pump open; thus, creating a negative pressure in the lacrimal sac that draws tears downward into the lacrimal sac. Obstruction of this system at any point can result in chronic tearing (epiphora).

Canalicular and Lacrimal System Trauma

Penetrating orbital injuries require a careful evaluation of the eyelids and the underlying soft tissues. The extent of the penetrating injury and the presence of foreign bodies are vital

N. Silverman · R. Shinder (✉)
Department of Ophthalmology, The State University of New York (SUNY) Downstate Medical Center, Brooklyn, NY 11203, USA
e-mail: shinder.roman@gmail.com

N. Silverman · R. Shinder
Kings County Hospital Center, Brooklyn, NY 11203, USA

S.C. Kaufman and D.R. Lazzaro (eds.), *Textbook of Ocular Trauma*,
DOI 10.1007/978-3-319-47633-9_7

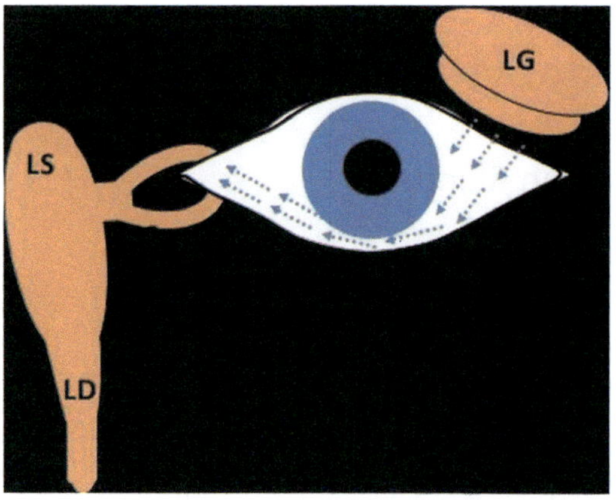

Fig. 7.1 Lacrimal system anatomy. Tears are produced in the lacrimal gland (LG) and spread over the surface of the globe. Tears accumulate as a tear lake along the eyelid margin and drain into the superior punctum (SP) and inferior punctum (IP). Tears then travel into the superior canaliculus (SC) and inferior canaliculus (IC) which come together to drain into the lacrimal sac (LS). Tears then flow into nasolacrimal duct (LD) and empty into the nasal cavity

determinations in the initial management. Sharp objects such as broken glass or knives are common causes of significant lid lacerations. Dog bites are also a common cause of lid lacerations, especially in children, and they have a propensity to involve the canalicular system. In a retrospective analysis of eyelid lacerations over the course of a decade, Savar et al. [2] found that 66% of patients who suffered dog bite injuries had resultant canalicular damage. The majority of these injuries involved damage to the inferior canaliculus [2]. Thus, a careful history detailing the timing and mechanism of injury in addition to a physical exam that rules out injury to the globe and assesses for changes in vision and diplopia are required. CT imaging without contrast can help to delineate the magnitude of any orbital injury.

During the initial patient encounter, tetanus status and inoculation history should be obtained. All patients should receive broad spectrum of antibiotics and pain management prior to wound exploration [3]. Soft tissue lacerations should be evaluated carefully to determine the extent of the damage. Eyelid lacerations can often be repaired at the bedside if the canalicular system is not involved. Canalicular injury can be presumed if the penetrating injury on the eyelid margin is full thickness and medial to the punctum [4, 5]. These patients can also present with displacement of the punctum laterally [5]. Lacerations can be the result of direct penetrating trauma or lid avulsion in the setting of tension forces inflicted on the eyelid. Avulsion injuries are more difficult to repair as shearing forces tend to impair easy visualization of the lacerated tissues [4]. Lacrimal system probing is required to confirm the diagnosis of a canalicular laceration. If lacrimal system injuries are not repaired, occlusion of the canalicular system will likely ensue, and a fistula tract may arise, as a result of scar formation. This may result in tearing, as each canaliculus provides approximately 50% of the tear drainage [4].

In the setting of lid avulsion, the medial canthal tendon will need to be reattached to its original anatomic insertion if disinserted (Fig. 7.2). The medial canthal tendon attaches anteriorly to the anterior lacrimal crest (the frontal process of the maxilla) and posteriorly to the posterior lacrimal crest (within the lacrimal bone). The canthal tendon hugs the lacrimal sac as it courses to its bony attachment. Proper apposition of the eyelid to the globe requires attachment of the posterior portion of the medial canthal tendon, and normal anatomic rounding of the lower lid requires attachment of the tendon to the anterior lacrimal crest. This alignment also helps to ensure proper positioning of the puncta in the tear lake.

Diagnosing Canalicular Trauma

Canalicular injuries are not always evident on cursory gross inspection, and it is prudent to evaluate all lid lacerations for canalicular involvement, after the globe is evaluated and it has been deemed safe to evaluate the lids and lacrimal system. Epidemiological reports have indicated that canalicular injuries are more common in young, male patients. One study revealed that almost 70% of canalicular lacerations were found in patients younger than 30 years old [6], and another study found that among young patients who suffered canalicular lacerations, 83% were male [7]. In order to

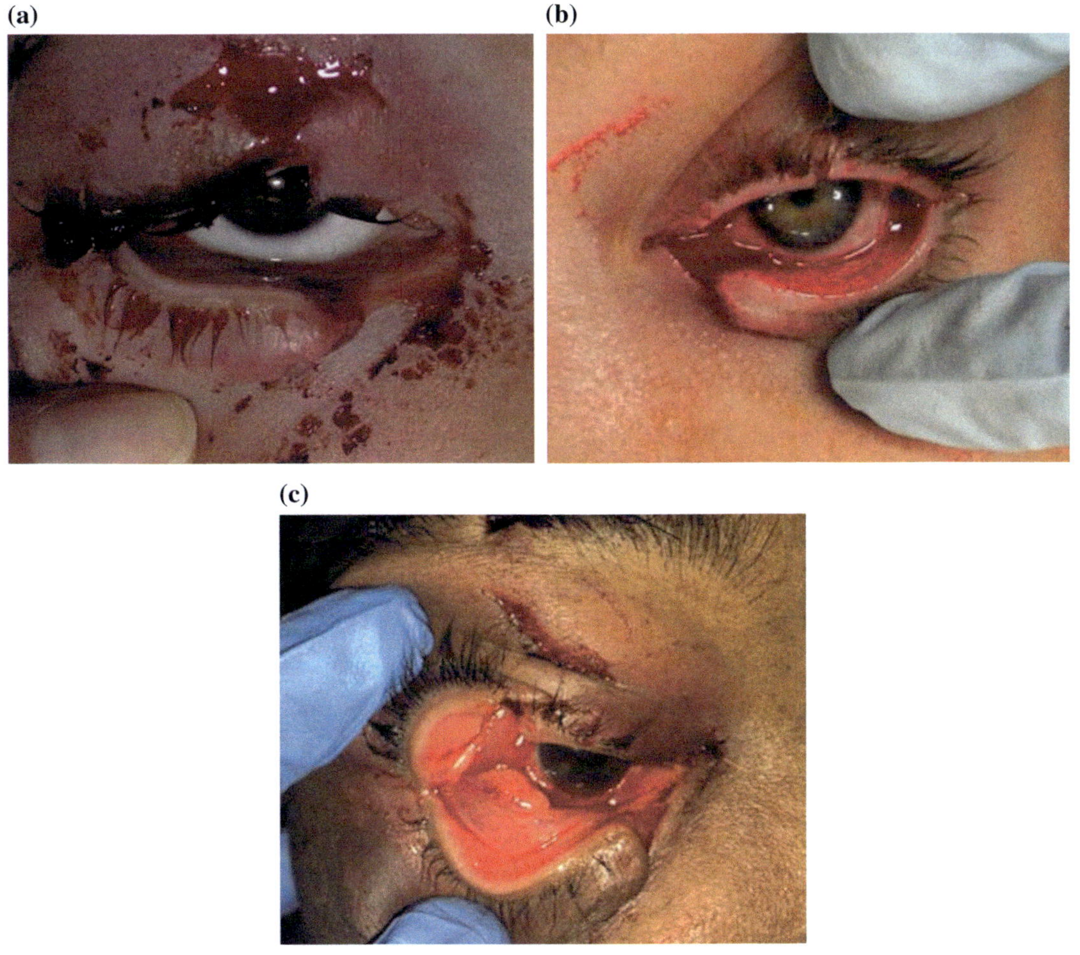

Fig. 7.2 Eyelid avulsion. The inferior crus of the medial canthal tendon was disinserted during traumatic avulsion type injuries that also resulted in an inferior canalicular lacerations (**a**, **b**, **c**)

diagnose canalicular trauma, punctal probing should be performed. A drop of topical anesthetic is instilled and a punctal dilator can be used initially to allow easier entry into the punctum if stenotic. Once a lacrimal probe is introduced into the punctum, the clinician should follow the anatomical path of the proximal lacrimal apparatus. The probe should be inserted perpendicular to the eyelid margin entering the punctum for approximately 2 mm, then turned at a sharp 90 degree angle to be parallel to the lid margin. At this point the probe can be advanced up to 8 mm through the canaliculus. If at any point the metal end of the probe can be visualized, a canalicular laceration is confirmed (Fig. 7.2). Lacrimal irrigation can also be used to confirm a canalicular laceration. After instilling topical anesthesia, a blunt lacrimal irrigation cannula attached to a 1 or 3 mL syringe, filled with normal saline, is inserted into the lacrimal apparatus entering the punctum and proximal canaliculus. Saline is injected slowly, and in a patient with an intact lacrimal system, saline will pass into the nasopharynx and the patient will feel and taste the fluid. In the setting of a canalicular laceration, the injected saline will exit in the area of the canalicular laceration and can be visualized. If punctal probing or lacrimal irrigation is not available, careful examination with magnification using a slit lamp or surgical magnifiers (surgical loupes) can be used to help identify canalicular lacerations (Fig. 7.3).

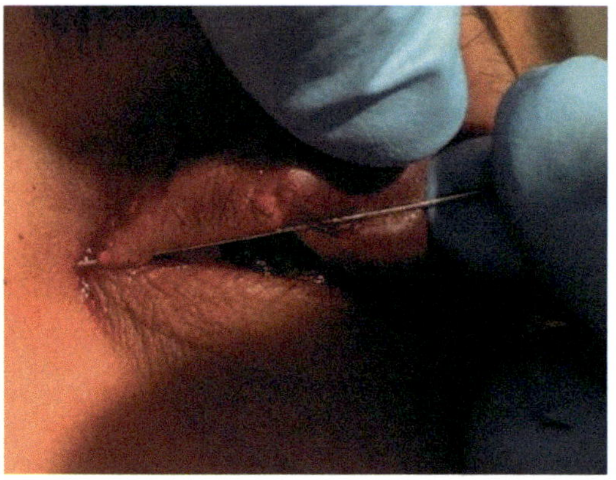

Fig. 7.3 Lacrimal system probing. A lacrimal probe is placed into the upper punctum and is seen exiting the proximal cut end of the canalicular laceration

Reconstruction

There are several methods that can be used to repair canalicular lacerations but this text will focus on two techniques that use silicone tube intubation. The advantage of such intubation is the reestablishment of normal anatomy [8]. Depending on the complexity and location of the trauma, canalicular lacerations can be repaired under either local or general anesthesia. Careful initial cleaning of the wound allows for better visualization of the extent of the injury. At this point, a thorough search for foreign objects within the wound should be performed. Canalicular repair should optimally be performed ideally within 24–48 h of the injury to prevent fibrosis and stenosis, which could lead to epiphora [9, 10]. The authors favor repair on the day of injury, whenever possible.

The first technique is repair using a monocanalicular stent (Mini Monoko stent, FCI Ophthalmics Inc., Pembroke, MA), and the second is bicanalicular intubation with a Crawford stent (FCI Ophthalmics Inc., Pembroke, MA). Bicanalicular intubation is more time-intensive and complex, and this text will focus on monocanalicular intubation. A benefit of monocanalicular stenting is that it involves only the injured canaliculus; bicanalicular stenting also passes through the uninjured canaliculus, and thus puts it at risk for injury [10]. The first step of intubation requires identification of the cut ends of the canaliculus, which often appear as small holes lined by mucosa [11]. As mentioned previously, this step can be challenging in the setting of a tractional injury. Use of magnification, either with a microscope or with surgical loupes can be helpful [11]. Other techniques that may aid in finding the distal cut end of the canaliculus include the use of phenylephrine or injection of either air, saline, or fluorescein into the lacrimal system. Application of phenylephrine 2.5% (Paragon Bioteck Inc, Portland, OR) to the tissue causes the edges of the cut end of the canaliculus to pout. Injection of air, saline or fluorescein solution into the uninjured canaliculus allows for visualization of a stream of air bubbles or fluid from the distal cut end [10–12].

Once the distal cut end of the canalicular laceration is identified, the Mini Monoka stent is cut to proper size to allow enough length for it to begin at the punctum, bridge the laceration, and end within the lacrimal sac. It is always prudent to cut the stent longer than anticipated and trim if needed, as a stent that is cut too short will have to be replaced. When cutting the stent the authors favor creating a sharp distal tip to allow for easier passage through the lacrimal system. The punctum is then dilated with a punctal dilator, and the Mini Monoka stent is passed from the punctum through the proximal cut end of the canaliculus. This process should be performed using non-toothed forceps to prevent injury to the silicone tubing. The tube is pulled and advanced until the proximal edge of the tube "locks in" and lies flush with the opening of the punctum. Next, the distal end of the tube is passed into the distal cut portion of the canalicular laceration and into the lacrimal sac. The authors favor a hand over hand technique with two forceps to gently advance the stent into the distal cut canalicular segment as the tubing has a tendency to roll up in the lacrimal sac and regurgitate back. Connecting the two cut ends of the system via the Mini Monoka stent is a challenging step in the surgery. The pericanalicular tissue must be sutured around the stent to ensure proper alignment and support of the system using 5-0 polyglactin suture.

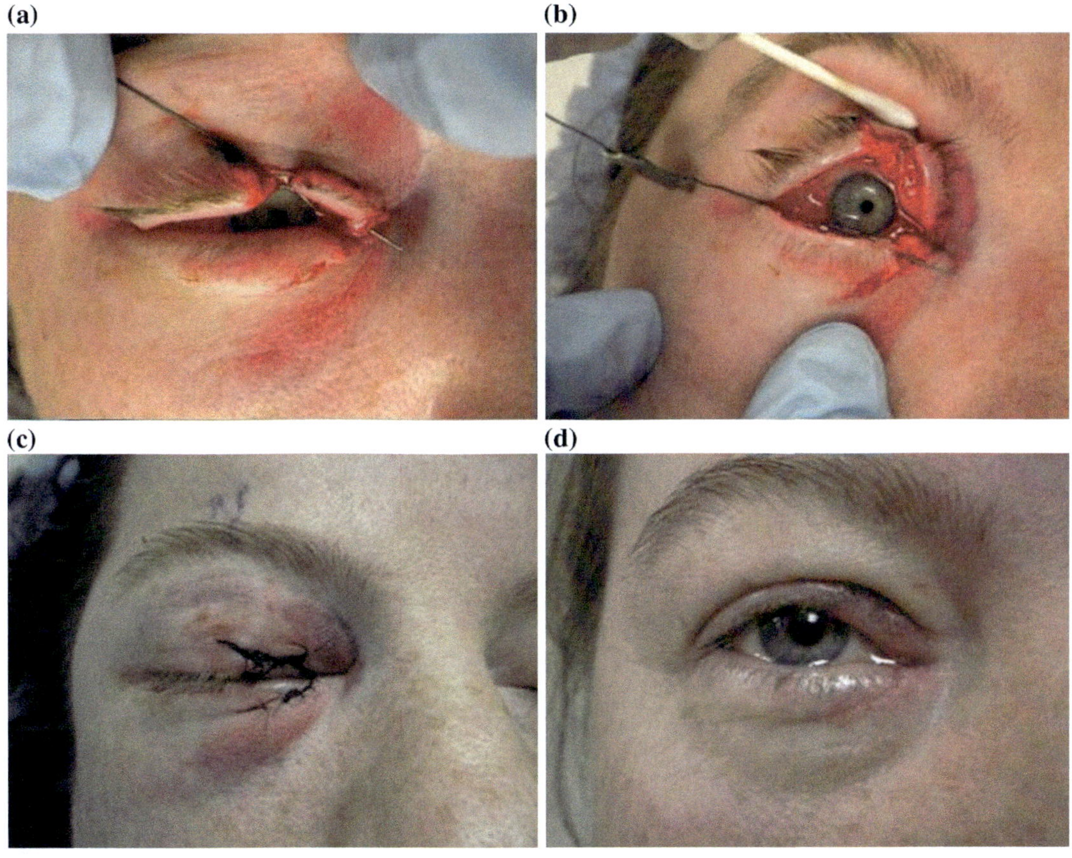

Fig. 7.4 Punctal probing revealing a bicanalicular laceration (**a**, **b**). Immediate postoperative photo of repair using a bicanalicular stent (**c**). Postoperative week 2 photo revealing proper orientation of lid margin and stent seen within puncta (**d**)

A suture is passed through both the proximal and distal portions of pericanalicular tissue. After the tube is in place and the suture is tied, the two ends of the cut canaliculus will come together and reestablish the lacrimal drainage apparatus. The authors suggest preplacing the pericanalicular suture and waiting to tie them until the stent is positioned in the subsequent step. This alleviates some of the challenge in securing the stent in the proper position. Once the suture is tied, the associated skin laceration can be repaired in typical fashion with the potential need for layered closure. When complete, the proximal end of the stent should be positioned within the tear lake in close apposition to the globe.

If using a bicanalicular stent, the aforementioned process is then repeated for the opposite canaliculus, which leaves a small portion of tubing between the superior and inferior puncta exposed. The two distal ends are retrieved in the nasal cavity where a securing procedure is needed to help maintain its position in the postoperative period [4]. If a patient has suffered a bicanalicular laceration then use of the bicanalicular stent is required.

If the medial canthal tendon has been avulsed from its bony attachment, it is at this point that it can be reattached either to periosteum using suture or a more complex reattachment to bone such as with drill holes (See lid laceration section). After the repair of all canalicular lacerations, patients are instructed to use topical antibiotic ophthalmic ointment three times daily for at least one week. The silicone tubes are

(a)

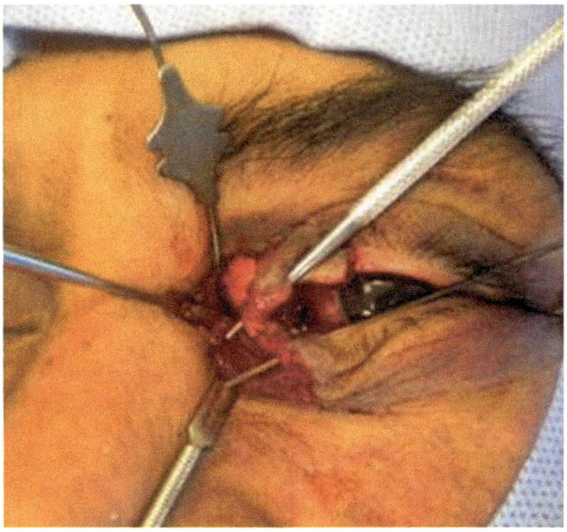

(b)

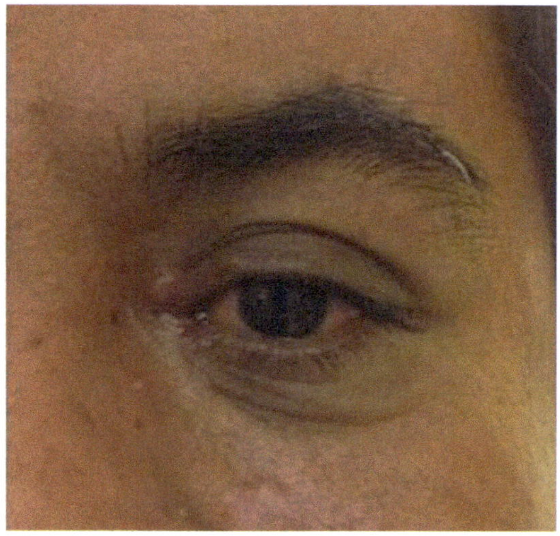

Fig. 7.5 Punctal probing reveals bicanalicuar laceration with medial canthal tendon avulsion, with third lacrimal probe noting the position of the superior distal cut canalicular end (**a**). Postoperative month 3 photo showing acceptable cosmetic result with puncta positioned in the tear lake after bicanalicular stenting and repair of laceration (**b**)

typically removed between 3 and 10 months after surgical repair to allow sufficient time for the body to generate a new canalicular tubing system around the stent [8, 10]. After a drop of topical anesthetic is placed on the eye, the proximal end of the Mini Monika stent is engaged with toothed forceps and simply pulled from the punctum. This process can be performed easily in an office setting [10]. The removal of a bicanalicular stent is more complex and typically done endonasally after the tubing is found and cut. The success of primary

(a)

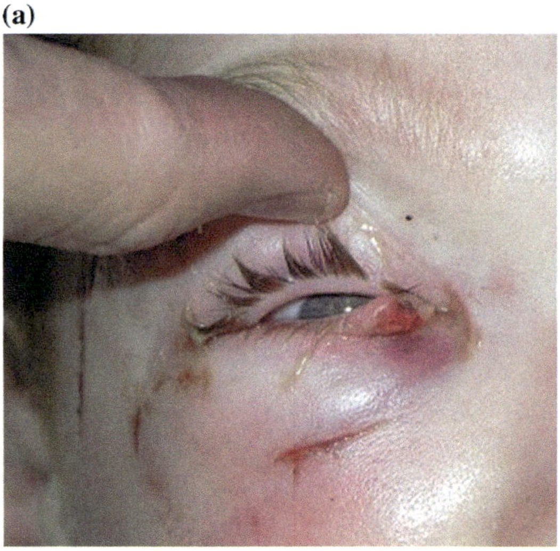

(b)

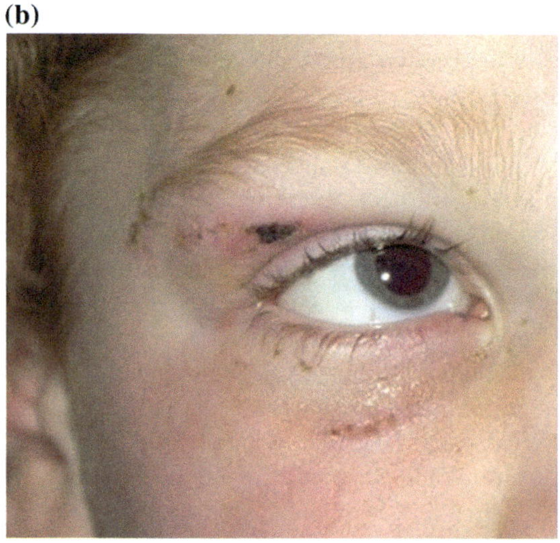

Fig. 7.6 An 8 year-old boy sustained a dog bite injury with resultant right lower lid canalicular laceration (**a**). Rabies status was assessed. The wound was repaired as described in this section. Postoperative week 1 follow up revealed appropriate apposition of lid to globe with Mini Monoka stent properly positioned within the tear lake (**b**)

canalicular repair has been cited as greater than 92% without distinction as to repair of the upper or lower canaliculus [8] [Figs. 7.4, 7.5 and 7.6].

References

1. Records RE. The conjunctiva and lacrimal system. In: Tasman W, Jaeger EA, editors. Duane's clinical ophthalmology (2005 Ed [CD ROM]). Philadelphia: Lippincott, Williams & Wilkins; 2010.
2. Savar A, Kirszrot J, Rubin PA. Canalicular involvement in dog bite related eyelid lacerations. Ophthal Plast Reconstr Surg. 2008;24(4):296–8.
3. Katowitz JA. Pediatric orbital trauma. In: Katowitz JA, editor. Pediatric oculoplastic surgery. 2nd ed. New York: Springer; 2002. p. 648.
4. Nerad JA. Eyelid and orbital trauma. In: Nerad JA, editor. Techniques in ophthalmic plastic surgery. New York: Saunders Elsevier; 2010. p. 356–67.
5. Rattan GH, Kulwin DR, Levine M, et al. Management of ocular adnexal trauma. In: Black EH, Nesi FA, Calvano CJ, Gladstone GJ, Levine MR, editors. Smith and Nesi's ophthalmic plastic and reconstructive surgery. 3rd ed. New York: Springer; 2012. p. 207–29.
6. Kennedy RH, May J, Dailey J, Flanagan JC. Canalicular laceration: an 11-year epidemiologic and clinical study. Ophthal Plast Reconstr Surg. 1990;6(1):46–53.
7. Naik M, Kelapure A, Rath S, Honavar SG. Management of canalicular lacerations: epidemiological aspects and experience with mini-monoka monocanalicular stent. Am J Ophthalmol. 2008;145(2):375–80.
8. Liang X, Lin Y, Wang Z, et al. A modified bicanalicular intubation procedure to repair canalicular laceration using silicone tubes. Eye. 2012;26(12):1542–7.
9. Jordan DR. To reconstruct or not. Ophthalmology. 2000;107(6):1022–3.
10. Kalin-Hajdu E, Cadet N, Boulos P. Controversies of the lacrimal system. Surv Ophthalmol. 2015.
11. Eo S, Park J, Cho S, Azari KK. Microsugrical reconstruction for canalicular laceration using monostent and mini-monoka. Ann Plast Surg. 2010;64(4):421–7.
12. Cho SH, Hyun DW, Kang HJ, Ha MS. A simple new method for identifying the proximal cut end in lower canalicular laceration. Korean J Ophthalmol. 2008;22(2):73–6.

Enucleation

8

Mamta Shah and Roman Shinder

Introduction

Loss of an eye to trauma can be damaging to a patient both physically through loss of binocular vision and depth perception, and psychologically due to reduced self-esteem. *Enucleation* is the removal of the entire globe while preserving the remaining adnexal and orbital tissues [1].

The role of primary enucleation in acute trauma remains controversial, particularly when a patient's mental status may be altered or when unable to consent. The authors strongly advocate for primary closure of a ruptured globe when surgically feasible regardless of preoperative vision or severity of ocular injury. This approach allows the patient to consider the options after the initial trauma and altered mental status has resolved and provides autonomy to elect this operation in the future if ever warranted. In select cases, where the eye is determined to have no visual potential and when repair of a ruptured globe is determined to be impossible by an ophthalmic surgeon (a *non-salvageable ruptured globe*), enucleation is the treatment of choice [2] (Fig. 8.1). In simplistic terms, a non-salvageable ruptured globe is one where there is no real hope to recover any vision in a badly traumatized eye due to severity of injury.

Enucleation in the setting of trauma requires considerate counseling and empathy from the ophthalmologist. The ophthalmologist also has the responsibility to outline postoperative care and expectations regarding the appearance of the patient. When done discerningly, these steps can help return the patient to a productive life.

The Ideal Anophthalmic Socket

The anophthalmic socket refers to an orbit that has had the globe removed. Characteristics of an ideal anophthalmic socket were outlined by Gougelman et al. and are as follows [3]:

(1) A well-centered, buried orbital implant that will minimize migration and extrusion
(2) Healthy conjunctiva and deep fornices to permit excursion of an ocular prosthesis
(3) Eyelids with normal position and tone
(4) An upper eyelid crease that is symmetric with that of the contralateral eyelid
(5) Normal position of the eyelashes and eyelid margin
(6) Good motility of overlying ocular prosthesis
(7) Comfortable ocular prosthesis that looks similar to the contralateral globe.

The goal of anophthalmic surgery is to attain a painless, noninflamed socket with an ocular prosthesis that looks and moves as close to the

M. Shah · R. Shinder (✉)
Department of Ophthalmology, The State University of New York (SUNY) Downstate Medical Center, 451 Clarkson Ave, E Bldg, 8th Floor, Suite C, Brooklyn, NY 11203, USA
e-mail: shinder.roman@gmail.com

M. Shah
e-mail: mamta.shah@downstate.edu

S.C. Kaufman and D.R. Lazzaro (eds.), *Textbook of Ocular Trauma*,
DOI 10.1007/978-3-319-47633-9_8

(a) (b)

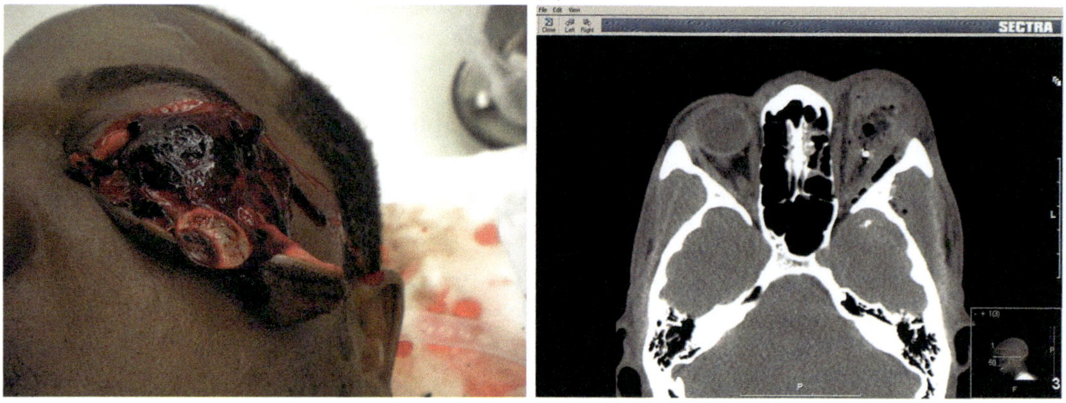

Fig. 8.1 **a** Gross external photograph of non-salvageable ruptured left globe with remnants of cornea and sclera visible along lower eyelid following penetrating periocular trauma. **b** Axial CT of the orbits showing disorganized left globe with inability to discern intraocular structures. The patient underwent a primary enucleation

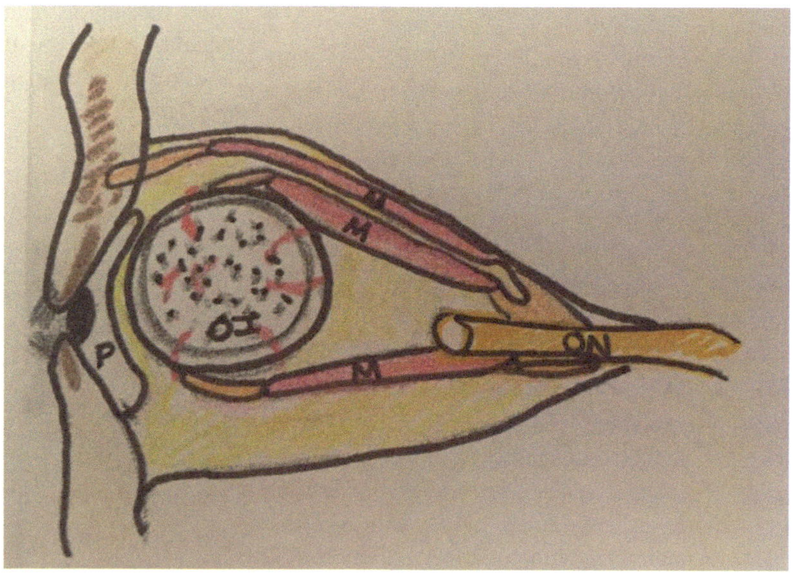

Fig. 8.2 Schematic of relationship between the anophthalmic socket, orbital implant, and ocular prosthesis. *P* = ocular prosthesis. *OI* = orbital implant. *M* = extraocular muscle. *ON* = optic nerve

unaffected eye as possible. Figure 8.2 illustrates the relationship between the anophthalmic socket, the orbital implant, and the overlying ocular prosthesis.

Preoperative Planning and Evaluation

The ophthalmologist should take a detailed ophthalmic history and perform a careful physical evaluation of the globe and surrounding soft tissues. The mechanism of injury, specifically blunt versus penetrating injury and the presence of possible foreign bodies are crucial steps in the initial management. The extent of penetrating injury is determined by the size of the object, its speed at the time of impact and its composition. Sharp objects such as broken glass or knives cause well-defined lacerations of the globe. Air gun pellets, although large, have a high kinetic energy and can thus cause considerable ocular damage. Esmaeli et al. [4] demonstrated that the predictors of excellent final visual acuity in penetrating ocular trauma included a sharp mechanism of injury. In contrast, blunt or missile injury was associated with poor visual outcome [4]. Finally, the factors predicting enucleation were similar to those predicting poor vision [4].

An intraocular foreign body may cause mechanical damage, introduce infection, or be toxic to intraocular structures as they can lodge anywhere in the anterior or posterior segment. Mechanical effects include cataract formation, vitreous liquefaction, and retinal tears. Stone and organic foreign bodies are associated with a higher rate of infection. Other substances such as glass, many plastics, gold, and silver are inert and less worrisome. CT of the orbits without contrast with thin axial and coronal cuts is used to detect and localize a metallic foreign body. MRI is contraindicated if there is a possibility of metallic foreign bodies. Patel et al. [5] showed that of 74 surgically confirmed intraocular foreign bodies in patients presenting with traumatic open globe injuries, clinical eye examination at presentation identified the foreign body in 34 (46%) of 74 patients and CT scan identified the foreign body in 56 (95%) of 59 patients.

Initial management of trauma patients should include a search for more serious or life threatening bodily injuries by clinical exam and imaging. Insults from head injuries and chest trauma are paramount and may require emergent surgical exploration that will take priority over globe exploration and repair. Medical history and surgical risk including cardiac risk factors should be assessed. The goals of anophthalmic surgery should be discussed with the patient and family, including the removal of the eye, restoration of orbital volume with an implant, and an aesthetically pleasing result with later prosthesis fitting [6].

The patient and family are informed about wearing a patch over the surgical site for about 5 days and use of an acrylic conformer until about 6 weeks after surgery when the patient can have a custom ocular prosthesis fitting with an ocularist. Postoperative pain, time away from work, and required follow-up visits should also be discussed. Finally, the ophthalmologist should review the risk of surgical complications such as infection, exposure, or migration of the implant, and the need for additional surgery [1, 6].

Finally, a porous or nonporous orbital implant must be selected. A porous implant refers to an implant with numerous interconnected pores or channels throughout its structure that permits fibrovascular ingrowth after surgery. Examples of such materials are hydroxyapatite, aluminum oxide, and porous polyethylene. A nonporous implant is solid and does not allow fibrovascular ingrowth. Examples include polymethylmethacrylate and silicone materials. The advantage of porous implants lies in the system of interconnecting pores that allow host fibrovascular ingrowth which potentially reduces the risk of migration and infection. The rough surface of porous implants can irritate and eventually thin the overlying tenons fascia and conjunctiva and thus produce higher rates of exposure of the anterior surface of the implant that carries risk of discharge and discomfort. The smoother nonporous implants have lower rates of exposure, but higher rates of migration. The biggest advantage of nonporous implants is that they are considerably less expensive than their porous counterparts. Porous polyethylene implants have a smoother surface than hydroxyapatite that allows for easier implantation and less irritation of the overlying tissues after placement [7, 8].

Indications for Enucleation and the Role of Sympathetic Ophthalmia

Sympathetic ophthalmia is a bilateral granulomatous panuveitis that can rarely occur after penetrating trauma to one globe. The injured eye is referred to as the exciting eye, whereas the uninjured fellow eye is termed the sympathizing eye. Intraocular uveal prolapse is often a feature of the initially traumatized ruptured globe. Specifically, the role of the penetrating wound appears important in sympathetic ophthalmia because of the access it provides for intraocular antigens to reach regional lymph nodes. The intraocular compartment has no lymphatic drainage, and it has been suggested that a penetrating wound exposes uveoretinal antigens to conjunctival lymphatics thereby inducing an immunopathologic response [9]. Although the precise autoantigen responsible is still inconclusive, the uveal pigment is thought to be the antigenic stimulus. Retinal S-antigen, interphotoreceptor retinoid binding protein, melanin associated antigens, and antigens derived from the retinal pigment epithelium and choroid have all been implicated as possibilities [9]. Histologically, a diffuse granulomatous nonnecrotizing inflammatory reaction appears within the uveal tracts composed of lymphocytes and epithelioid histiocytes containing phagocytosed melanin pigment [9]. Immunohistochemical techniques have been used to show that CD4+ T lymphocytes are important early in the disease with CD8+ T lymphoyctes evident later [9]. Presentation in trauma-induced cases is typically between 2 weeks and 3 months after initial injury but has been reported as late as 50 years following trauma [9]. The incidence of sympathetic ophthalmia is 0.2–0.5% after ocular trauma from a penetrating wound, but these estimates are based on retrospective studies [10], A prospective study estimated that 3 out of every 10 million cases of penetrating injury or surgery resulted in sympathetic ophthalmia [10]. Enucleation traditionally has been the surgical technique used to decrease the risk of sympathetic ophthalmia as the entire globe is removed including any possible inciting uveal antigens. Conversely, evisceration (removal of intraocular contents while leaving the scleral shell) carries a theoretical risk of not removing all the uveal tissue and thus not eliminating the potential for sympathetic ophthalmia. Primary enucleation should be considered within the first 2 weeks following trauma and ideally as soon as possible once the globe is judged to be non-salvageable [1, 2]. A comprehensive chapter on sympathetic ophthalmia is included in this textbook.

Enucleation: Surgical Technique and Points to Consider in Trauma

Figure 8.3 outlines the steps of enucleation. An enucleation is performed as an outpatient procedure typically under general anesthesia. If general anesthesia is contraindicated, intravenous sedation with a local retrobulbar block can be utilized. Intravenous antibiotic therapy should be administered if not given in the emergency room, and the authors also prefer to give intravenous steroids to decrease orbital edema and inflammation postoperatively. After a time-out is performed to confirm the correct operative eye with the entire operating room team, the face is prepared and draped in sterile fashion. An eyelid speculum is placed to retract the eyelids. A limbal conjunctival peritomy is performed with Wescott scissors for 360° (Fig. 8.3a). Blunt dissection in the sub-Tenon's plane is then carried out in each of the oblique quadrants between the rectus muscles using blunt Stevens tenotomy scissors. Each rectus muscle is then identified, isolated with muscle hooks, secured with 6-0 polyglactin suture, and cut. The vertical rectus muscles are cut at the insertion to the globe while the horizontal rectus muscles are cut a few millimeters from the globe so as to leave a short stump of tendon attached to the globe (Fig. 8.3

b). Prior to cutting the muscle tendon an application of bipolar cautery can aid in hemostasis. The ends of the suture for each rectus muscle can be held out of the surgical field with the aid of a bulldog or small clamp. The superior and inferior oblique muscles are isolated in similar fashion and transected in a similar manner without suture imbrication and allowed to retract into the orbit. When working on the extraocular muscles during surgery, it is crucial to be aware of the physiologic oculocardiac reflex. This reflex can cause bradycardia when traction is applied to extraocular muscles. The anesthesiologist should be warned preoperatively of this possibility and again just before rectus muscle stimulation as intravenous anti-muscarinic acetylcholine antagonists such as atropine or glycopyrrolate may be needed. If bradycardia does occur, removal of the stimulus is immediately indicated. This often results in the restoration of normal sinus rhythm of the heart. If not, the use of atropine or glycopyrrolate will usually be successful and permit continuation of the surgical procedure.

The horizontal rectus tendon stumps are grasped with toothed forceps and the globe is rotated to help break up soft tissue attachments until able to rotate freely. With the medial rectus stump rotated laterally, the optic nerve is identified, strummed, and clamped for one minute entering the orbit medially with a long surgical clamp to encourage hemostasis prior to transection with enucleation or other long scissors (Fig. 8.3c). The globe is then tented out of the orbital cavity and any last soft tissue attachments are carefully cut paying close attention not to cut the previously placed sutures. The globe is typically sent for histopathologic analysis. Additional hemostasis is then achieved for a couple of minutes with direct pressure in the intraconal space with gauze soaked in cold saline until the cut central retinal artery within the optic nerve has quieted. Of note, in the setting of a

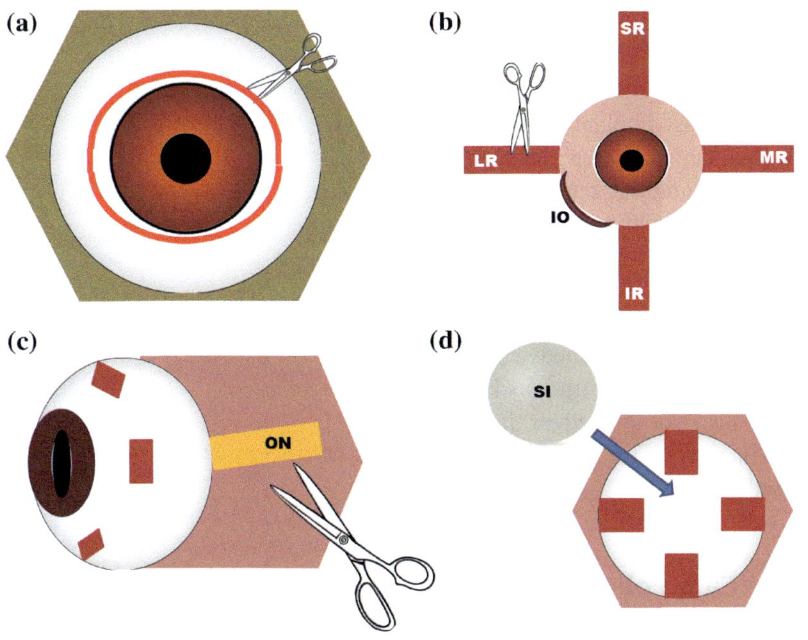

Fig. 8.3 **a** A limbal conjunctival peritomy is performed for 360 degrees. **b** After identification and isolation of each rectus muscle, the four recti and the superior and inferior oblique muscles are cut. **c** The optic nerve is identified, strummed, and clamped before transection with long scissors. **d** An orbital implant is placed in the intraconal space with gentle posterior pressure. *LR* = lateral rectus. *SR* = superior rectus. *MR* = medial rectus. *IR* = inferior rectus. *SO* = superior oblique. *IO* = inferior oblique

non-salvageable ruptured globe, the intraocular contents may not be identifiable and the anatomy may be distorted resulting in no formed globe to perform all the standardized steps mentioned, making the surgery more challenging.

An orbital implant is then placed in the intraconal space and then "seated" by applying gentle posterior pressure (Fig. 8.3d). The largest implant that can be properly placed is chosen to maintain adequate orbital volume with a 20 mm implant being a typical size chosen in adults. The authors at this point choose to secure the rectus muscle sutures after passing them through Tenon's fascia and conjunctiva. The more conventional way secures them to the anterior portion of the implant just anterior to their normal anatomic insertion sites.

Tenon's capsule is then meticulously closed with buried 5-0 polyglactin suture in interrupted fashion for robust protection against implant exposure. It is very important that Tenon's fascia is not closed under tension. If tension exists, the implant should be positioned more posteriorly in the orbit, and if already sitting posteriorly this would indicate that the implant chosen is too large and should be replaced with a smaller implant to guard against implant exposure and extrusion. The conjunctiva is then closed with a running 6-0 plain gut suture. A retrobulbar block of bupivicaine with epinephrine is administered to aid in postoperative pain management. Antibiotic ointment is applied to the conjunctiva. An acrylic vented conformer is placed within the palpebral fornices over the conjunctiva. A pressure patch is then placed over the socket and either benzoin or mastisol applied to the cheek and forehead skin aids in the patch remaining secure for several days.

Postoperative Care Following Enucleation

Postoperative pain is managed with analgesic medications such as acetaminophen with or without codeine and hydrocodone. Severe pain may be treated with more potent oral narcotics. Postoperative nausea occurs in approximately one-third of anophthalmic surgery patients, and this can be treated with antiemetic therapies intraoperatively and in the recovery room [1].

Some surgeons prescribe a course of oral antibiotics but the authors defer this unless the tissues are contaminated from the trauma. A rapid course of oral steroids is given to decrease tissue edema and increase patient comfort. The patient is seen back at postoperative day 5 at which point the patch is removed and topical combined antibiotic-steroid ophthalmic ointment is begun three times daily over the conformer for several weeks. If the conformer falls out during the healing phase, it can be replaced either by the patient or the surgeon into the lid fornices. If considerable edema and chemosis are present then the conformer may not be able to stay in and can be removed until it can be placed back. Once the patch is removed, the patient is given a prescription for spectacles containing polycarbonate lenses to protect the other eye for the remainder of the patient's life.

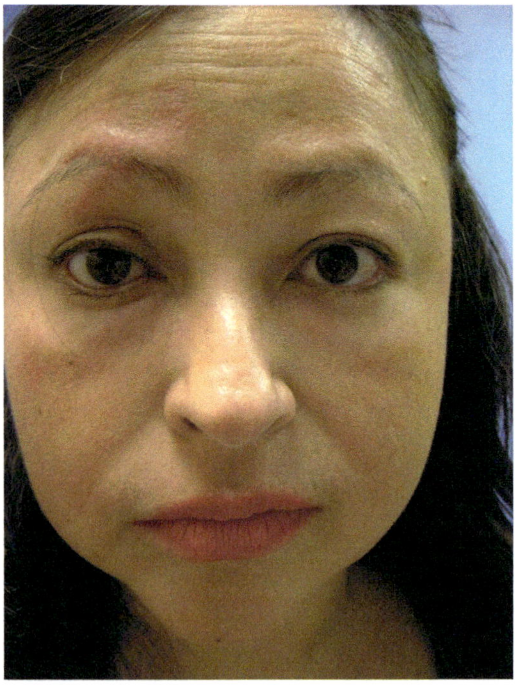

Fig. 8.4 Postoperative patient following right enucleation with fitted ocular prosthesis

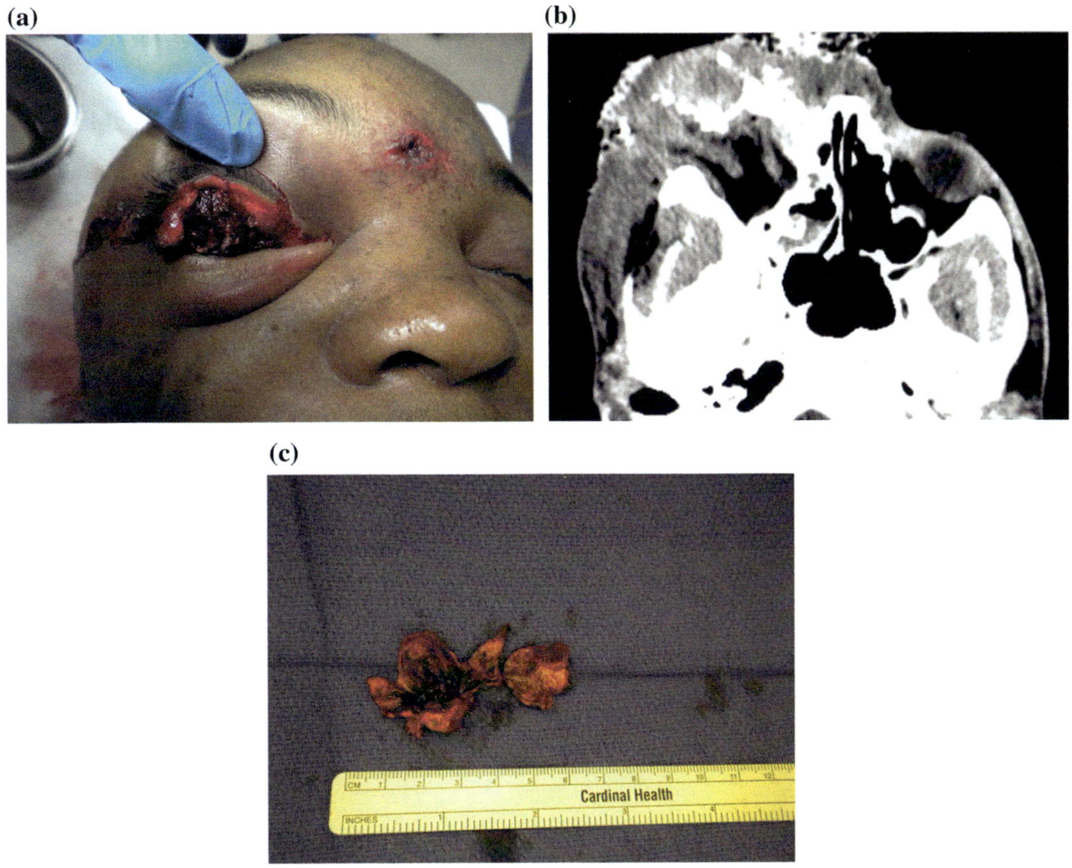

Fig. 8.5 **a** External photo of patient on presentation showing badly ruptured right globe. **b** Axial CT orbits showing disorganized right globe. **c** Enucleation specimen showing severity of globe rupture

Patients are given appointments to visit with the ocularist 6 weeks following surgery for evaluation and fabrication of the ocular prosthesis that will sit over the conjunctiva and within the lid fornix and replace the conformer. At 3 months following surgery the patient is checked wearing the ocular prosthesis for comfort, fit, cosmesis, and the underlying tissues are examined for health. Socket irritation and discomfort and chronic socket discharge may be caused by a poorly fitting prosthesis. Modifying the prosthesis at an annual checkup or refitting the socket with a new prosthesis, approximately every 5 years, may help prevent mucous production, pyogenic granuloma formation, or implant exposure. The upper and lower eyelid as well as the superior sulcus may change with time during the postoperative course. Ptosis, lower eyelid laxity with retraction or ectropion, and a deep superior sulcus may require a prosthetic adjustment or surgical intervention. Yearly follow-up thereafter is suggested to continue to monitor the comfort and fit of the prosthesis as well as the underlying ocular tissue examining for implant exposure at each visit. Minor exposure can be treated conservatively with topical antibiotics, but more severe exposure requires patching the exposed area or replacement of the orbital implant. A deep superior sulcus deformity can be managed with hyaluronic acid filler or an inferior subperiosteal implant to add orbital volume. Figure 8.4 depicts a patient after enucleation and prosthesis fitting.

Case

A 21-year-old male presented to the emergency room after suffering gunshot wounds to his right globe and face. Exam disclosed a badly ruptured right globe that was deemed non-salvageable along with other periocular injuries (Fig. 8.5a). Orbital CT scan demonstrated a severely ruptured right globe with disorganization of the globe anatomy (Fig. 8.5b). He underwent a right primary enucleation and periocular reconstruction. The enucleated globe was badly ruptured on inspection (Fig. 8.5c).

References

1. Rattan GH, Kulwin DR, Levine M, et al. Management of ocular adnexal trauma. In: Black EH, Nesi FA, Calvano CJ, Gladstone GJ, Levine MR, editors. Smith and Nesi's ophthalmic plastic and reconstructive surgery. 3rd ed. New York: Springer; 2012. p. 207–29.
2. Moshfeghi DM, Moshfeghi AA, Finger PT. Enucleation. Surv Ophthalmol. 2000;44(4):277–301.
3. Timothy NH, Freilich DE, Linberg JV. Evisceration versus enucleation from the ocularist's perspective. Ophthal Plast Reconstr Surg 2003;19(6):417–20.
4. Esmaeli B, Elner SG, Schork A, Elner VM. Visual outcome and ocular survival after penetrating trauma: a clinicopathologic study. Ophthalmology. 1995;102:393–400.
5. Patel SN, Langer PD, Zarbin MA, et al. Diagnostic value of clinical examination and radiographic imaging in identification of intraocular foreign bodies in open globe injury. Eur J Ophthalml. 2012;22(2):259–68.
6. Custer PL. Enucleation: past, present, and future. Ophthal Plast Reconstr Surg. 2000;16(5):316–21.
7. Perry AC. Advances in enucleation. Ophthal Plast Reconstr Surg. 1991;4:173–82.
8. Blaydon SM, Shepler TR, Neuhaus RW, et al. The porous polyethylene (Medpor) spherical orbital implant: a retrospective study of 136 cases. Ophthal Plast Reconstr Surg. 2003;19:364–71.
9. Ramadan A, Nussenblat R. Visual prognosis and sympathetic ophthalmia. Curr Opin Ophthal. 1996;7:39–45.
10. Kilmartin D, Dick A, Forrester J. Prospective surveillance of sympathetic ophthalmia in the UK and Republic of Ireland. Br J Ophthal. 2000;84:259–63.

Orbit

9

Reshma Mehendale and Roman Shinder

Introduction

The orbit is a socket in the skull in which the globe and its appendages are situated. The orbit has many important anatomical landmarks and a knowledge of their relationships with the surrounding vital structures is crucial for accurate diagnosis in the event of trauma.

Anatomy

The orbit has a volume of 30 ml of which the globe occupies approximately 6.5 ml. It is shaped like a trapezoid with its apex directed posteriorly. It is comprised of seven bones (Fig. 9.1). The roof is formed by the frontal bone and lesser wing of sphenoid. The roof houses the lacrimal gland fossa, the fossa for the trochlea of the superior oblique tendon and the supraorbital notch. The anterior cranial fossa and the frontal sinus are just posterior and superior to it, respectively. The zygoma and the greater wing of sphenoid form the lateral wall of the orbit. The important anatomic relations of the lateral wall include the lateral orbital tubercle of Whitnall, the attachment for the lateral horn of the levator aponeurosis, lateral canthal tendon, ligament of Lockwood, and the check ligament of the lateral rectus. It is the strongest of the orbital walls with the middle cranial fossa posterior and the temporal fossa lateral to it. The ethmoid, lacrimal, maxilla, and the lesser wing of sphenoid form the medial wall. The ethmoid bone (lamina papyracea) is the thinnest orbital bone and is a common site for medial orbital wall fracture. The ethmoid and sphenoid sinuses lie just medial to the medial orbital wall. The maxilla, zygoma, and palatine bones form the orbital floor. The maxilla is the second thinnest orbital bone and a common site for orbital floor fracture. The floor harbors the infraorbital canal and infraorbital groove that transmit the infraorbital artery and the maxillary division of the trigeminal nerve (V_2). The orbital floor is synonymous with the roof of the maxillary sinus.

The orbit contains the optic nerve (II), the globe, orbital fat, the extraocular muscles and their corresponding innervating nerves [oculomotor (III), trochlear (IV), abducens (VI)], trigeminal nerve (V_2), blood vessels and nerves, and the lacrimal gland. The greater and the lesser wing of sphenoid form the superior orbital fissure. The superior orbital fissure transmits cranial nerves III, IV, VI, and the ophthalmic division of trigeminal nerve (V_1), superior orbital vein, and sympathetic fibers. The inferior orbital fissure lies between the lateral orbital wall and the floor of the orbit. It transmits V_2, the zygomatic nerve, and inferior ophthalmic vein. The optic canal is located in the lesser wing of sphenoid and is approximately 8–10 mm long. It transmits the

R. Mehendale · R. Shinder (✉)
Department of Ophthalmology, The State University of New York (SUNY) Downstate Medical Center, 541 Clarkson Ave, E Bldg, 8th Floor, Suite C, Brooklyn, NY 11203, USA
e-mail: shinder.roman@gmail.com

S.C. Kaufman and D.R. Lazzaro (eds.), *Textbook of Ocular Trauma*,
DOI 10.1007/978-3-319-47633-9_9

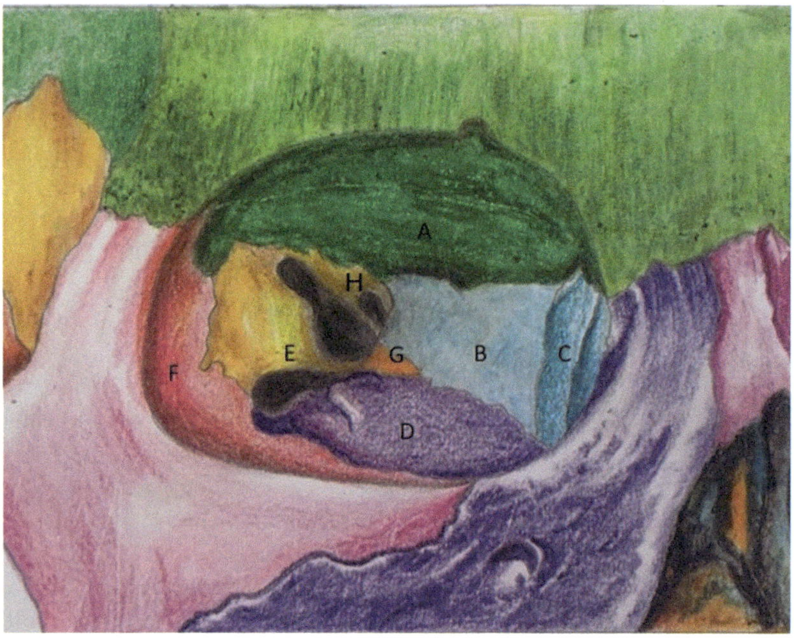

Fig. 9.1 Bones of the right orbit *A* Frontal, *B* Ethmoid, *C* Lacrimal, *D* Maxillary, *E* Greater wing of sphenoid, *F* Zygoma, *G* Palatine, *H* Lesser wing of sphenoid

optic nerve, ophthalmic artery, and sympathetic nerve fibers. Traumatic fracture of the optic canal can result in optic nerve damage and vision loss. The paranasal sinuses are located just outside the orbit (Fig. 9.2).

The annulus of zinn is an important anatomical landmark of the orbit formed by the common origin of the superior, inferior, medial and lateral rectus muscles. The optic foramen and the central portion of the superior orbital fissure are enclosed within the annulus. This part of the orbital apex is called the oculomotor foramen. The superior and inferior divisions of CN III, CN VI, and the nasociliary branch of CN V pass through this foramen (Fig. 9.3). The lacrimal, frontal and trochlear nerve and the superior ophthalmic vein pass through the superior part of the fissure outside the annulus.

The orbit is divided into different compartments by virtue of the location of the extraocular muscles, periorbita (periosteum lining the orbital bones), and the tenons fascia that form five

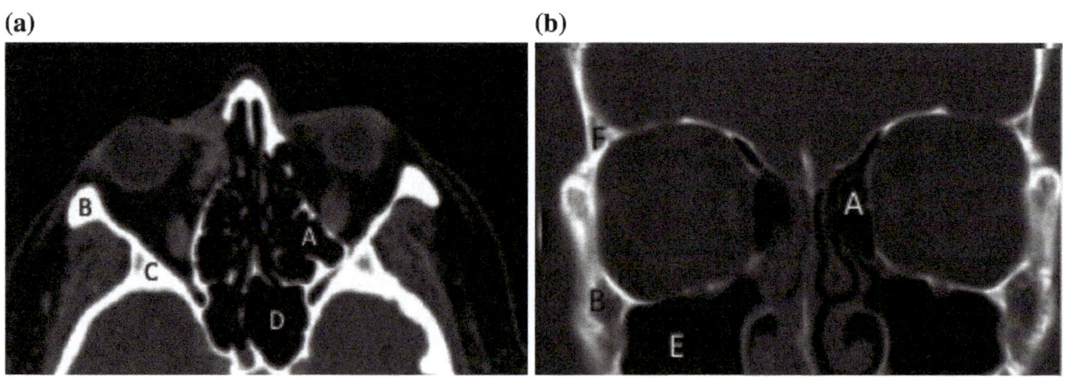

Fig. 9.2 Axial (**a**) and coronal (**b**) orbital CT showing relationship of sinuses to orbit: *A* Ethmoid sinus, *B* Zygoma, *C* Greater wing of sphenoid, *D* Sphenoid sinus, *E* Maxillary sinus. *F* Frontal bone

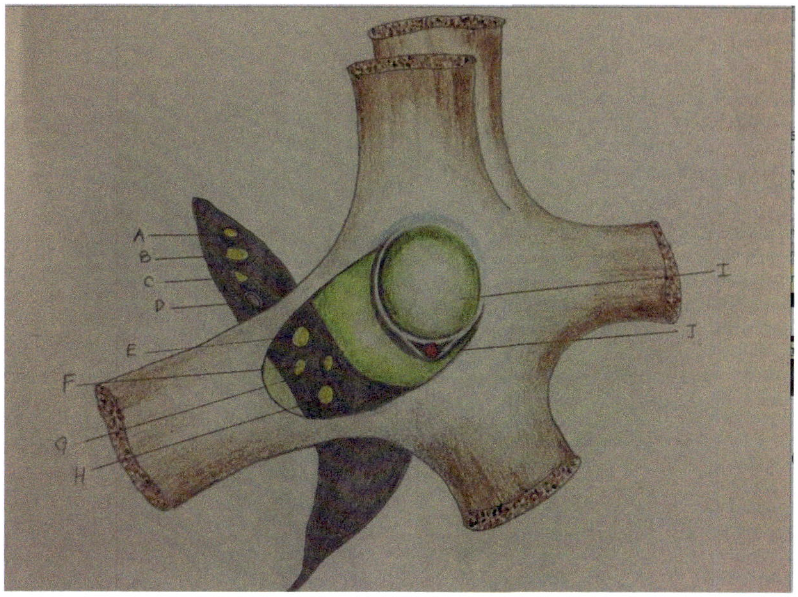

Fig. 9.3 Structures passing through the right orbital apex and superior orbital fissure: *A* Lacrimal nerve, *B* Frontal nerve, *C* Trochlear nerve (CN IV), *D* Superior ophthalmic vein, *E* Superior division of oculomoter nerve (CN III), *F* Abducen nerve (CN VI), *G* nasociliary nerve, *H* Inferior division of CN III, *I* Optic nerve, *J* Ophthalmic artery

surgical spaces within the orbit. The extraconal space lies between the periorbita and rectus muscle cone. The intraconal space lies within the rectus muscle cone. The subperiosteal space lies between bone and periorbita. The episcleral space lies between Tenon's capsule and the globe. Lastly, the subarachnoid space lies between the optic nerve and the optic nerve sheath (Fig. 9.4). The optic nerve is within the intraconal space. Any traumatic event that causes a compartment syndrome, either due to accumulation of air or blood within the intraconal space, poses a risk for optic nerve compression and possible long-term vision loss. The intermuscular septum is a membranous ring that connects the rectus muscles in the anterior portion of the orbit. This ring divides the orbit into intraconal and extraconal compartments.

The orbital blood supply arises primarily from the ophthalmic artery, a branch of the internal carotid artery. A small portion of the supply is also derived from the internal maxillary and facial arteries which are branches of the external carotid artery. The venous drainage for the orbit is provided mainly by the superior ophthalmic vein. The vein runs from the superonasal quadrant of the orbit, through the superior orbital fissure draining into the cavernous sinus.

Orbital Trauma

Evaluation

A detailed history and examination is essential to guide the clinician in determining the extent of trauma and potential need for emergent surgical intervention to prevent long-term morbidity including permanent visual loss [1]. It is important to ascertain the timing and mechanism of trauma, and blunt versus penetrating mechanisms. Changes in visual acuity or double vision, if present, provide a valuable clue that the injury to the globe or orbit may be of a serious nature. Their absence, however, does not rule out the potential for severe trauma. Nausea or vomiting in the setting of a suspected orbital wall fracture is highly suspicious of possible muscle entrapment, which is an ocular emergency. Examination of a patient with orbital trauma involves careful evaluation of visual acuity and extraocular movements in all cardinal positions of gaze. Confrontation visual fields can be valuable to determine the presence of optic nerve trauma. Once a ruptured globe has been ruled out, intraocular pressure should be assessed in a standard fashion.

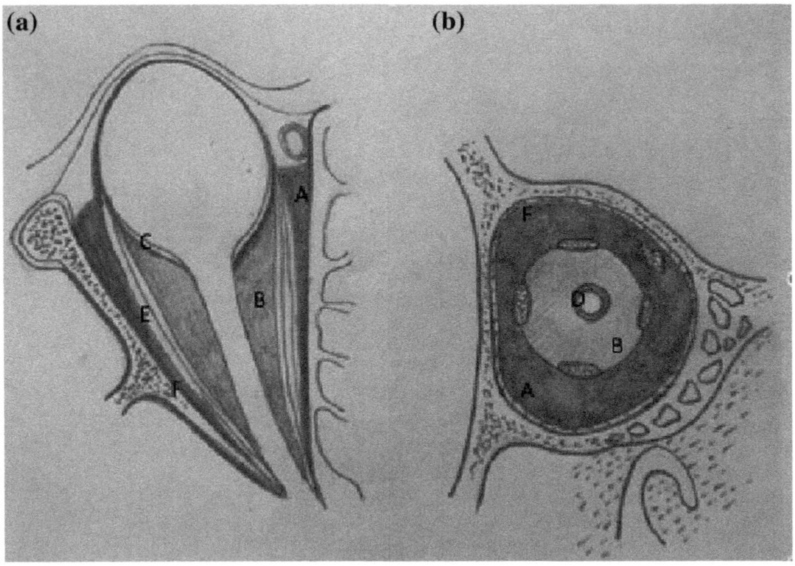

Fig. 9.4 **a** Axial and **b** Cornonal view of the orbital spaces: *A* Extraconal space, *B* Intraconal space, *C* Sub Tenon space, *D* Subarachnoid space, *E* Extraocular Muscle, *F* Subperiosteal space

Imaging

Orbital CT without contrast is a useful study for a quick evaluation of pathology and is the standard imaging modality used in the setting of trauma. It exposes the patient to a low dose of radiation (1–14 mSv) [2]. Coronal sections are best for evaluating orbital fractures. CT is also the study of choice when an orbital or intraocular foreign body is suspected [3].

MRI allows better visualization of the orbital soft tissue, does not involve radiation exposure, but is contraindicated if a metallic foreign body is a possibility, and is rarely used in traumatic patients in the acute setting.

Different Presentations of Orbital Trauma

1. **Orbital Contusion:**
   Orbital contusion occurs secondary to blunt trauma and can present with variable amounts of pain, blurry vision, proptosis, periorbital edema and ecchymosis. Radiography shows preseptal edema in the absence of fractures and other signs of severe injury. Treatment is typically conservative and consists of elevation of the head of the bed and cold compresses, and analgesics as needed. Some advocate the use of oral steroids to alleviate swelling and inflammation. In most cases the signs and symptoms are self-limiting and resolve within days to weeks.
2. **Orbital Fractures:**
   Orbital blowout fractures account for 18–50% of all maxillofacial trauma [4]. Common presenting signs in patients with blowout fractures include periocular edema and ecchymosis, diplopia with decreased extraocular movements, and hypoesthesia. Large orbital fractures can sometimes lead to noticeable enophthalmos (>2 mm) once the initial periorbital edema subsides. Thin-cut orbital CT, especially coronal sections, is essential to investigate the extent of the fracture.

Orbital Floor Fracture

Orbital floor fractures account for 65–80% of all orbital fractures. Fractures are classified as either "Pure" or "Impure". The more common pure fractures have no rim involvement and are caused by blunt impact on the globe causing secondary fracture of the floor via retropulsion. The less common impure fractures are caused by direct impact to the rim causing fracture of the rim and floor via buckling.

Two theories predominate to describe the pathophysiology of an orbital blowout fracture: the hydraulic or retropulsion, and the buckling theories. The hydraulic theory suggests trauma, with a significant impact to the globe, results in a retropulsion force that results in a blow out fracture [5–7]. In the buckling theory, traumatic forces are conducted along the orbital rim to the orbital bones resulting in fracture [5–7].

Patients with an orbital fracture may present with edema, ecchymosis, enophthalmos, and diplopia. It is important to palpate the area for any crepitus, or bony step off of the orbital rim if a displaced fracture is present [8]. Extraocular movements may be limited due to chemosis, orbital hemorrhage or inflammation, muscle or nerve trauma. Floor fractures involving the infraorbital canal can result in numbness of the V_2 distribution including the cheek, lower eyelid, upper lip, upper gums, and teeth on the affected side. This typically resolves over weeks to months of observation. Patients can present with limitation of both supra- and infraduction with diplopia in up- and/or down gaze. If the fracture site is large, typically more than 50% of the entire floor and especially when in conjunction with large medial wall fractures, it may cause enophthalmos due to herniation of orbital soft tissues into the adjacent sinuses. The great majority of orbital floor fractures do not require surgical intervention.

Entrapment is more commonly seen in trapdoor, orbital floor fractures in the pediatric population due to higher elasticity of bones in the younger population. Orbital bones in children are more elastic and tend to instantly snap back into normal position after trauma, hence allowing the trapping of orbital soft tissues within the fracture plane. Patients may present with nausea, vomiting, diplopia, and bradycardia. This should be suspected when there is restriction of globe movements in both supra- and infraduction, often with the globe failing to elevate vertically past the midline. Globe movement, in acute trauma, maybe limited due to muscle trauma, hematoma, edema, or pain. True entrapment can be confirmed by clinical exam, and careful review of radiography. In the authors' experience, radiologists may at times miss an entrapped fracture and the CT findings can be subtle. It is therefore paramount for surgeons to carefully review thin cut CT imaging of all orbital trauma patients. If an entrapped fracture is suspected, the patient must be placed on cardiac monitoring and instructed to relax without extreme eye movements, which may trigger the oculocardiac reflex, with urgent preparation for surgical repair. The oculocardiac reflex, a reflex arc of the trigeminal and vagus nerves, can cause bradycardia or cardiac arrhythmia in patients with an entrapped orbital fracture [3, 9–12].

Figure 9.5 depicts a schematic of an entrapped floor fracture detailing the complex network of fascia that exists in the orbit and that has an intimate relationship with the inferior rectus muscle. It is important to note that an entrapped fracture can result from the incarceration of any orbital soft tissue including the fat, and does not require the inferior rectus muscle being at or inferior to the plane of the fracture. It is this fascial network that is a key in making the orbital soft tissues a single functional unit.

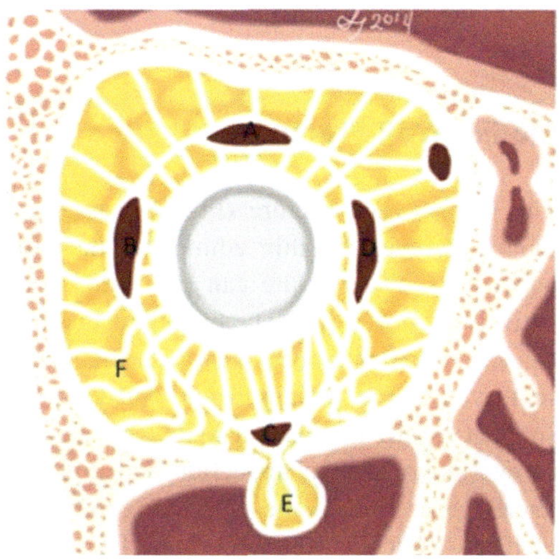

Fig. 9.5 Schematic of a right orbital floor fracture with entrapment (Courtesy Sunny Tang). *A–D*. Extraocular muscles, *E* entrapped soft tissue, *F* Fascia

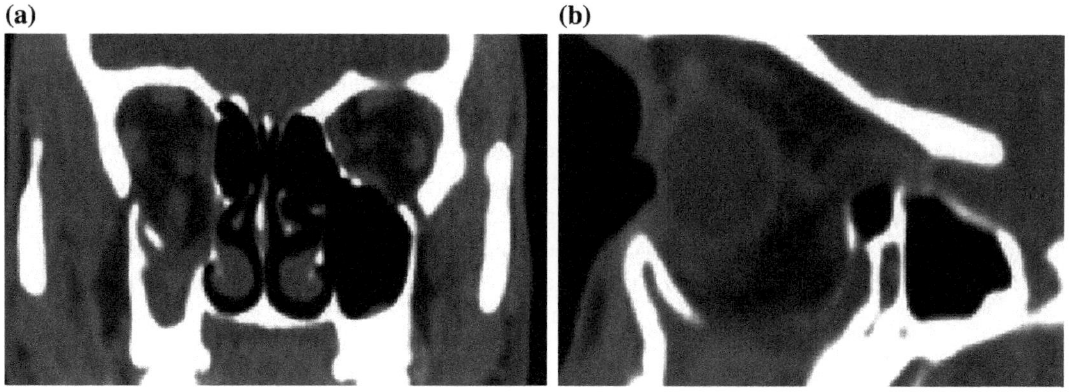

Fig. 9.6 Coronal (**a**) and sagittal (**b**) orbital CT scan showing a large displaced right orbital floor fracture with prolapse of orbital soft tissues into the maxillary sinus

The maxilla in the posteromedial aspect of the orbital floor is the thinnest part of the floor and commonly the site of fractures (Fig. 9.6). Rarely an orbital fracture may present as a "white-eyed blowout" fracture especially in children under the age of 16 [13]. Patients with these kinds of fractures show minimal signs of soft tissue injury, minimal enophthalmos, and minimal prolapsed tissue or fracture area on CT scans. However, they do show marked restriction in both supra- and infraduction with possible bradycardia on eye movements. In these presentations, it is recommended that surgical intervention be prompt once entrapment is confirmed.

Medial Wall Fracture

The medial wall fracture (Fig. 9.7) most commonly involves the thin ethmoid bone (lamina papyracea). The fracture can be treated conservatively in most cases. The medial rectus muscle can rarely get entrapped within the fracture and in that case the patient would need emergent surgical repair. The patient may show limitation of eye movement on abduction and diplopia in lateral gaze. Due to the close proximity of the medial wall to the ethmoid sinus, fractures can cause orbital emphysema which, if severe, can cause a compartment syndrome. Patients with both large medial and floor fractures are at increased risk of developing enophthalmos and should be monitored for this potential finding on serial clinical exams with Hertel exophthalmometry.

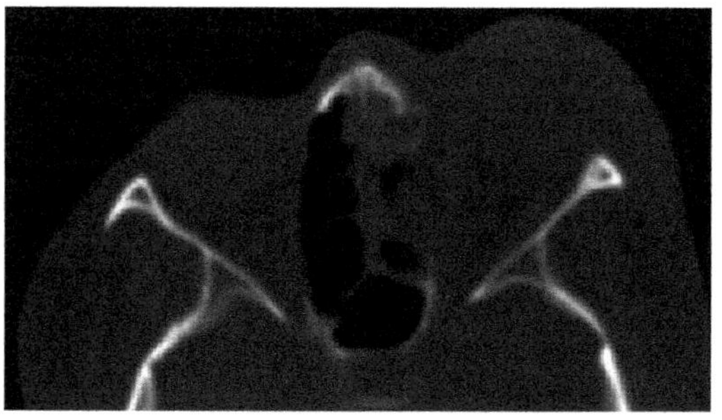

Fig. 9.7 Axial orbital CT scan showing fracture of the left medial wall

Orbital Roof Fractures

Fractures of the orbital roof are usually caused by blunt trauma or projectile missile injuries. They are more common in children as they do not have formed pneumatized frontal sinuses to absorb the impact of the trauma. The majority of roof fractures do not require surgical repair. Any patient who presents with a fracture of the roof warrants a neurosurgical consultation, and intracranial injury must be evaluated and ruled out. If repair were warranted, such as in cases of severe intracranial injury or hematoma, the surgical approach would be done in conjunction with a neurosurgeon. Pulsating proptosis may occur as a delayed complication of severe comminuted orbital roof fracture resulting from the transmission of cerebrospinal fluid pulsations through the bony defect.

Orbital Apex Fracture

Orbital apex fractures involve the optic canal and/or the superior and inferior orbital fissures. This type of fracture can cause traumatic optic neuropathy, multiple cranial neuropathies, and long-term visual morbidity.

Lateral Wall Fracture

Lateral wall fractures are rare given the strength of the zygoma and greater wing of sphenoid. A specific type of fracture known as the zygomaticomaxillary complex (ZMC) or tripod fracture involves the lateral wall. It is a constellation of fractures that includes the zygoma in two locations, the inferior orbital rim and the maxillary sinus wall (Fig. 9.8). Severe ZMC fractures can cause globe dystopia, trismus and malar flattening. Large and displaced fractures especially when in conjunction with a symptomatic patient may warrant surgical repair that typically involves open reduction of the fractures with fixation with titanium plates and screws. Displaced zygoma fractures without surgical repair can lead to an antimongoloid slant of the lids if the lateral canthal tendon attachment to the zygoma becomes displaced.

LeFort Fractures

LeFort fractures are midfacial fractures and are classified into three types. LeFort type 1 fracture involves a break through the alveolar ridge, inferior wall of the maxillary sinus, and lateral wall of nose, separating the upper face from the teeth. LeFort type 2 fracture involves a break through the lateral wall of the maxillary sinuses, inferior orbital rims, nasal bones, and posterior alveolar area. LeFort type 3 fracture involves a break through the nasofrontal suture, maxillofrontal suture, lateral and medial orbital walls and zygomatic arches. LeFort type 3 fractures are a craniofacial disjunction.

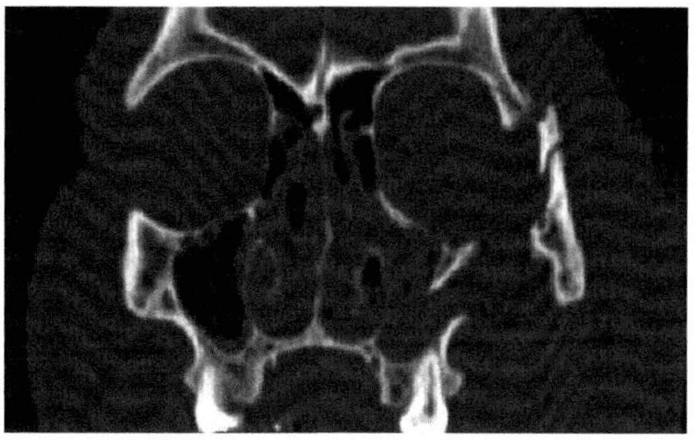

Fig. 9.8 Coronal CT scan showing left zygomaticomaxillary complex fracture including the zygoma in two places, inferior orbital rim and maxillary sinus wall

Nasoorbitoethmoidal Fractures (NOE)

These are fractures involving the nose, orbit, ethmoid sinus, frontal sinus, and the insertion of the medial canthal tendon. If this fracture is suspected, the nasolacrimal outflow system should be evaluated through lacrimal irrigation. Unrepaired NOE fractures can lead to telecanthus when the medial canthal tendon attachment becomes medially displaced.

Management of Fractures

Medical Management

Once it is established that a patient has an orbital fracture that does not need emergent surgical intervention, medical management should be initiated. Patients with blowout fractures without entrapment can be managed clinically with medical management in most cases. Patients with medial wall fractures are ordered to avoid nose blowing and to only sneeze with their mouths open to avoid orbital emphysema that can lead to compartment syndrome and visual loss. Cold compresses should be initiated, 20 minutes on and 20 minutes off and continued for the first 48–72 hours to help reduce soft tissue swelling that typically accompanies orbital trauma. Many studies have looked at the benefit of prophylactic antibiotics in patients with orbital or facial fractures, and have found no substantiation to support their use [14]. The authors do not typically give systemic antibiotics to patients with orbital fractures. A rapid course of oral steroids of 1 mg/kg per day for a few days or a methylprednisolone dose pack can help reduce swelling and development of scar tissue. Steroids can provide a more rapid improvement in periorbital and orbital edema, which permits a more accurate assessment of extraocular movements, diplopia, and enophthalmos at the post injury week 1 visit and more rapid surgical planning when warranted. Use of oral steroids is contraindicated in patients' with intracranial injury [15]. The authors routinely give oral steroids unless contraindicated at the initial patient encounter. Adjunctive use of analgesics and nasal decongestants can be recommended for initial medical management. Decongestants such as phenylephrine nasal spray directly stimulate the alpha-adrenergic receptors on the nasal mucous membrane and cause vasoconstriction which decreases the likelihood of orbital emphysema and potential compartment syndrome if the patient blows their nose.

Surgical Management

Indications for surgical intervention in an orbital fracture include entrapment, symptomatic diplopia within 30° of primary gaze that is not improving with observation, enophthalmos of >2 mm that bothers the patient, and a large floor fracture or multiple large fractures typically more than 50%, or an orbital wall with considerable tissue herniation into the adjacent sinuses. The authors do not consider a fracture >50% alone as a surgical indication (as some do) because many patients will not develop noticeable enophthalmos with this single radiographic finding alone. Patients in certain professions, such as truck or school bus drivers, may be more troubled by diplopia and thus the profession and hobbies of the patient should be taken into account when assessing the degree of diplopia and possible surgical intervention.

As patients are observed after trauma and edema and inflammation subside, diplopia typically improves with time while enophthalmos becomes more apparent. These are important points to keep in mind while following a patient with a fracture and surgical consideration is being contemplated.

The timing for non-emergent fracture repair is controversial and advocates for both rapid repair and delayed repair exist. The authors attempt to perform repair within 2 weeks of injury when warranted as orbital scar tissue increases after this period [16–18]. This 2-week window allows improvement in periorbital and orbital edema, inflammation and hematoma, allowing better surgical exposure and a more straightforward surgical experience. Access to orbital radiography is valuable intraoperatively to correlate operative and radiographic findings. Image-guided systems are also available in some centers that perform endoscopic fracture repair.

The surgical approach is surgeon and fracture site dependent. For floor fractures, an inferior transconjunctival approach is preferred as it does not leave a cutaneous scar and has a lower rate of causing lower eyelid malposition as compared to a transcutaneous infraciliary approach. Potential approaches to repair a medial wall fracture include transcaruncular, transcutaneous, or endoscopic. The authors prefer a transcaruncular approach to a transcutaneous approach as the cosmetic result is superior without a facial scar and exposure is adequate in most cases.

The authors herein describe repair of an orbital floor fracture, which is the most common orbital fracture to require surgical intervention, and is typically an outpatient procedure. The patient is placed under general anesthesia and prepped and draped in typical sterile oculoplastic fashion. Local anesthetic containing a 50:50 mixture of lidocaine with epinephrine and bupivacaine with epinephrine is injected into the inferior extraconal orbit for hemostasis and postoperative pain. Intravenous corticosteroid is given to combat orbital inflammation and edema. The lower lid is retracted inferiorly with a Desmarres retractor and the globe is protected with a malleable retractor. An inferior transconjunctival incision is made with needle tip monopolar cautery from lateral to medial cutting conjunctiva, lower lid retractors, and periosteum along the inferior orbital rim. Care must be taken in the medial area of the orbital rim to dissect anterior to the origin of the inferior oblique muscle. A lateral canthotomy and inferior cantholysis may aid in exposure for very large fractures but the authors have found that it is typically not needed if an assistant provides good retraction. A subperiosteal plane is created and followed using a freer periosteal elevator. Blunt dissection is continued with the Freer repositing any orbital soft tissues that have herniated or become entrapped in the maxillary sinus. Care must be taken to preserve the infraorbital neurovascular bundle containing the maxillary nerve if it is visualized to avoid postoperative hypoesthesia. For cases with entrapment, it is sometimes necessary to enlarge and displace the fracture site into the maxillary sinus to be able to free and reposition the entrapped tissue. When manipulating the orbital tissues it is possible to stimulate the oculocardiac reflex and the anesthesiologist must be made aware of this possibility preoperatively and intraoperatively before traction is placed on the orbital tissues if bradycardia occurs. If the heart rate does decrease, the surgeon should stop and remove all orbital instruments, and the anesthesiologist may either wish to observe or give medication to bring the heart rate back up. Once all the tissues have been reposited, the surgeon should be able to see the entire fracture for 360°. This is especially important posteriorly as persistent diplopia and/or enophthalmos can remain if the entirety of the fracture is not exposed and repaired.

The fracture dimensions are viewed and the desired implant is measured and cut to fit the defect appropriately to be able to lie flat on sturdy bone for 360°.

Various surgical implants are available including alloplastic (porous polyethylene, titanium, supramid, gortex, Teflon or silicon) or autogenous (bone, cartilage or fascia) materials [19–21]. The Iliac crest and the calvarium are the most commonly used bony cadaveric donor sites [19–21], whereas auricular and septal donor sites can be used to harvest cartilage. Bone offers good strength and is radio opaque but is not flexible for a contoured floor surface. Bone also undergoes resorption, which could cause undercorrection over a period of time. Cartilage, on the other hand is more flexible, but offers limited structural support and can also be resorbed over time. Autogenous grafts also require a separate surgical site with potential morbidity in the donor area. Porous polyethylene and titanium reinforced porous polyethylene sheets are widely used for their biocompatibility, highly pliable property, and long-term stability due to high tensile strength and low infection rates. These sheets can be cut to proper size and shape with a large surgical scissor. The titanium-strengthened sheets are radiologically opaque, enabling exact postoperative positioning evaluation with radiography if warranted for implant migration or infection. The authors favor the use of titanium embedded porous polyethylene sheets that come in various thicknesses (Fig. 9.9).

Once the implant is fashioned it is positioned to cover the entire fracture using a thin clamp, and final position adjusted with forceps and Freer. Care must be taken to avoid any orbital soft tissues being trapped between the implant and the orbital floor. A forced duction test is utilized after implant placement to confirm the globe is freely mobile without any restriction. This is especially important to confirm in cases of entrapped fractures. Implant fixation to the orbital rim is an option utilizing screws but the authors choose to defer fixation and allow the orbital soft tissues to tamponade the implant against the orbital floor which typically maintains stable position until eventual tissue fibrosis stabilizes it permanently. Once the implant is placed, the cut conjunctival edges are positioned in their normal anatomical plane and allowed to

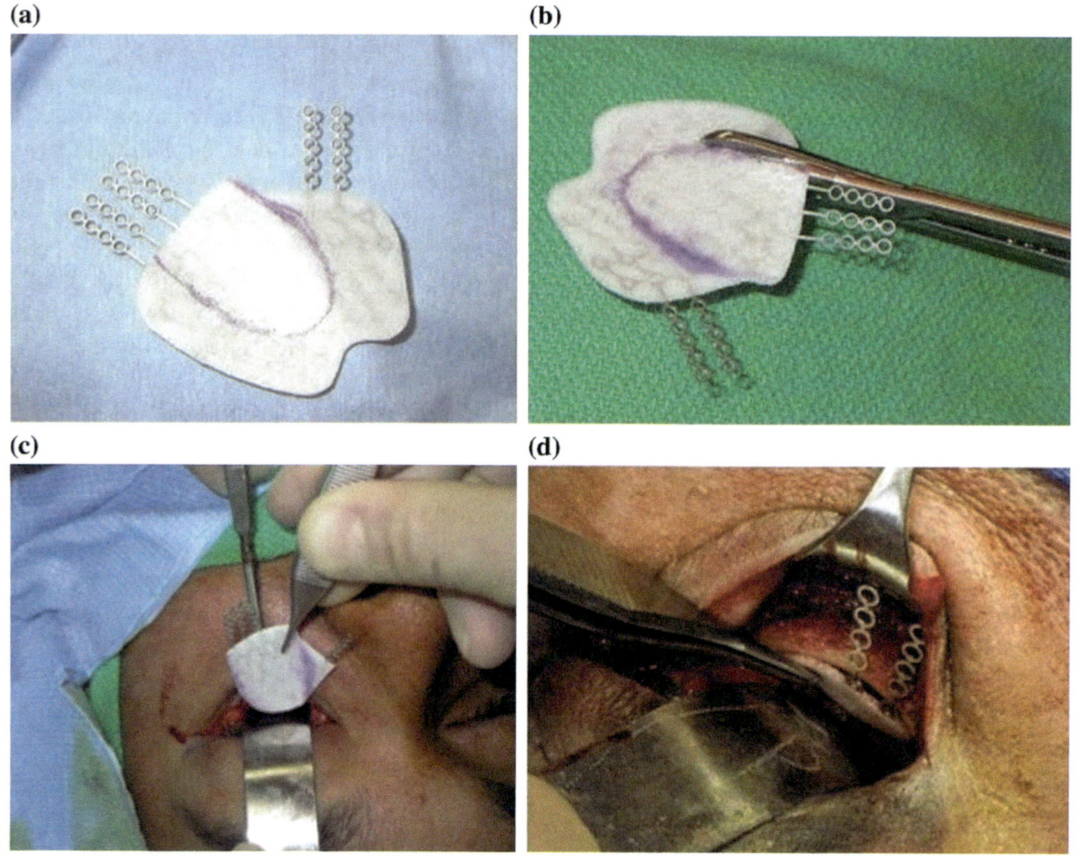

Fig. 9.9 Implant placement during orbital floor fracture repair. **a** Titanium embedded porous polyethylene implant marked based on fracture size. **b** Implant is cut with heavy scissors. **c** Placement of the implant with careful tissue retraction. **d** Implant is positioned over fracture site

heal by secondary intention. Some surgeons will close the conjunctiva with a running fast absorbing 6-0 plain gut suture. Antibiotic ophthalmic ointment is placed on the conjunctival wound. Throughout the case hemostasis is maintained with a 7 French suction tip, and exposure is optimized with Desmarres and malleable retractors. Surgical repair of medial wall, lateral wall and roof fractures, ZMC, NOE, and LeFort's fractures are beyond the scope of this text.

Postoperative care after orbital surgery involves measures to reduce soft tissue edema by recommending head of bed elevation, ice packs, and rapid course of oral steroids. Analgesics as needed are suggested but use of nonsteroidal anti-inflammatory agents should be avoided to reduce chances of bleeding. Antibiotic ophthalmic ointment to the conjunctival wound is given three times daily for one week. Although the authors choose not to, some surgeons give a course of oral antibiotics. Some hypoesthesia and diplopia can follow fracture repair and is typically transient. Patients are typically seen one week following surgery and followed subsequently to evaluate improvement in ocular movements, diplopia, and enophthalmos (Fig. 9.10).

Orbital Compartment Syndrome

Orbital compartment syndrome is a rare but very important condition that can occur in a trauma setting when either blood or air is trapped in the closed orbital compartment. Blood can cause a compartment syndrome after blunt or penetrating

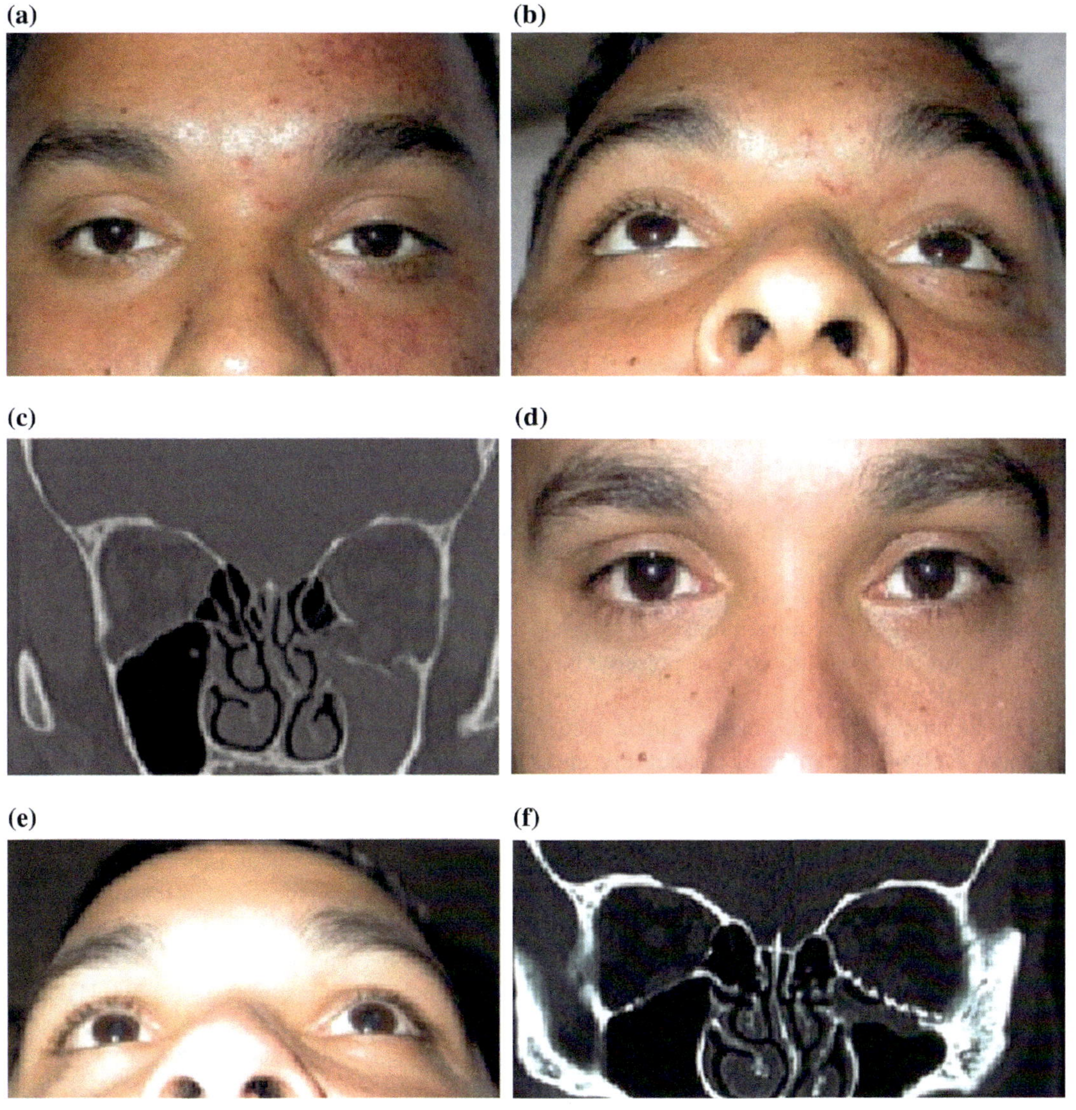

Fig. 9.10 **a**, **b** Preoperative clinical frontal and worm's eye photos of a patient with significant left enophthalmos. **c** Coronal CT orbits confirms a large displaced left orbital floor fracture with herniation of orbital soft tissue into the maxillary sinus. **d**, **e** One month postoperative clinical frontal and worm's eye photos showing improved globe position. **f** Coronal CT orbits showing properly placed orbital implant

trauma with or without orbital fracture. If a patient has a medial orbital wall fracture and forcefully blows their nose or sneezes with their mouth closed, air can move in a retrograde direction from the ethmoid sinus through the fracture site and become trapped in the orbit. Orbital compartment syndrome is a surgical emergency, and without prompt intervention, permanent visual loss may ensue from a compressive optic neuropathy or retinal vascular occlusion. Compartment syndrome should be suspected in any patient who has suffered orbital trauma that presents with pain, decreased visual acuity with relative afferent pupillary defect, proptosis, elevated intraocular pressure, tense lids and adnexa, chemosis and possibly

(a) (b)

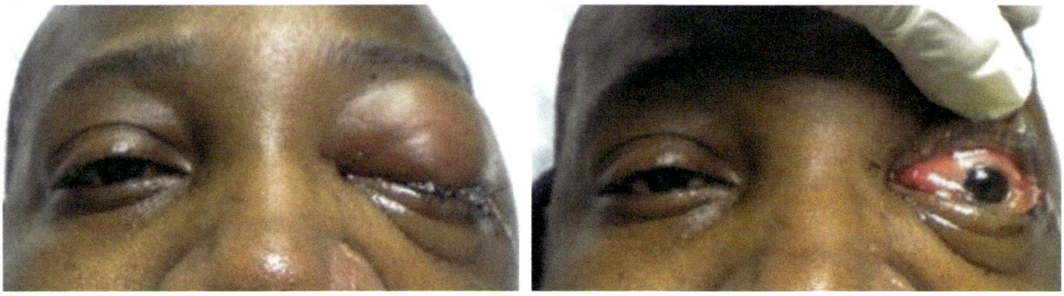

Fig. 9.11 A patient with left orbital compartment syndrome due to a motor vehicle accident. **a** Clinical frontal photograph showing significant periorbital edema and tense eyelids. **b** Mechanical left upper lid retraction reveals proptosis, and significant chemosis

decreased ocular movements (Fig. 9.11). Orbital CT will reveal retrobulbar hemorrhage or air depending on the mechanism of the syndrome. If clinical suspicion of a compartment syndrome is high, radiography should be deferred and surgical intervention initiated in urgent fashion in an attempt to improve or preserve the visual function.

The surgery needed in patients with a compartment syndrome is a lateral canthotomy and cantholysis. The initial steps require a prompt preparation of the surgical site with cleaning off any blood, topical anesthetic to the globe and prepping the periocular area with Betadine. Local anesthesia with epinephrine is given subcutaneously in the area of the lateral canthus. A thin clamp can be used to clamp the lateral canthal angle to achieve further hemostasis. The lateral canthus is then cut down to the zygoma with scissors for 1–2 cm finalizing the canthotomy (Fig. 9.12a). Using toothed forceps, the lower lid is pulled inferiorly and the inferior crus of the lateral canthal tendon is cut with scissors in a posterior and inferior direction until the entire tendon has been severed from its bony attachment. Strumming the tissues can aid the surgeon in finding the crus and confirming it has been properly cut. This should make the lower lid freely mobile (Fig. 9.12b). At the end of the procedure, the vision, pupil, and intraocular pressure are rechecked for signs of improvement. If adequate decompression is not achieved based on exam and the tissues remain tense, a superior cantholysis can be performed in similar fashion. A canthotomy and cantholysis can reduce the intraorbital pressure by 30–40 mm Hg, thus allowing reperfusion of the intraorbital tissues including the optic nerve. When warranted,

(a) (b)

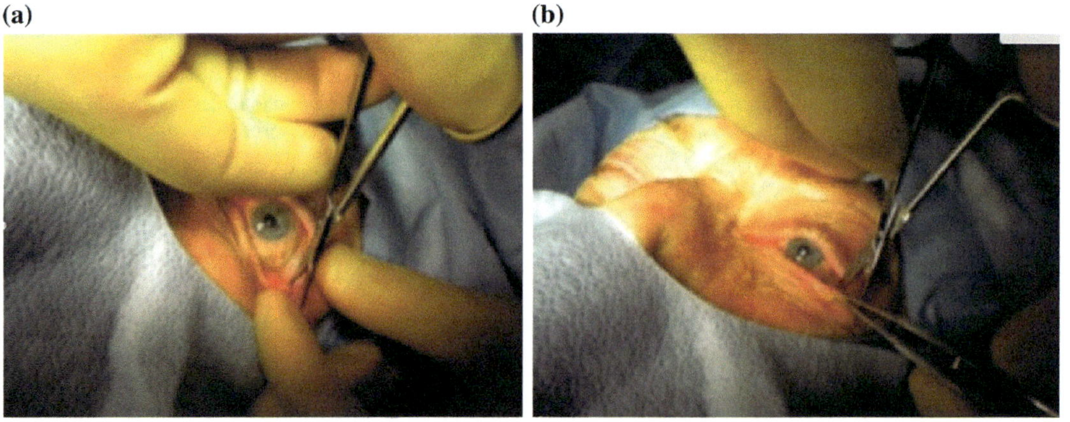

Fig. 9.12 Technique showing incision for a lateral canthotomy (**a**) and inferior cantholysis (**b**)

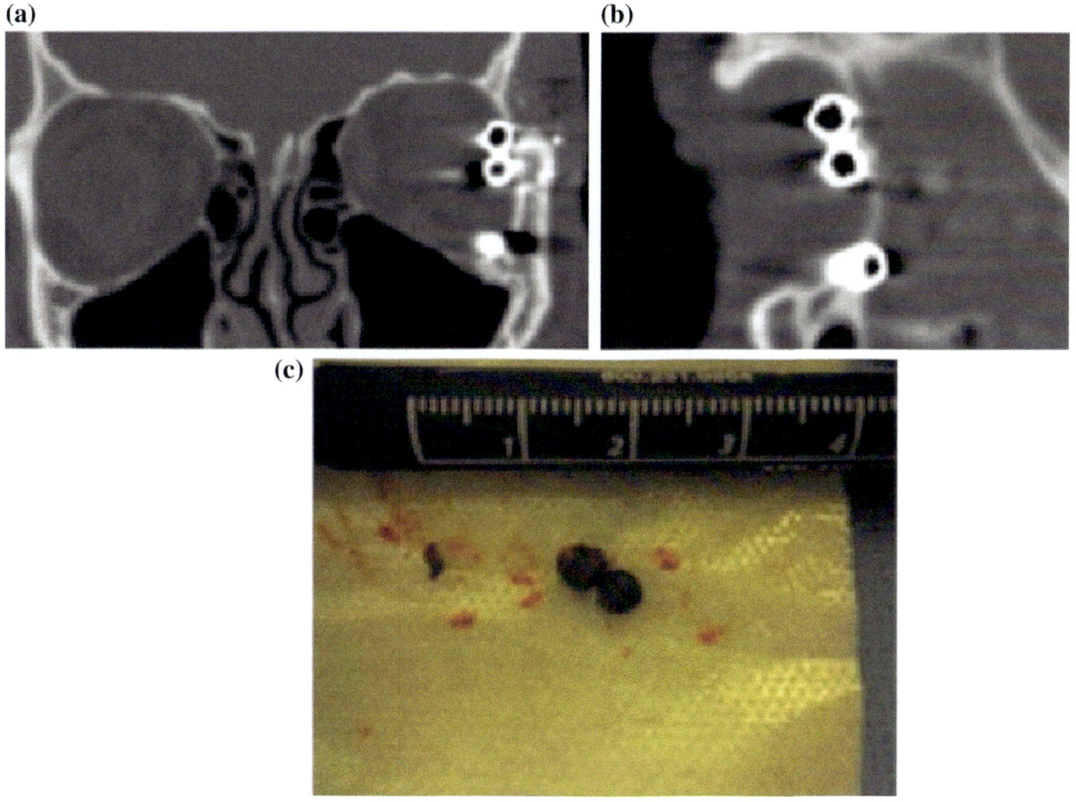

Fig. 9.13 Coronal (**a**) and sagittal (**b**) orbital CT scans showing bullet casings lodged in the lateral extraconal orbit causing fracture of the lateral orbital wall. The foreign bodies were removed via orbitotomy (**c**)

adjuvant medical management including high-dose intravenous steroids, mannitol, or acetazolamide can help decrease orbital and intraocular pressure, but should not be used as single modality therapy. Postoperatively, the wound is left open with a dressing to drain any bleeding, antibiotic ointment is applied, and steroids can be given to decrease pressure and edema. The cutaneous wound will typically heal in an acceptable fashion via secondary intention and rarely requires reconstruction. Visual improvement is possible if the syndrome is diagnosed early and surgical intervention instituted in a timely fashion.

Orbital Foreign Body

Orbital foreign bodies may present without obvious external evidence of trauma and can be missed by clinicians if not vigilant. Foreign bodies made of iron, copper, wood, vegetative material, or those causing penetrating injury to contiguous structures need urgent surgical removal. Foreign bodies made of inert materials like glass, gold, silver, platinum, porcelain, plastic, sand, cilia, or rubber should be treated conservatively with observation, especially if the patient is asymptomatic and/or the foreign body is in a difficult to access orbital location. Orbital radiography confirms the diagnosis, although depending on the material of the foreign body this can be challenging. Intraorbital wooden foreign bodies (IOWFB) present a particular diagnostic challenge to physicians. It is important to inform the radiologist if a history and mechanism of injury is suggestive of an IOWFB, as routine CT settings may allow the IOWFB to masquerade as air or fat [22–25]. Complications from retained IOWFB may present anytime from

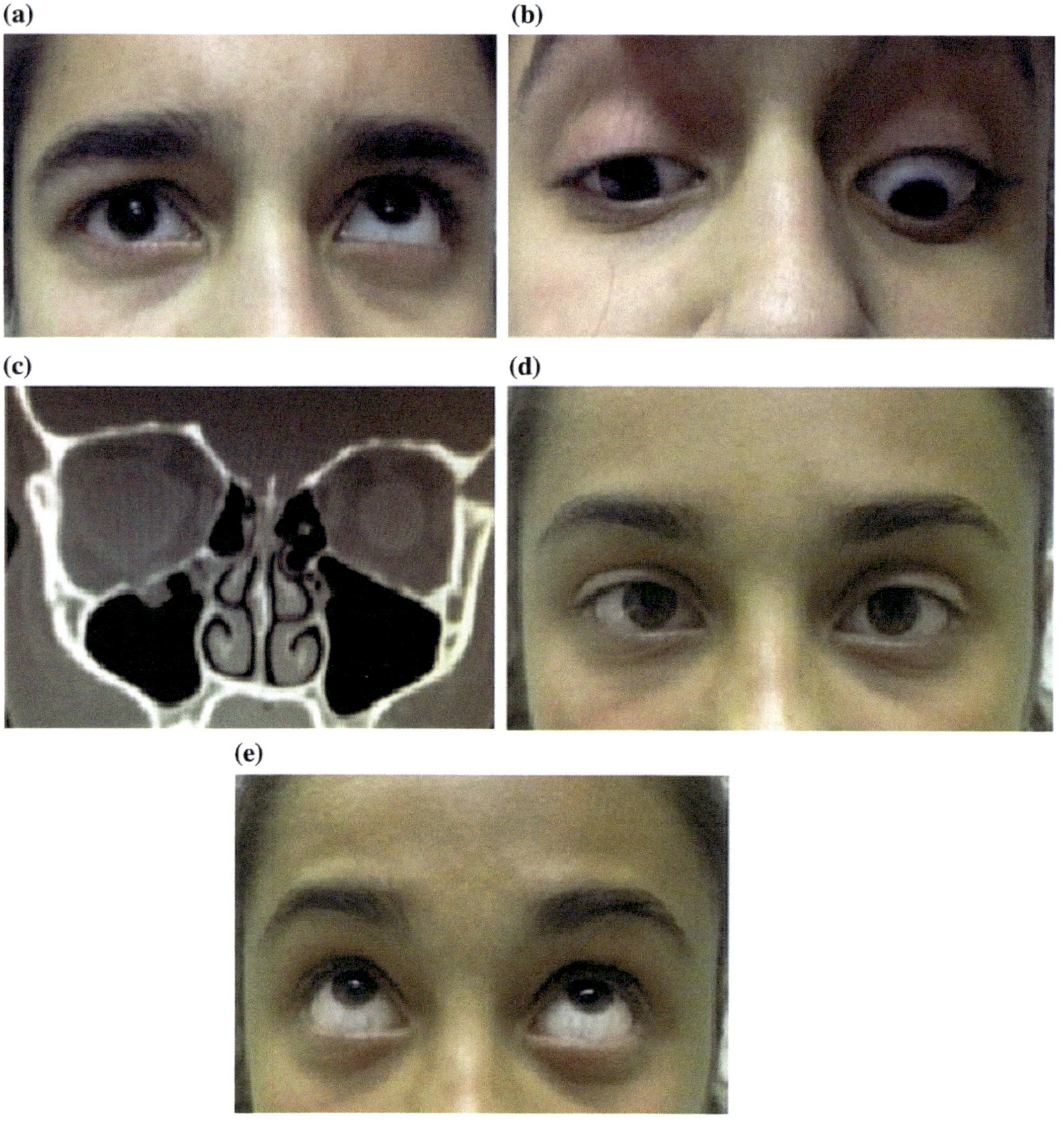

Fig. 9.14 Clinical photographs at presentation of a young girl who suffered blunt periocular trauma showing restricted right supraduction (**a**) and infraduction (**b**). **c** Coronal orbital CT scan confirming an entrapped right trapdoor floor fractures. Clinical photographs one week following fracture repair showing normal globe position (**d**) and full supraduction (**e**)

1 day to 1 year after injury [24]. Delay in recognition and treatment may lead to serious complications such as orbital abscess or cellulitis.

Tracking the entry wound via an anterior orbitotomy by retraction and dissection along the path of trajectory is the preferred method for surgical removal of orbital foreign bodies so as not to incur any additional trauma to adjacent orbital structures (Fig. 9.13). All patients should receive systemic antibiotic treatment and retrieved foreign bodies should be sent for culture and sensitivity especially if felt to be contaminated.

Case Presentation

A 9-year-old girl presented to the emergency department with complaints of double vision and nausea following accidental injury to the right periocular area with a basketball a few hours earlier. On examination, there was restricted supra- and infraduction of the right eye with pain and binocular diplopia. Orbital CT scan confirmed an entrapped trapdoor fracture of the orbital floor (Fig. 9.14a–c). The patient was urgently taken to the operating room where the entrapped tissues were freed and the fracture repaired with an implant. Postoperatively, the patient had complete resolution of all signs and symptoms and returned to baseline (Fig. 9.14d, e).

References

1. Babineau MR, Sanchez LD. Ophthalmologic procedures in the emergency department. Emerg Med Clin North Am. 2008;26(1):17–34, v–vi.
2. McCollough CH, Primak AN, Braun N, et al. Strategies for reducing radiation dose in CT. Radiol Clin North Am. 2009;47(1):27–40.
3. Merali FI, Grant MP, Mahoney NR. Orbital floor fracture with atypical extraocular muscle entrapment pattern and intraoperative asystole in an adult. Craniomaxillofac Trauma Reconstr. 2015;8(4):370–4.
4. Joseph JM, Glavas IP. Orbital fractures: a review. Clin Ophthalmol. 2011;5:95–100.
5. Nagasao T, Miyamoto J, Nagasao M, et al. The effect of striking angle on the buckling mechanism in blowout fracture. Plast Reconstr Surg. 2006;117 (7):2373–80.
6. Adeyemo WL, Aribaba OT, Ladehinde AL, Ogunlewe MO. Mechanisms of orbital blowout fracture: a critical review of the literature. Niger Postgrad Med J. 2008;15(4):251–4.
7. Bullock JD, Warwar RE, Ballal DR, Ballal RD. Mechanisms of orbital floor fractures: a clinical, experimental, and theoretical study. Trans Am Ophthalmol Soc. 1999;97:87–110.
8. Huempfner-Hierl H, Bohne A, Wollny G, Sterker I, Hierl T. Blunt forehead trauma and optic canal involvement: finite element analysis of anterior skull base and orbit on causes of vision impairment. Br J Ophthalmol. 2015;99(10):1430–4.
9. Reddy SS, Landry JP, Douglass K, Venugopalan PP. A case of ocular cardiac reflex in a child with blunt ocular trauma. BMJ Case Rep. 2014;2014.
10. Kasi SK, Gorovoy IR, Vagefi MR, Kersten RC. The oculocardiac reflex in an adult with a non-displaced orbital floor fracture. Orbit. 2014;33(4):286–8.
11. Wartak SA, Mehendale RA, Lotfi A. A unique case of asystole secondary to facial injury. Case Rep Med. 2012;2012:382605.
12. Bagheri A, Tavakoli M, Khosravifard K, Yazdani S. Clinical and radiologic characteristics of inferior rectus muscle sheath entrapment in orbital blowout fracture. J Craniofac Surg. 2015;26(7):e633–5.
13. Jordan DR, Allen LH, White J, et al. Intervention within days for some orbital floor fractures: the white-eyed blowout. Ophthal Plast Reconstr Surg. 1998;14(6):379–90.
14. Zix J, Schaller B, Iizuka T, Lieger O. The role of postoperative prophylactic antibiotics in the treatment of facial fractures: a randomised, double-blind, placebo-controlled pilot clinical study. Part 1: orbital fractures in 62 patients. Br J Oral Maxillofac Surg. 2013;51(4):332–6.
15. Millman AL, Della Rocca RC, Spector S, et al. Steroids and orbital blowout fractures—a new systematic concept in medical management and surgical decision-making. Adv Ophthalmic Plast Reconstruct Surg. 1987;6:291–300.
16. Brucoli M, Arcuri F, Cavenaghi R, Benech A. Analysis of complications after surgical repair of orbital fractures. J Craniof Surg. 2011;22(4):1387–90.
17. Burnstine MA. Clinical recommendations for repair of isolated orbital floor fractures: an evidence-based analysis. Ophthalmology. 2002;109(7):1207–10.
18. Yu DY, Chen CH, Tsay PK, et al. Surgical timing and fracture type on the outcome of diplopia after orbital fracture repair. Ann Plast Surg. 2016;76 (Suppl 1):S91–5.
19. Baino F. Biomaterials and implants for orbital floor repair. Acta Biomater. 2011;7(9):3248–66.
20. Banica B, Ene P, Vranceanu D, Ene R. Titanium preformed implants in orbital floor reconstruction—case presentation, review of literature. Maedica. 2013;8(1):34–9.
21. Bratton EM, Durairaj VD. Orbital implants for fracture repair. Curr Opin Ophthalmol. 2011;22 (5):400–6.
22. Adesanya OO, Dawkins DM. Intraorbital wooden foreign body (IOFB): mimicking air on CT. Emerg Radiol. 2007;14(1):45–9.
23. Hansen JE, Gudeman SK, Holgate RC, Saunders RA. Penetrating intracranial wood wounds: clinical limitations of computerized tomography. J Neurosurg. 1988;68(5):752–6.
24. Shelsta HN, Bilyk JR, Rubin PA, Penne RB, Carrasco JR. Wooden intraorbital foreign body injuries: clinical characteristics and outcomes of 23 patients. Ophthal Plast Reconstr Surg. 2010;26(4):238–44.
25. Dalley RW. Intraorbital wood foreign bodies on CT: use of wide bone window settings to distinguish wood from air. AJR Am J Roentgenol. 1995;164 (2):434–5.

Retina and Posterior Segment Injuries

10

Andrew Hou and Eric M. Shrier

Trauma to the posterior segment can drastically impact visual acuity and result in disability and permanent visual loss. In US emergency rooms, the annual incidence of ocular injuries is roughly 3.2 per 1000 people [1, 2]. This translates to approximately 650,000 patients with eye trauma seen by New York City area physicians each year. Considering those numbers, and the fact that nearly all irreversible vision loss due to eye trauma results from posterior segment or retinal damage, it is important to recognize the signs early on. Obtaining an accurate history is vital in accurately triaging patients. Identifying the nature and etiology of trauma, with concern for velocity of impact, size of impacting object, and composition of materials help to determine the amount of traumatic forces that are transferred to the eye. Whether or not the trauma victim was wearing eye protection should be ascertained and documented for a variety of reasons. The incident specifics, coupled with important symptoms such as new onset floaters, flashes of light, or the vision loss effect of a "curtain coming down" on a patient's vision are red flags for significant retinal injury which should be expertly evaluated and appropriately referred.

The retina is a multilayered, laminar structure with a definite center, the macula, where most of our critical vision is concentrated. Injury to the macula often leads to permanent "legal blindness" (20/200 best-corrected visual acuity (VA) or worse). The product of visual signal transduction in the macula and peripheral retina is ultimately delivered via the nerve fiber layer to the optic nerve head, and onward to the brain via projections of axons. When describing various pathological processes and injuries that come to afflict the eyeball, the eye is often likened to a photographic instrument, a "film-camera." In this demystified paradigm, the retina is the "film" in that camera. As with a fine and precise instrument such as a vintage camera, the various parts are quite delicate and intricate. They are also prone to jarring and accidental trauma. Like "film" in the camera, the retina is paper thin and easily susceptible to permanent damage. Further, the retina requires nourishment from intrinsic blood vessels (the retinal vascular circulation of arteries and veins) located within the inner retina and a deeper encapsulating vascular choroid layer. The inner two-thirds of the retina is supplied by the retinal blood vessels while the outer one-third is supplied by the choroidal circulation. The choroidal circulation encircles the outer sensory retina and along with its pigment and pigmented cellular layers is also known as the posterior uveal layer. The anterior portion of this uveal tissue forms the ciliary body, which produces aqueous humor and contains the muscles that change the shape of the lens for near viewing (accommodation). A relatively thick, durable fibrous protective layer called the sclera covers and protects this uveal vascular layer. This white

A. Hou (✉) · E.M. Shrier
Department of Ophthalmology, The State University of New York (SUNY) Downstate College of Medicine, 450 Clarkson Avenue, Brooklyn, NY 11203, USA
e-mail: andrewchenhou@yahoo.com

S.C. Kaufman and D.R. Lazzaro (eds.), *Textbook of Ocular Trauma*,
DOI 10.1007/978-3-319-47633-9_10

scleral layer is remarkably resilient, deformable, and elastic. It does not, however, provide much protection to the retina and choroid from jarring injury and sharp penetration.

The eye is filled posteriorly with vitreous gel, a complex, thick jelly-like structure composed mostly of fluid (90%) and loosely organized collagen fibrils. The vitreous body is relatively dense (similar to the body of a clear jellyfish) until middle age, and is firmly adherent to the retina, optic nerve, and retinal blood vessels. The vitreous is ordinarily fully adherent to all regions of the retina until the fourth or fifth decade of life, when the process of separation from the retina begins to occur. The points of attachment on the retina at the time of injury are areas that act as target points for traumatic energy forces. This can result in various consequences that will be described later.

Unlike traumatic damage to the anterior segment, visualizing posterior eye injuries is not always simple and the extent of injury is far less obvious. Emergency room and acute care primary physicians are often not comfortable using the direct ophthalmoscope to examine the retina in routine patients, and even less so in patients with acute eye trauma. Therefore, it is best to approach eye trauma methodically and with great thought. In severe trauma, as patients are medically stabilized, the eye can be simultaneously stabilized and properly imaged. In less severe trauma cases, time should be spent thinking of the correct diagnosis, and managed with an urgent retinal service consultation.

Ocular trauma can present with a wide spectrum of symptoms. Depending on the region of injury, there may be severe pain, or none at all. Importantly, the retina itself has no somatic pain fibers, thus trauma and damage in this area may be totally painless. In contrast, the anterior portion of the eye is densely innervated with somatic fibers and patients with very mild injury may be in excruciating pain (e.g., corneal abrasion). When triaging patients with ocular trauma, it is important to refer to Ophthalmology, as the complexity of the trauma may be dramatic. However, there are multiple steps that can be taken to provide some relief for the patient. Upon examining the patient, if the eye is intact with relative certainty that the patient does not have an open globe, there are a variety of medications physicians can use to provide relief for patients.

There is an ocular trauma "cocktail" consisting of cycloplegic agents and steroids that can be used for patients with evidence of uveitis, or inflammation of the eye, after trauma. Traumatic insult and inflammation of the uveal tract, or uveitis causes the iris and ciliary muscles to spasm, triggering painful photosensitivity and tissue damage that can create synechiae, or adherence of the muscle to the lens capsule. Mydriatic (pupil-dilating) agents such as 1% tropicamide, 2.5% phenylephrine, and 1% cyclopentolate drops can be used to both help examine the eye and reduce the spasm of the iris and ciliary muscles (cycloplegia). This can provide some temporary relief for patients, and will also aid in examination of the posterior pole of the eye; however, pharmacologic pupil dilation should not be used prior to a neurological examination, since large, immobile, or asymmetric pupil size may signal central nervous system (CNS) damage. In addition, topical steroid drops (prednisolone acetate 1%) can reduce or prevent an inflammatory reaction from developing in the eye. Steroid drops are only relatively contraindicated if the cornea is largely abraded, especially if acute or recurrent herpetic (HSV) keratitis is considered in the differential diagnosis. HSV has a characteristic-staining pattern with fluorescein under a cobalt blue light at the slit lamp and can be evaluated if steroids are considered.

Perhaps, the most crucial step in management is placing the patient on surgical precaution as the ophthalmology team may decide on emergent surgery for the patient. Some of the simplest steps in preparing the patient on triage are vital signs, labs, IV fluids, and having the patient on *nil per os* (NPO) status. This is a logical step if surgery is a possibility and can potentially limit the extent of nausea and emesis.

Examination

The previous chapters have detailed the examination of the anterior segment of the eye. Here, we will discuss how to approach the examination of the posterior eye and retina. Vital signs, both systemic and ocular, are the most important in initial triage. Checking the three ocular vital signs of visual acuity, pupil reactivity, and ocular pressure are key in assessing the patient. In assessing the state of the retina, determining how the vision differs from the patient's baseline vision is important. The penlight exam is a simple and noninvasive test that provides some information about the neurologic function of the eye. When light is shined into the eye, unreactive pupils or dilation indicates acute or prior damage to the optic nerve, central nervous system (CNS), or severe iris sphincter damage.

Ocular Vital Sign Check

(1) Check left and right eye visual acuity independently by occluding one eye at a time.
(2) Use a penlight or other light source to examine the pupil for reactivity and symmetry.
(3) Ocular pressure: use a tonometry pen or Goldmann applanation tonometer to measure the pressure in each eye. This step should be immediately avoided if an open globe injury is suspected.

After grossly examining the eye, if no obvious penetrating trauma is noted, a detailed examination with a slit lamp bio-microscope is the next step. Slit lamp examination is crucial in looking for penetrating trauma or the presence of entry wounds. Chemosis (swelling) of the conjunctiva should be noted, as well as the presence of subconjunctival hemorrhage. Often, patients do not complain of feeling anything entering their eye, but focal conjunctival findings such as a large conjunctival laceration or iris distortion may be seen. Very small penetrating objects may provide minimal irritation acutely, but can cause severe damage long term, and should be searched for carefully on exam. For more details, see the Cornea Trauma chapter.

Continuing in a front to back systematic examination, it is important to visualize the fundus and ensure the status of the retina. For a detailed and thorough examination, dilation of the pupil is crucial. However, once dilated, the effects last for several hours and makes near vision difficult to assess unless reading glasses are utilized. Pupillary reexamination is then impossible to perform for several hours, so some care must be taken initially. Typical dilating drops administered in the setting of trauma are 1% tropicamide, 2.5% phenylephrine (4 h), and 1% cyclopentolate, which will last approximately 8 h. Atropine (1%) drops should not be used first-line for examination as its effects can last for 1–2 weeks. Therefore, detailed assessment and documentation is important for communication with other physicians when discussing the case at hand. Neurosurgical staff monitoring patients in the ICU for head trauma and changes in intracranial pressure must be made aware of pupillary dilation, as the presence of a pharmacologically dilated pupil will confound their examination.

There are two common methods ophthalmologists use to examine the fundus of the eye. Hand-held glass 78 diopter or 90 diopter lenses are used to view the posterior pole out to the mid-periphery at the slit lamp bio-microscope. Indirect ophthalmoscopy (lighting and viewing source is worn on the viewer's head) with a 20 or 28 diopter lens will help get a detailed view of the mid-periphery and far retinal periphery of the eye and the retina. However, direct ophthalmoscopy is the basic modality more commonly taught and available to primary care and emergency physicians. First, observing the red reflex provides significant information concerning the state of the posterior eye. An asymmetric or absent red reflex could indicate traumatic lens damage, the presence of retinal detachment, bleeding in the vitreous, or other forms of damage to the posterior eye. It will never, however, be a definitive test in ruling out significant posterior segment trauma.

Good visualization during the exam is key to deciding management. However, when there is a barrier to visualizing the back of the eye, it is important to identify the cause. Anterior obstructions could be due to corneal edema, or lens clouding (cataract) from trauma. The iris may be prolapsed or the pupil may be irregular and unreactive. Blunt trauma can tear blood vessels and produce a collection of blood in the anterior chamber of the eye called a hyphema. Hyphemas also can seep into the vitreous cavity, resulting in obstruction of the fundus exam. Complete filling of the anterior chamber of the eye by the hyphema, known as an "eightball hyphema" (grade IV hyphema), is especially problematic because it completely obstructs the direct visualization of the posterior segment [3].

Trauma involving the macula, the central part of the retina that houses the majority of photoreceptors (cones), may jeopardize a patient's central vision. If the peripheral retina is torn and/or detached, and the macula remains attached, urgent surgical repair of the detachment is indicated within approximately 48 h of injury. The same holds true for recent macula-off non-traumatic retinal detachments. This limits the amount of damage that invariably occurs from oxidative damage and apoptosis due to/of photoreceptors in the macula from vitreous fluid accumulation under the macula [4].

When vitreous or anterior segment bleeding has occurred, ultrasonographic examination should be performed (B-scan ultrasound of the eye) in order to better determine the state of the posterior pole [5]. Ultrasound can help determine the gross integrity of the retina (if it is detached), and relatively easily identify the presence of acoustically solid (radio-dense) intraocular foreign bodies. Acute retinal detachment or intraocular foreign bodies seen on ultrasound will require emergent surgical intervention. Ophthalmic ultrasound units are the equipment of choice but "in a pinch," a conventional abdominal/obstetrical ultrasound unit can also be used in the emergency department, especially if the staff is experienced and comfortable with their operation.

However, placing a B-scan ultrasound probe places some pressure on the globe and is relatively contraindicated by an inexperienced operator. If there is any suspicion of an open globe, realize that, pressure on the eye can cause prolapse of intraocular contents through an open wound. If structural integrity is possibly compromised in penetrating or perforating trauma, care should be taken to immediately place an eye shield for protection. The shield will prevent examiners from unnecessarily touching the eye, and patients from touching and further damaging their own eye. The goal is not to put any pressure on the eye, and therefore no patching or excessive force should be placed on the eye. This shield must rest on the orbital rim bones in order to keep the globe and soft tissue guarded from physical contact. In these scenarios, other imaging techniques such as CT can be used to study the state of the damaged eye. Anti-emetics can be used if nausea is present, as vomiting can lead to expulsion of intraocular contents in the case of larger globe ruptures.

CT imaging is highly useful in determining the presence of fractures and small intraocular foreign bodies [6]. It is a fast and highly sensitive test that is often first-line in ocular imaging. CT is also highly useful in identifying the integrity of the anterior chamber, retinal detachments, and evidence of globe rupture. However, CT has a lower sensitivity for soft-tissue injury in the orbit. Despite this limitation, CT is an excellent tool to image the orbit and the eye. MRI on the other hand, may provide greater detail for soft tissue, however it is not preferred emergently due to the time required for scanning. In addition, any possibility of metallic foreign objects in the eye is a contraindication to using MRI as it can cause secondary damage through induced movement of a metallic foreign body by the MRI's magnet. MRI is avoided if metallic objects are considered. Plain X-ray orbital (scout) films will always reveal metallic bodies and can be used to clear for orbital MRI (see Plastics Trauma chapter).

Ophthalmologists also have other imaging modalities that provide greater detail of the status of the eye and document the changes that occur over time. Color photography of the fundus can provide good two-dimensional (2-D) imaging of the back of the eye. Although this may result in loss of detail compared to the structures in a three-dimensional perspective, fundus photos are invaluable in long-term followup of gross structural changes. Newer imaging systems provide a view of the posterior pole through a non-dilated pupil, and others provide wide-field viewing through a dilated pupil. Expertise is required to assimilate this imaging data, integrate it with the clinical exam and provide treatment recommendations.

Fluorescein angiography is another tool ophthalmologists commonly use to look closely at the vasculature in the posterior pole. Done on an outpatient basis, vessel leakage or occlusions are evident and can pinpoint areas in the eye that may require treatment. Fluorescein angiography is not performed in the acute trauma setting.

One final imaging modality ophthalmologists can use is optical coherence tomography (OCT). This test allows for visualization of individual layers of the retina, the state of the macula, optic nerve head, and provides significant detail in guiding therapy and assessing the visual prognosis. Hand-held OCT devices have recently been commercialized, however, the equipment is not yet readily available to triaging physicians.

Retina

In this section, we will talk about the various forms of retinal trauma you may see in an acute care facility. We will also give an overview of the various medical and ocular conditions that may predispose people to have severe retinal damage and poor outcomes.

The thin film-like layer of the sensory retina is attached to the nourishing layer of the retinal-pigmented epithelium (RPE). In sum total, the layers are only about 400 microns thick. These thin layers can separate from one another from increased subretinal fluid, vitreous, or blood, and display retinal detachment. Once this occurs, the retina is cut off from its blood supply and source of nutrients and will quickly begin to die. There are important other effects to consider as well.

Any eye trauma necessarily disturbs the vitreous gel, which will cause pulling on the retina, to some extent. This is more problematic in younger individuals, as the vitreous gel is less likely to have already liquefied and separated from the retina, a process called syneresis (liquefaction) and Posterior Vitreous Detachment (PVD). In any person, the vitreous base always remains attached near the front of the eye (at the *ora serrata*) and pulling of the vitreous body can induce retinal tears at the posterior portion of its insertion. In younger persons, traumatic PVD often induces bleeding from the retina, optic nerve head, and sometimes the retinal blood vessels under the retina. This traumatic pulling on the retina by the vitreous body can also induce tears, holes, and subsequently induce rhegmatogenous retinal detachment (RRD).

There are preexisting conditions that make the retina more susceptible to holes, tears, and detachment. Therefore it is vital to obtain a history and determine whether patients have had prior eye trauma or a diagnosis of retinal thinning or holes. Additionally, it is important to discern whether the patient has had prior retinal detachments, prior eye surgery, or family members with a history of retinal detachment. Patients with eye complaints consistent with retinal detachment such as new floaters, flashes of light, or curtain/veil coming down on the eye should be addressed urgently. However, many patients with an initial retinal detachment are unaware of their preexisting risk factors.

The first risk factor is a condition that is extremely common, known as myopia. The eye is extremely fragile in high myopia (Fig. 10.1). Myopia is optical "nearsightedness" due to a long-shaped (elongated axial length) eyeball, causing light to focus in front of the retina and at distance, objects appear blurry. The retina is paper-thin, and anatomical stretching of the eye leads to thinning. In high myopia (greater than eight diopters) the eyeball is so long that it not only causes great blurring of vision at distance, but also stretches the contents inside the eye creating tension on the retina. Naturally, this puts the retina at high risk for detachment. Low amounts of myopia (three diopters) have a higher incidence of lattice degeneration (discussed later). Having an eyeglass or contact-lens prescription for moderate myopia of more than six diopters (−6.00D) is a major risk factor for developing retinal detachments [7]. For patients

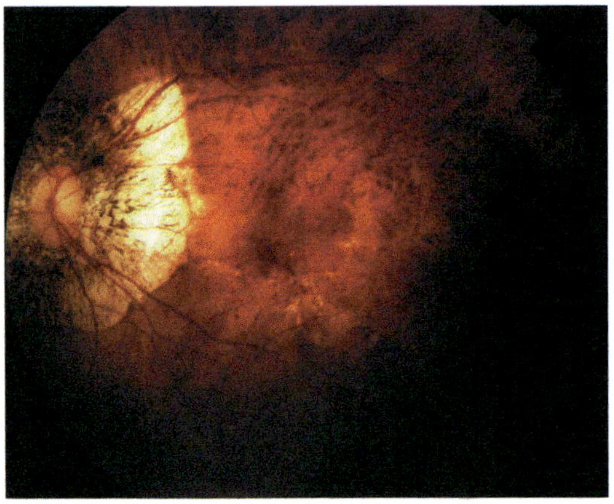

Fig. 10.1 Posterior pole of a highly myopic individual. The optic disc is somewhat tilted. There is broad peri-papillary atrophy and macular pigmentary mottling

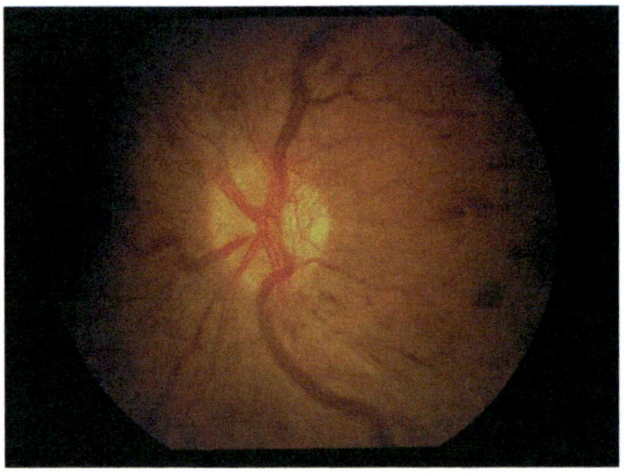

Fig. 10.2 New vessels (neovascularization) are seen to proliferate on the optic disc. These fine vessels are often missed on casual examination

with high myopia (>8 diopters) coming in with complaints of vision changes or loss, there is a high index of suspicion for retinal detachment.

Another condition that affects the integrity of the retina and predisposes the patient to retinal and vitreous cavity bleeding is diabetic retinopathy. Patients with significant or active proliferative diabetic retinopathy (PDR) (Fig. 10.2) with the aberrant and uncontrolled blood vessel growth along the posterior eye, are at high risk of bleeding with trauma as seen in Fig. 10.3a-c. Though there is no way of knowing whether a patient has PDR until you thoroughly examine the back of the eye, since the visual acuity may be very good; if there are vision complaints consistent with a retinal detachment in a diabetic patient, the physician's suspicion should be high.

Finally, lattice degeneration (Fig. 10.4) is another common condition that places people at higher risk of retinal detachment. Lattice degeneration is a common condition, takes many forms and is a disease where thinning in the peripheral retina appears to form a lattice like structure. These thin areas predispose to the development of holes, tears, and detachments after an increase in tension forces in the back of the eye [8]. However, as lattice degeneration is asymptomatic, patients presenting for trauma may not have been diagnosed with the disease. Instead, gathering a good history and performing a good eye exam will help determine the status of the retina. Many retinal detachments are due to lattice degeneration, but not all persons with lattice degeneration develop retinal detachment. In the setting of trauma, it is the trauma itself that leads to retinal detachments in areas of preexisting weakness (concept of *locus minoris lesestencia*).

So-called, "White without pressure" change (Fig. 10.5a, b) from zonal vitreous base traction on the retina predisposes to retinal tears with blunt eye trauma. This is a common phenomenon, more so in myopic eyes [9]. This condition is so-named because it appears whitened in contrast to the appearance of adjacent areas of retina. The predominant theory is that traction from the peripheral vitreous base area contributes to the appearance of the retina. These patients can be referred for outpatient monitoring with a retinal specialist. White without pressure predisposes to retinal tears in general and is more prevalent in moderate myopia and with trauma.

When examining the back of the eye, it is important to look at the vitreous space. Based on the history of the trauma, the presence of intraocular debris is an emergency and can require surgical intervention. In addition, the type of debris or foreign body will determine the severity of secondary damage inside the eye. This will be expounded upon in later sections.

The next step in evaluating posterior segment trauma should be looking for the presence of bleeding in the back of the eye. There are four major areas where bleeding can arise, each with their own distinct appearance and implications.

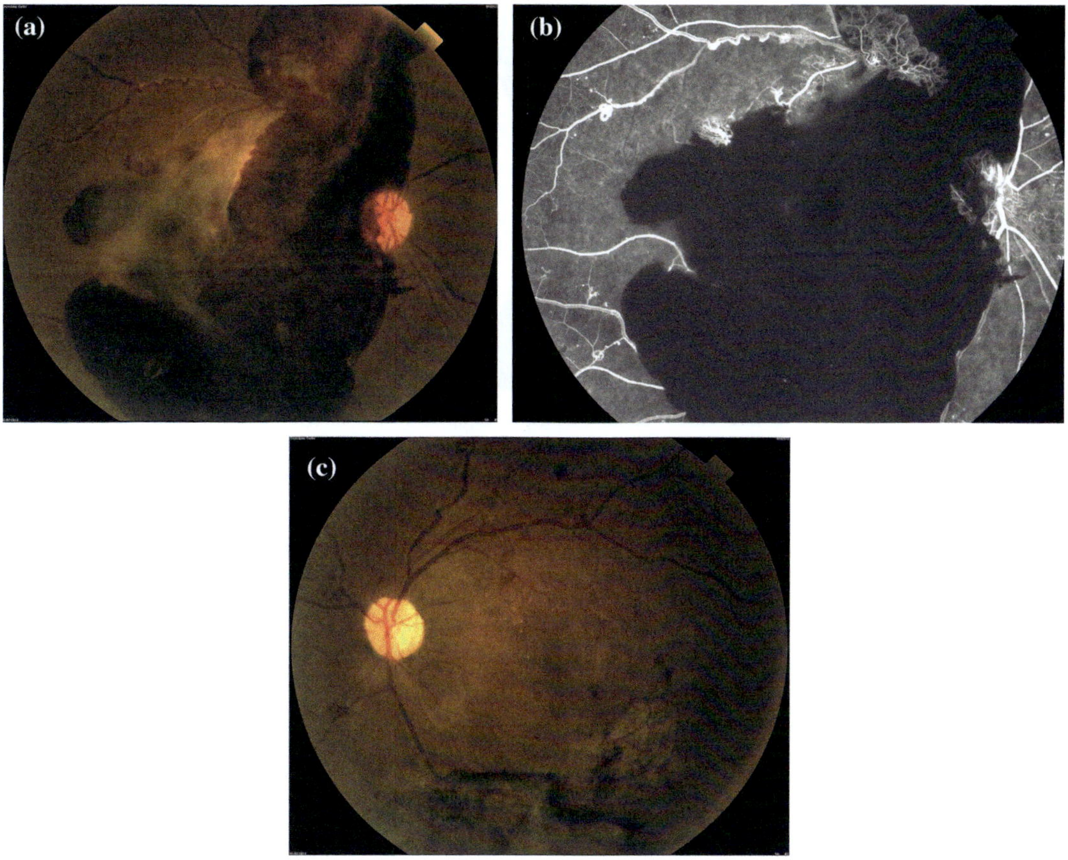

Fig. 10.3 **a** Severe diabetic retinal neovascularization has led to massive preretinal hemorrhage. The white area is an opacification of the posterior hyaloid of the vitreous. Note also the tortuosity of the retinal vasculature due to hypoxia. **b** Early fluorescein angiographic image of the fundus in (**a**). There is hypofluorescence centrally due to blockage by blood. There is hyperfluorescence superiorly due to neovascularization elsewhere (NVE). **c** The fellow eye of the patient depicted in (**a**, **b**) shows fibrovascular proliferation and sparse neovascularization of the optic disc

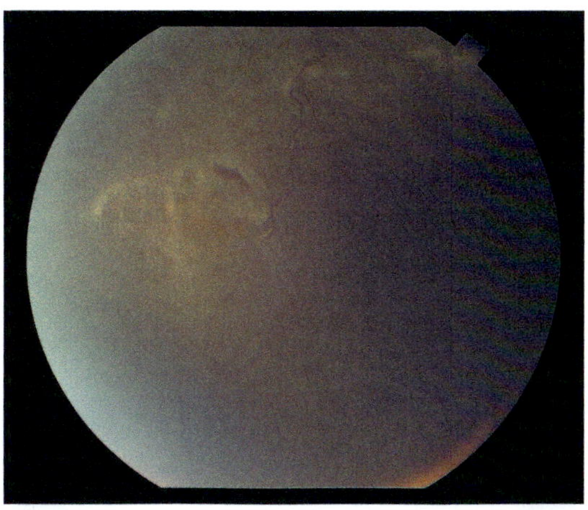

Fig. 10.4 An area of lattice is seen to the left of a slit-like retinal break. The retina is detached as a result

Though trauma does not adhere to the patterns often described in text, recognizing bleeding patterns can help with triaging patients. Small, round dot-shaped hemorrhages are usually deep within the retina, and when seen in isolation, are not commonly associated with trauma (Fig. 10.6). Flame-shaped hemorrhages are created from the damage of vessels in the superficial retinal fiber layer and are more concerning. Large hemorrhages called boat-shaped preretinal hemorrhages (Fig. 10.3a) are areas of bleeding that have not (yet) broken into the vitreous cavity. Finally, vitreous hemorrhages can be especially worrisome as the murky blood can reduce the ability to examine the state of the posterior eye as seen in Fig. 10.7a, b. A vitreous hemorrhage should be considered

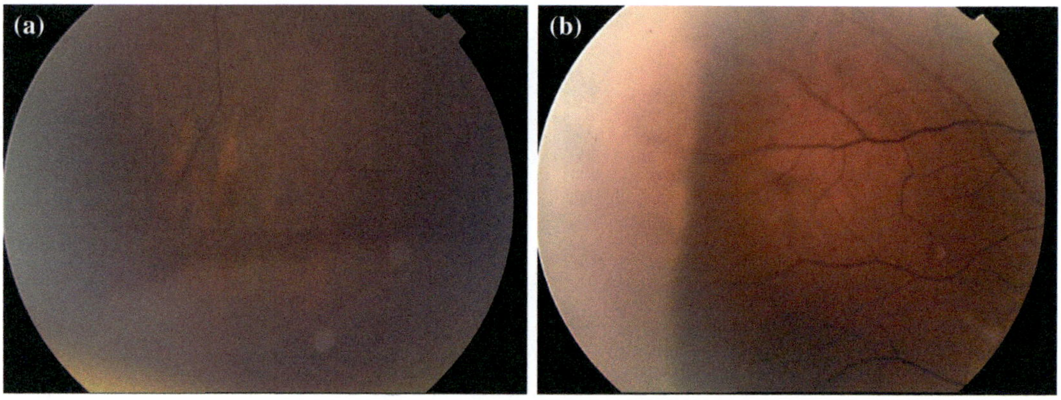

Fig. 10.5 a White without pressure vitreo-retinal change is depicted in the inferior portion of the photo. b White without pressure vitro-retinal change is depicted to the left of the photo

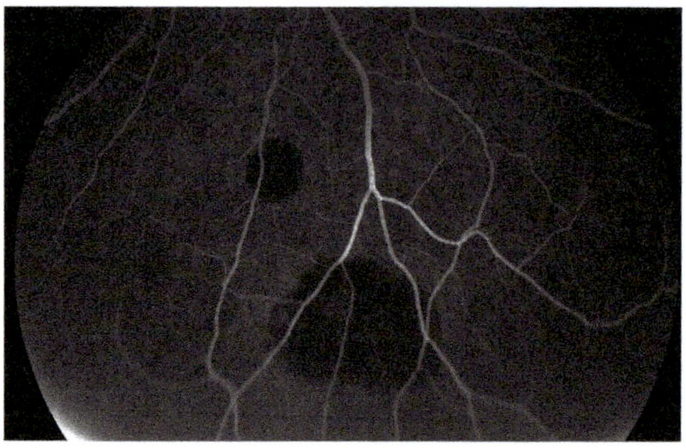

Fig. 10.6 Deep retinal hemorrhages are depicted as hypofluorescence on the angiographic image

due to a retinal tear until proven otherwise (i.e., it cannot be simply blamed on a systemic condition, such as diabetes mellitus and related retinopathy). By becoming comfortable with identifying these patterns of bleeding, the physician can get a better idea of the forces and concepts involved in the trauma and plan further examination and therapy.

On examination, the presence of new visual field loss is very worrisome concerning retinal detachment. This can sometimes be ascertained, but of course not proven with finger counting in all four visual field quadrants with the eyes tested independently. Using an Amsler grid (straight line grid) (Fig. 10.8a), if the patient states they experience distortion or curving of the lines, this could indicate problems in the macular area as depicted in Fig. 10.8b. It is important to understand the process that leads to retinal detachment.

In the posterior portion of the eye, the vitreous body is attached firmly to the retina and in the presence of traumatic tension forces, the vitreous pulls on the retina, potentially causing a hole or a tear and result in acute retinal detachments as

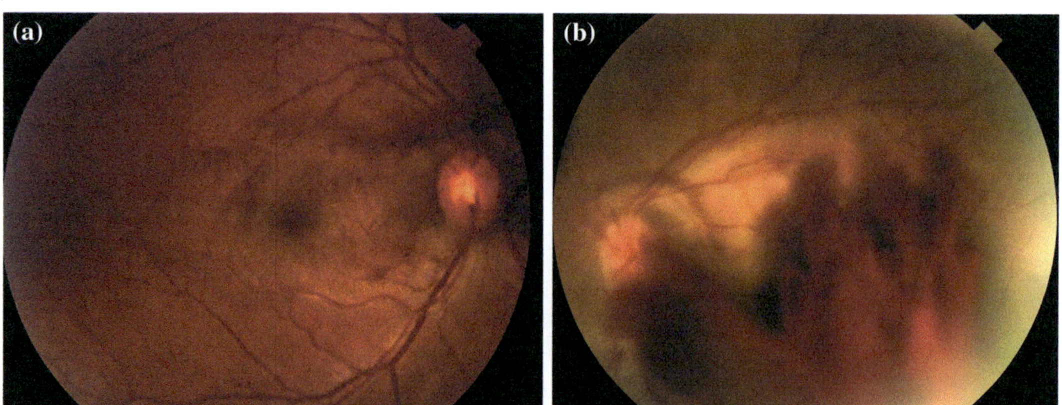

Fig. 10.7 a Mild vitreous hemorrhage and commotio retinae is shown. b Significant preretinal hemorrhage has broken into the vitreous cavity and become a vitreous hemorrhage. Severe commotio is seen as well

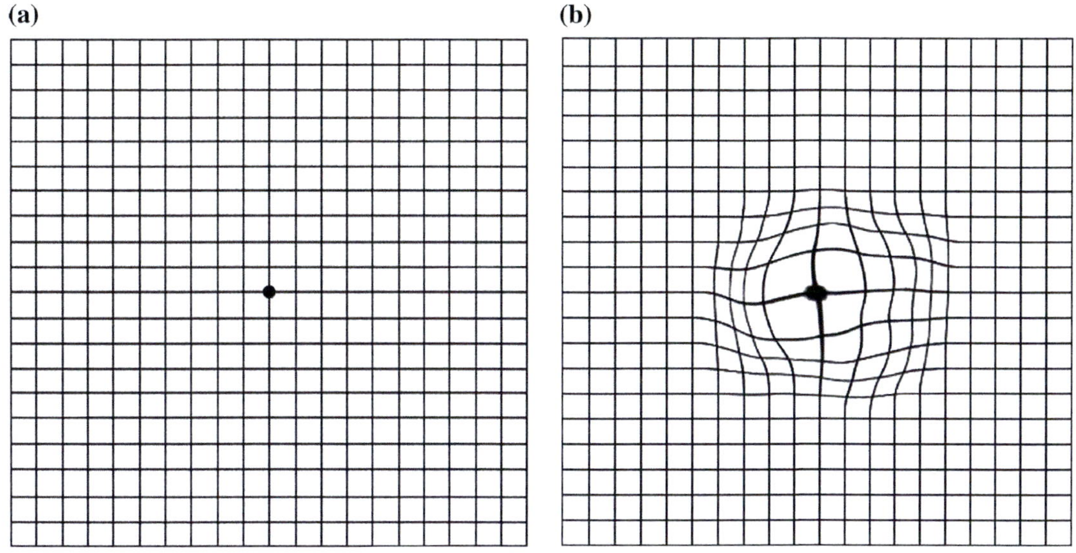

Fig. 10.8 **a** Amsler grid used for macular testing. **b** Abnormal Amsler grid test showing metamorphopsia (distortion)

seen in Figs. 10.9 and 10.10. This is called a rhegmatogenous retinal detachment (RRD). An area of focal vitreous traction causes tears. Pieces of retina can avulse and come off, leaving small round holes called operculated holes. There can also be small tears in the far periphery of the retina usually in older individuals who have previously undergone cataract surgery. However, more worrisome are flap tears or horseshoe tears, which usually lead to RRD. This is because the vitreous gel remains attached to the flap, exerts anterior-posterior traction, and lets vitreous fluid pass underneath to detach the neurosensory retina. A large flap tear with subretinal fluid and low-bullous retinal detachment is seen in Fig. 10.11. These tears are usually located in the mid-periphery of the retina at the posterior aspect of the vitreous base and will certainly be missed with direct ophthalmoscopy or at the slit lamp. Ultrasound can also help identify tears in the periphery, but only by a very experienced ultrasound operator.

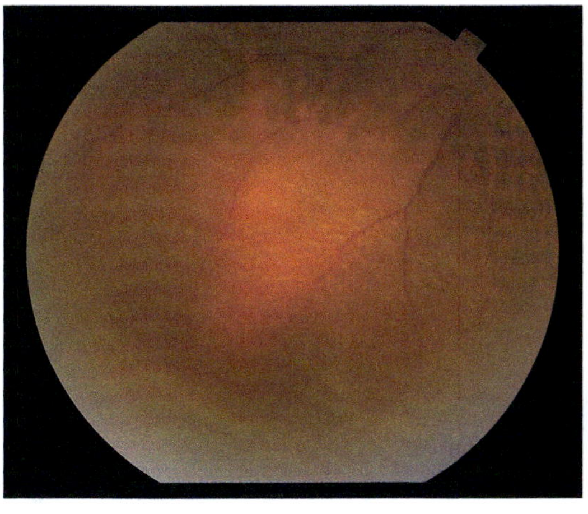

Fig. 10.9 Rhegmatogenous retinal detachment (RRD). A causative small round hole is seen to the right of the photo

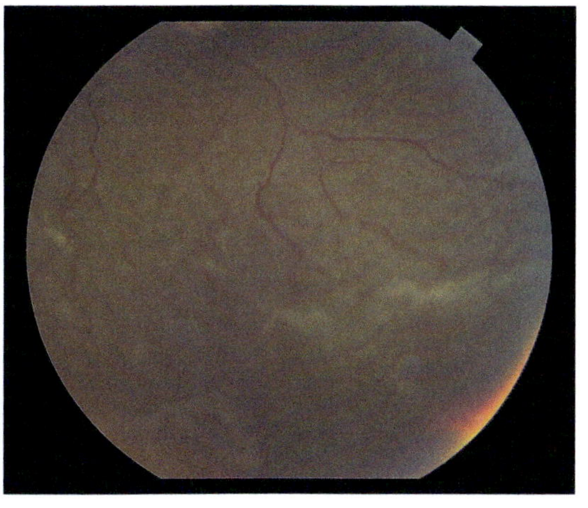

Fig. 10.10 Rhegmatogenous retinal detachment (RRD). A double-horseshoe break is seen inferiorly

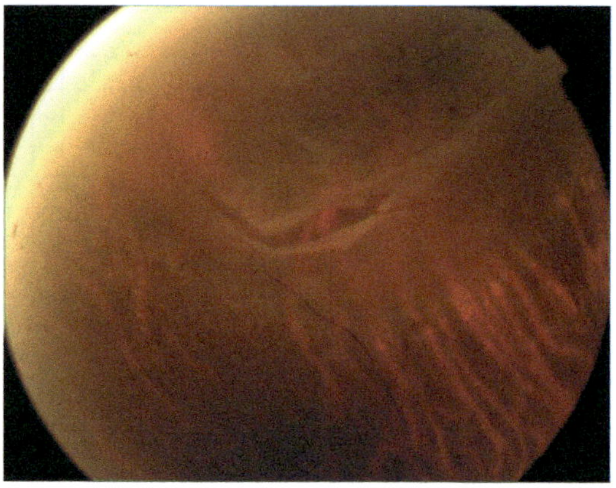

Fig. 10.11 A large horseshoe tear has caused detachment. Laser pexy hyperpigmented marks are seen below the detachment

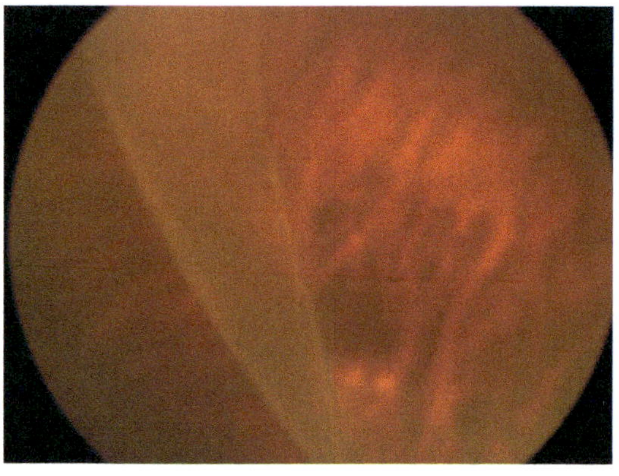

Fig. 10.12 A giant retinal tear is depicted

Giant tears are those which involve three clock hours or more (Fig. 10.12). They are particularly tricky to manage surgically, requiring pars plana vitrectomy, use of perfluorocarbon liquid, and usually primary lensectomy for successful repair.

Retinal dialyses (Fig. 10.13a, b) are radial anterior slit tears, which are usually seen to occur inferiorly. They are seen in younger individuals and are concentric to the ora serrata. They are usually managed with scleral buckling if significant detachment is associated, but sometimes are just treated with observation, laser (as seen in this case) and/ or cryotherapy if pathology is more anterior.

The management of retinal trauma can also vary dramatically depending on the state of the eye. Small retinal tears or detachments in the peripheral retina may not require a trip to the operating room. They may be treated in the eye clinic with laser or cryotherapy at the site of tears or minimal detachment to seal the area and prevent further damage. This will be discussed later.

In younger patients with traumatic detachments, scleral buckling is another commonly used technique (Fig. 10.14). By inserting a silicone band around and suturing the element(s) to the sclera, underneath Tenon's capsule and the conjunctiva, the structural outer layers of the eye are imbricated/pushed toward the retina, returning the contact of the neuro-retinal tissue with the pigment epithelium; thus restoring the gross structural integrity and allowing proper vascular perfusion.

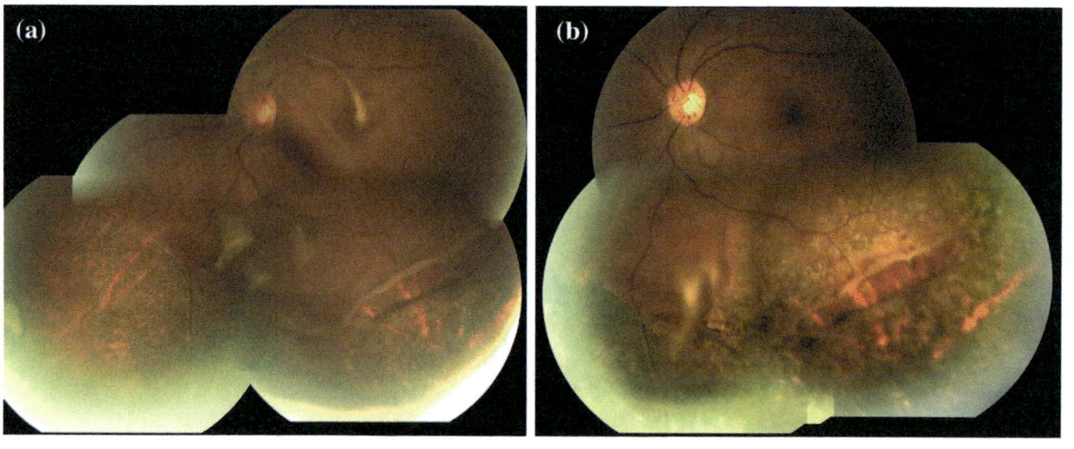

Fig. 10.13 **a** Retinal dialysis seen. There is chorioretinal scarring anteriorly connoting chronicity. Some preretinal ochre-colored opacities in the vitreous is due to prior vitreous bleeding. **b** Retinal dialysis seen in (**a**) after laser treatment has been applied posteriorly

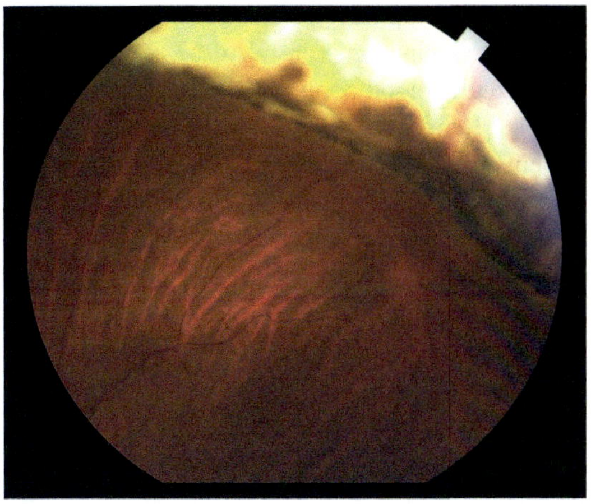

Fig. 10.14 Appearance of a scleral buckle in place. Its appearance is blurred as it is elevated in relation to the normal retina posterior to it. The buckled area has a sclopteric appearance from cryotherapy

External drainage of subretinal fluid is sometimes simultaneously performed using various means. Either cryotherapy or laser treatments at the time of scleral buckling surgery are also necessary to seal the areas of detachment, preventing recurrence. Laser treatment cannot be performed in areas of detached retina, so it is sometimes used in the acute postoperative period when the retina has reattached. Although its sealing-effect is more immediate, cryotherpy is more pro-inflammatory to the eye than is laser treatment.

More severe retinal tears or detachments may require the injection of long acting gases such as sulfur hexafluoride (SF6) or perfluoropropane (C3F8) to tamponade the retina and push the neuronal film back onto the RPE. These gases work to potentiate the efficacy of laser and cryotherapy treatments by holding the retina in place while they heal together. Gas bubbles sometimes require strict postoperative positioning to ensure proper placement and tamponade, ranging from lying forward on their face, to their side, or remaining upright for several days depending on the location of the pathology. They cannot fly in an airplane or travel to elevated altitudes for any reason with the bubble in place. At higher altitudes (lower atmospheric pressures) and the resulting pressure elevation in the eye will cause severe pain and occlusion of the central retinal artery. Patients who may be unable to properly position are poor candidates for cryotherapy/gas treatments (and pneumatic retinopexy).

Silicone oil is an alternative treatment for severe traumatic detachment or extensive inferior-retinal detachment in patients who may not tolerate gas therapy. The silicone oil acts similarly as a tamponade to push the retina in place, with a shorter time needed for rigid positioning. In contrast, gas is a better tamponade than silicone oil, due to the surface tension intrinsic to a gas. However, with oil, patients may only require one day of lying in a particular position to help with reabsorption of subretinal fluid and may move about normally thereafter. Finally, silicone oil will probably require extraction at a later time, and a secondary procedure will present with its own inherent risks, whereas gas will always reabsorb spontaneously.

Trauma frequently causes inflammation, and thus it can trigger severe fibrous proliferation and scarring in the vitreous and further secondary damage. Coincident vitreous hemorrhage, anterior segment damage, lens damage, and retinal trauma almost always sets in motion a chain of inflammatory event that will usually leads to loss of the eye. For this reason, retinal surgeons often perform pars plana vitrectomy (PPV), which removes some or most of the vitreous body from the eye. This is done in order to cut out and remove sources of tension that pull the retina. Then the surgeon can reposition the retina back onto the underlying structures. Primary PPV is now preferred to scleral buckling in most cases. Luckily, people do not require vitreous humor to see. After the vitreous humor is removed from the posterior segment of the eye, aqueous humor will proceed to fill the space. Many of the procedures mentioned earlier require postoperative time in certain positional states that may not be tolerable for an older patient.

It is important to inform the patient that any damage to the retina results in a guarded prognosis. Patients may be left with permanent visual deficits. If these deficits are in the far periphery of the eye, patients may not notice a change in their vision and will be able to cope easily. However, if the damage is near or involves the macula, the deficit in central vision can be highly disabling, and may require significant coping skills and rehabilitation to manage their impairment.

The macula has the highest density of vision sensing neurons (cones) in the eye and is situated in the central area of the retina. These neurons aggregate and form the crux of a person's central and color vision. Therefore, damage to the macula can be debilitating to a patient. As a very thin film of neurons in the back of the eye, the macula is susceptible to damage in numerous ways. Significant lasting and demonstrable anatomical and visual defects usually occur with significant trauma to the eye. The macula is highly susceptible to neuronal injury and to bleeding secondary to blunt trauma.

Foveal and macular photoreceptor and RPE damage is irreparable and even minor trauma, from a finger, a pencil, automobile airbag, paintball, soccer or tennis ball can lead to severe injury and be permanently blinding and disabling.

After injury, weakening or breaks in Bruch's membrane of the choroid layer can trigger bleeding under the macula [10]. This is known as traumatic sub-macular hemorrhage and patients will notice a severe, sudden loss of their vision. Unfortunately, this condition has a poor prognosis as the blood pooling behind the macula is toxic to the tissues due to iron in the hemoglobin. Bleeding underneath the macula can also lead to neovascularization of choroid vessels, worsening the visual acuity. The trauma to the retina and the damage to the macular area can also lead to fibrosis [11].

The fundus exam reveals a red elevation under the macular area, varying in color based on chronicity. Optical Coherence Tomography (OCT) examination can also be performed to visualize the blood pooling underneath the macular region. Retinal specialists may then decide if patients require immediate surgical intervention. Patients with sub-macular hemorrhage can be treated with a combination of vitrectomy, gas tamponade, and injections of tissue plasminogen activator (t-PA) directly into the vitreous cavity [12]. The usage of recombinant t-PA (rt-PA) has been shown to have good outcomes in clearing the sub-macular bleed and has become more accepted as a viable form of treatment. An example of this treatment effect is seen in Fig. 10.15a, b.

This subretinal hemorrhage is very important to note as the changes from the accumulation of blood beneath the retina is toxic and will kill the cone photoreceptors. However, as it is not in the central visual area, patients may not notice changes in their central vision if there is a small area of subretinal bleeding. This damage is time sensitive as well. As the clot organizes, it takes on an ochre-yellow color seen in Fig. 10.16 [13]. The treatment of acute subretinal hemorrhage is the same as sub-macular hemorrhages, but it is important to follow these patients long term.

Cracks in the tissue of Bruch's membrane that led to the bleed can cause slow degeneration of the vision, if they expand. These cracks can be spotted on examination as linear streaks in the subretinal space or as small spots of hyperpigmentation (known

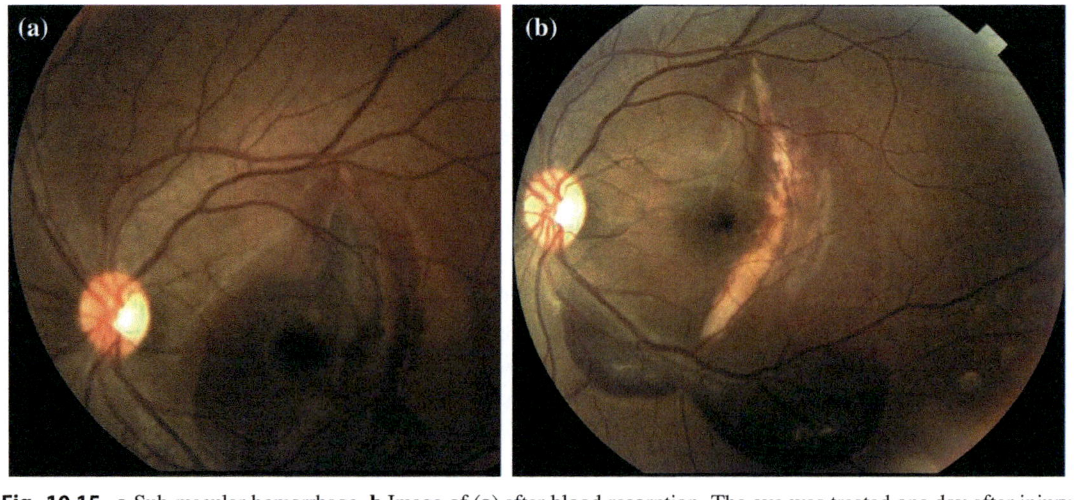

Fig. 10.15 **a** Sub-macular hemorrhage. **b** Image of (**a**) after blood resorption. The eye was treated one day after injury with intravitreal t-PA injection, PPV and SF6 gas tamponade

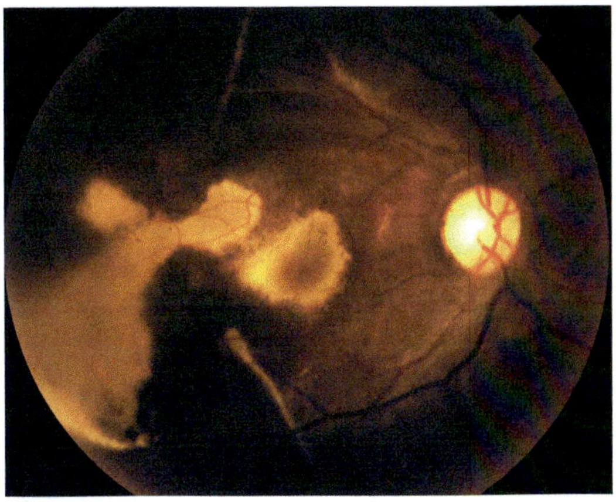

Fig. 10.16 Sub-acute sub-macular hemorrhage is seen. It has an ochre-yellow appearance

as Fuch's spots in the case of myopia) (Fig. 10.17a, b) [14]. If these signs are spotted on exam, patients tend to have a poorer prognosis. They often exhibit a degree of associated subretinal fibrosis and scarring (Fig. 10.18a, b). They commonly spawn subretinal neovascular membranes later that also can cause significant bleeding under the retina (Fig. 10.19a, b, c). Choroidal ruptures tend to be circumlinear, can be multiple and are usually concentric in relation to the optic disc (Fig. 10.20a, b).

Holes in the macula can be created secondary to trauma from acute vitreous traction, with a hole forming in the neuronal layer responsible for central vision, one can expect the patient to complain of distortion in their central vision. Less severe holes

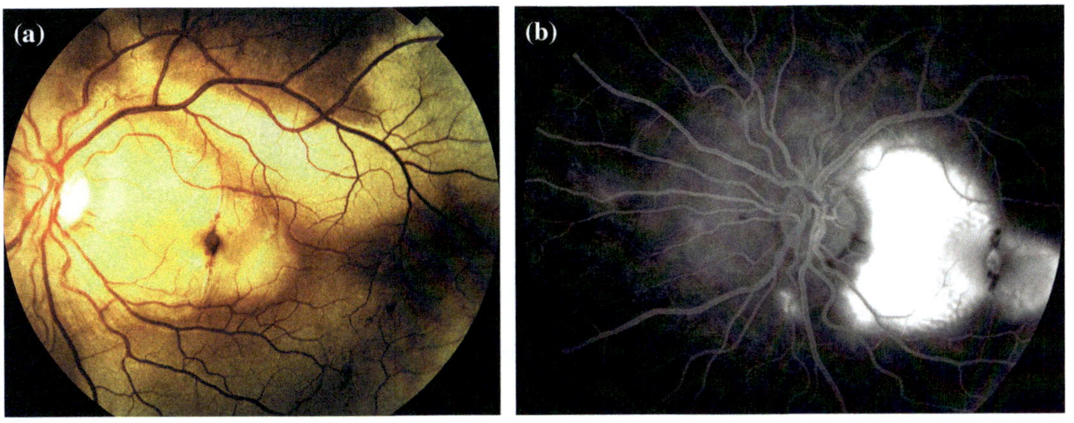

Fig. 10.17 **a** Fuch's-like spot due to trauma. It is highlighted by severe commotio and retinal edema. **b** Late-phase angiographic appearance of (**a**) showing hyperfluorescence due to extensive dye leakage and pooling due to dye extravasation from injury

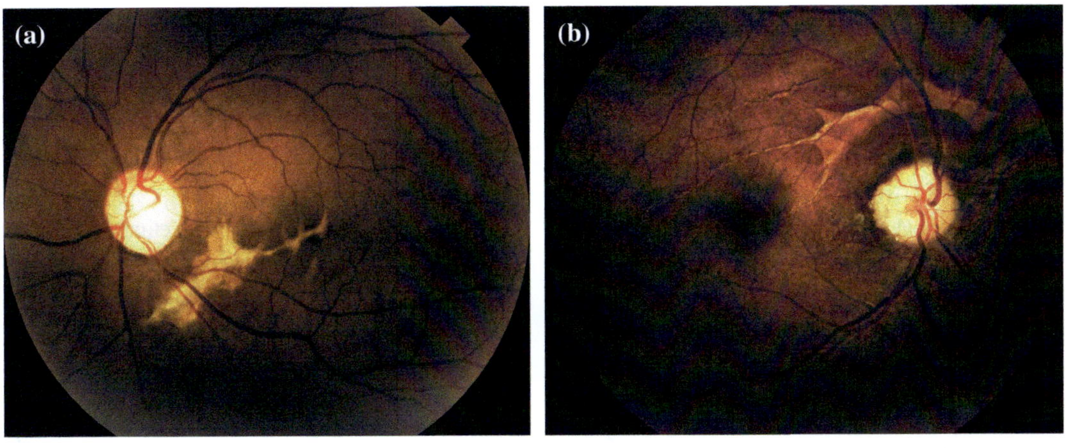

Fig. 10.18 **a** Bruchs membrane (lacquer) cracks with mild subretinal fibrosis. **b** Bruchs membrane cracks (lacquer) cracks with extensive subretinal fibrotic scarring reaction. The appearance of the optic disc is typical of buried optic disc drusen

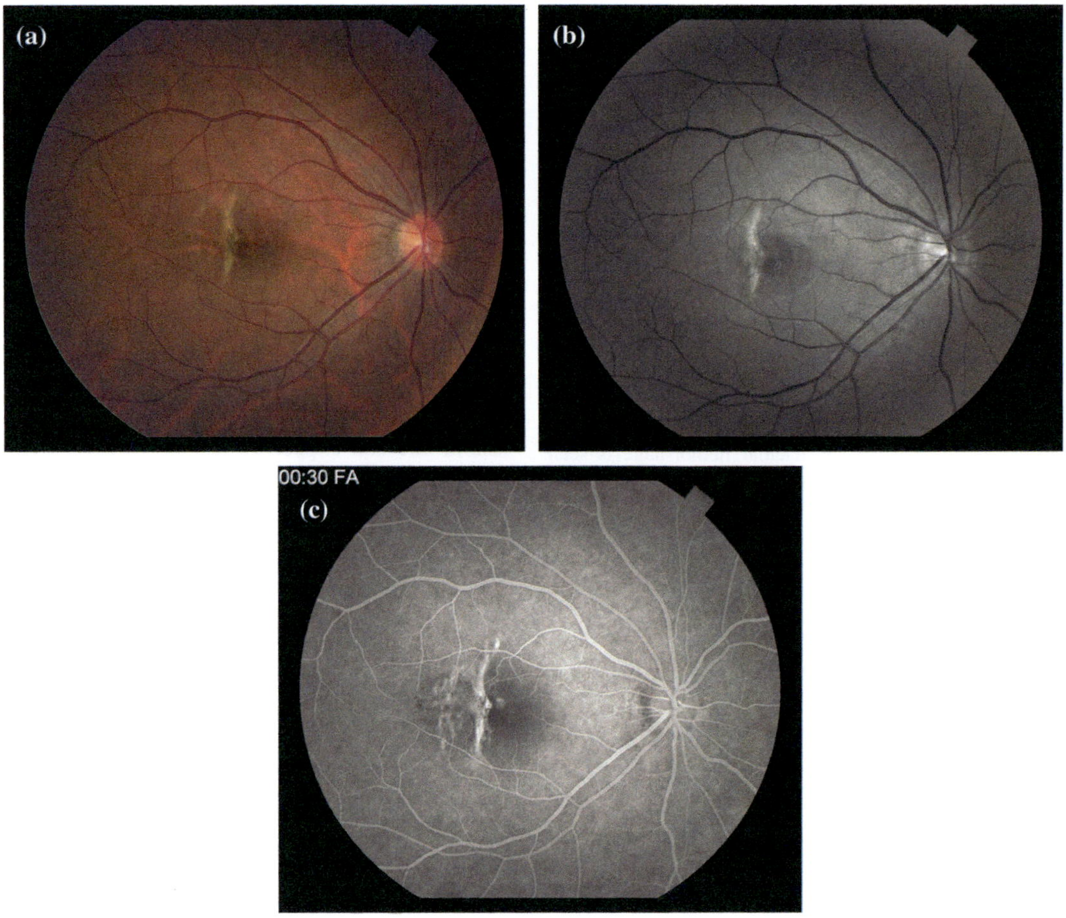

Fig. 10.19 **a** Choroidal rupture with subretinal neovascular membrane. It has been recently treated with intravitreal injection of bevacizumab (Avastin) and is now quiescent. **b** Red-free photos (left eye) of (**a**). **c** Recirculation (mid-phase) angiographic image of (**a**, **b**). There is hyperfluorescence due to window defects in the areas of the Bruchs membrane/RPE defects. Late dye leakage (not shown) or occurrence of bleeding would indicate activity of the subretinal neovascular membrane

may simply cause metamorphopsia, or distorted vision, with complaints of warped images [15]. The diagnosis of macular holes can be confirmed with a fundus exam. An older large traumatic hole in the macula is seen in Fig. 10.21. Smaller holes are harder to detect (Fig. 10.22). For physicians with access to optical coherence tomography (OCT), a near histopathologic-microscopic finding confirms the presence of the hole and the diagnosis (Fig. 10.23a, b). Fortunately, small macular holes like this, especially if the overlying vitreous (posterior hyaloid) is separated, can heal with close outpatient observation indicated. Eventually, the macula will seal and the patient's vision will often return to some extent. However, if there is no spontaneous resolution over a period of time, Retinal surgeons can proceed to surgery and perform a pars plana vitrectomy and internal-limiting membrane peeling with gas tamponade to seal the hole.

Another common type of retinal damage is caused by shockwave damage from blunt trauma to the eye, also called commotio retinae or Berlin'e edema (Fig. 10.24). Commotio (which is anatomic commotion) to the macula generally only occurs in younger individuals where a posterior hyaloid–vitreous separation-detachment (PVD) does not yet exist. Shockwaves from traumatic impact are

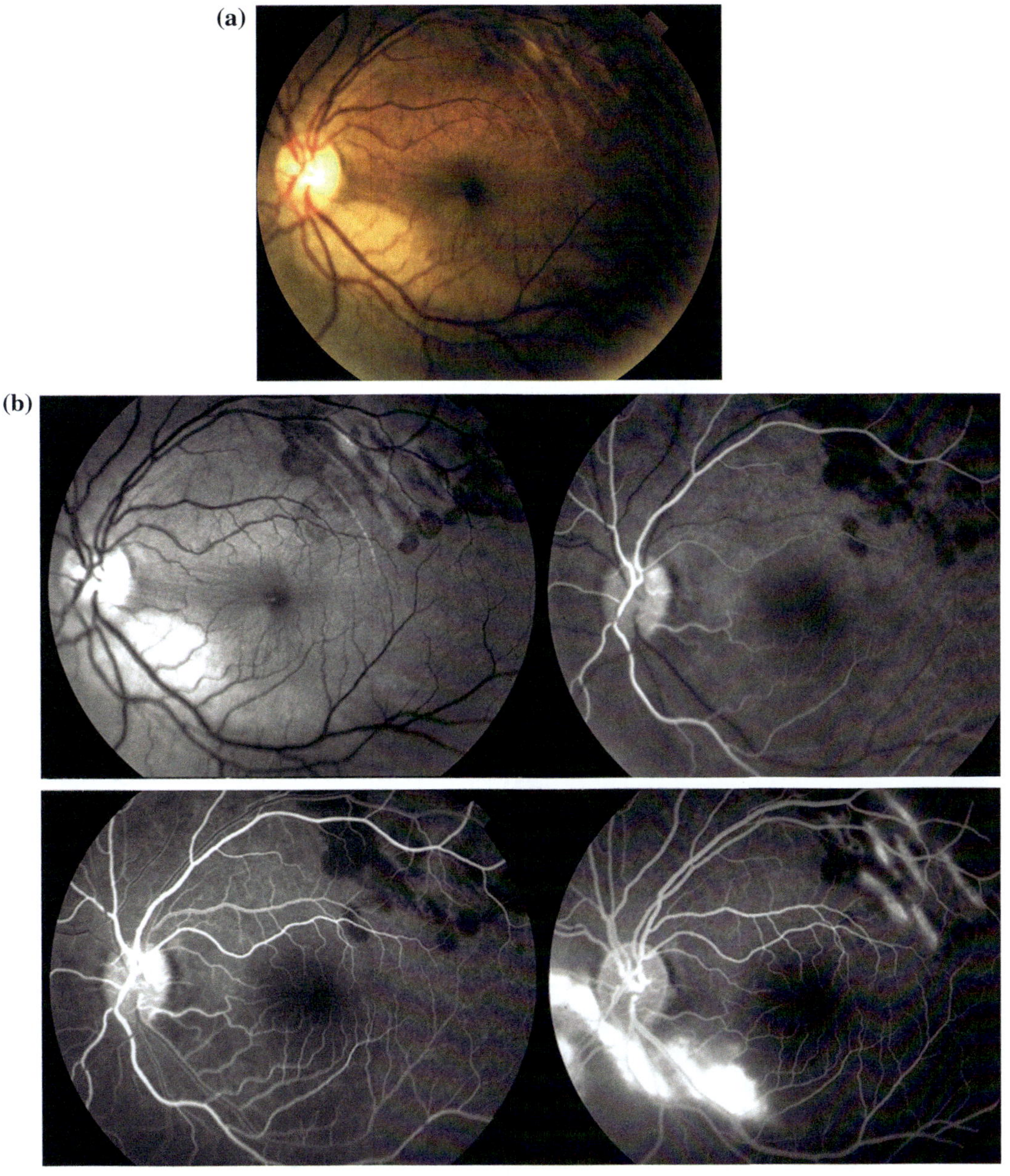

Fig. 10.20 **a** Multiple circumlinear choroidal ruptures at top right, associated deep-retinal hemorrhages, an area of retinal edema infero-temporal to the optic nerve and stellate maculopathy due to hypotony. **b** Angiographic frames of patient in (**a**). The *top left* is the red-free. *Top right* is the early arterial phase, showing hypofluorescence due to blockage of dye transmission due to blood. *Bottom left* is the laminar venous phase of the angiogram. *Bottom right* is the mid-phase of the angiogram showing hyperfluorescence due to leakage from the choroidal ruptures superiorly. Below the disc shows profuse leakage due to occult ruptures allowing dye extravasation

transmitted to the macula from the attachment of the vitreous triggering shearing of neuronal layers from the nerve fiber layer (Berlin's edema) all the way down to the photoreceptor layer of the retina [16]. Milder shockwaves may cause poor visual acuity and may only partly resolve. Commotio retina can permanently damage the macula, affecting the ellipsoid (inner-outer segment) junction of the

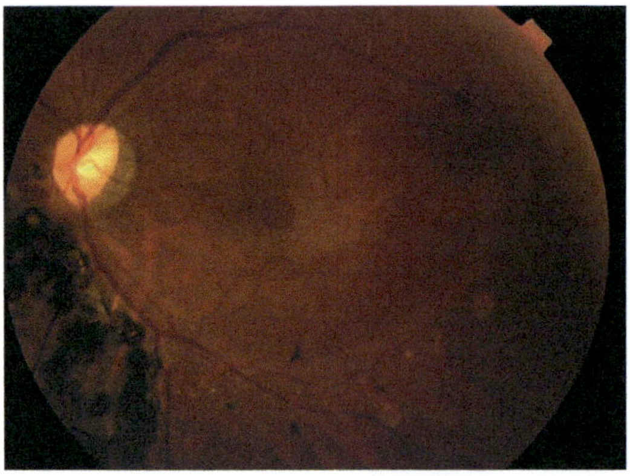

Fig. 10.21 An older traumatic full-thickness macular hole is seen. There is chorioretinal hypertrophic scarring inferior to the nerve

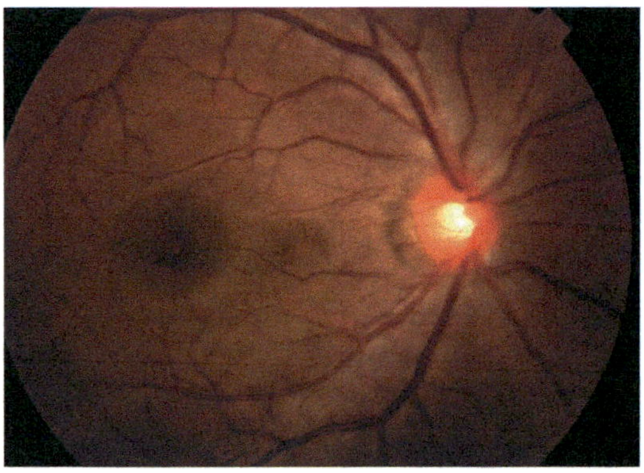

Fig. 10.22 Color fundus photo of a small, traumatic macular hole. There is peri-papillary atrophy and mild tilting of the optic disc due to moderate myopia

photoreceptors and also the underlying pigmented epithelium (Fig. 10.25a, b). More severe late macular (outer retinal) damage is shown in Fig. 10.26. In this latter instance, with no good treatment options, visual outcomes are quite poor. Ophthalmologists use OCT to look at the state of the layers of the retina and guide followup. Fortunately however, many patients with commotio will recover with time. Monitoring changes to the macular ellipsoid junctional zone and signs of atrophy/RPE hyperpigmentation can help physicians determine the prognosis.

Vitreous

Before detailing the various types of vitreous damage that can occur, it is important to understand a fundamental concept of blunt injury to the eye. The eye is a globular structure encased in layers of tissues, each possessing a unique function. At the core of the eye, the vitreous jelly retains the shape and structure. However, these tissues are non-compressible liquids and thus will not deform and disperse energy when under impact. As the eye is situated in a closed and confined space, there is little leeway for impact energy to be absorbed by surrounding orbital fat or soft tissues. This becomes very important, as

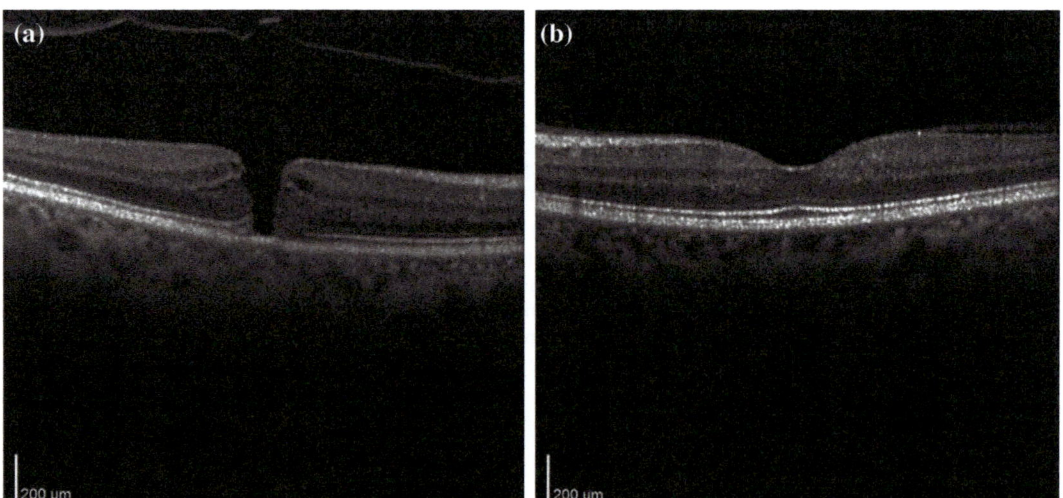

Fig. 10.23 **a**, **b** OCT image of the new full-thickness, small macular hole in the right eye. The normal fellow eye is shown next to it for reference

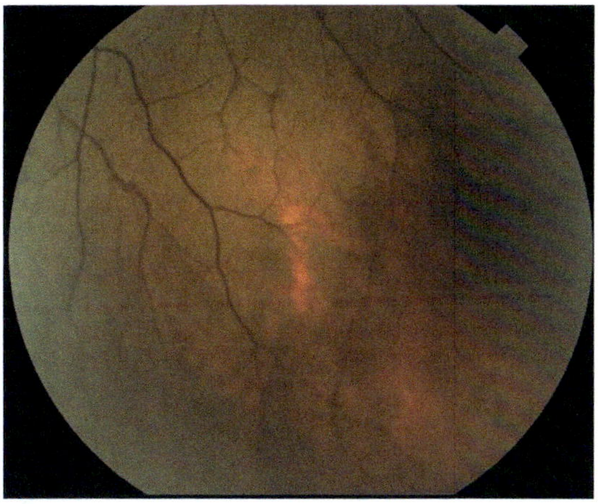

Fig. 10.24 Mild mid-peripheral retinal whitening indicative of comotio retina (Berlin's edema). See also Figs. 10.7 and 10.8. This will resolve without visual sequela, leaving mild pigment alterations

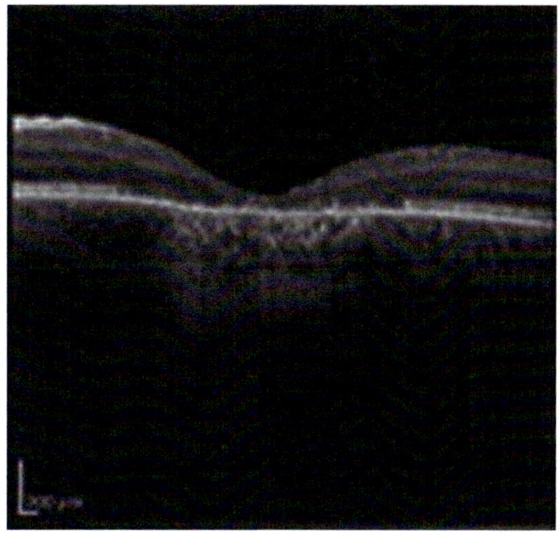

Fig. 10.26 Severe outer retinal damage and RPE hypertrophic scarring seen on OCT. This patient was felt to have also suffered a traumatic macular hole which self-sealed. Vision is only CF

blunt force trauma will create damage through three mechanisms.

With blunt impact to the eye, there can be coup injuries, contre-coup injuries, and compressive injuries. Coup injuries are due to the direct impact of the injury to the eye. This more commonly affects the anterior segment of the eye as the structures are in direct contact on impact. Contre-coup injuries are due to the shockwave forces in the posterior segment as the eye stops short after impact. These injuries spread through the posterior pole and can result in tears, bleeds, holes, fracture in nearby structures, and commotio [17]. Finally, compressive injuries occur due to the deformation of the eye as it adjusts to the forces of

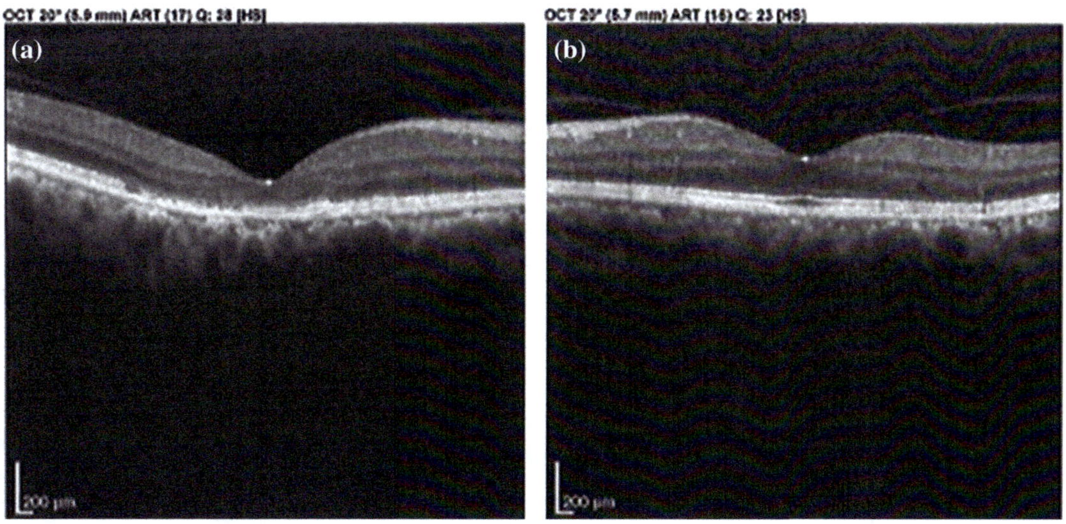

Fig. 10.25 Late OCT image after severe macular commotio. There is disruption of the ellipsoid (IS-OS) layer and the outer nuclear layer. The vision is 20/40 in the damaged eye, with significant metamorphopsia. At right is the normal fellow eye for reference

impact. Like bouncing a rubber ball on the ground, the eye will compress and deform to an elliptical shape, then rebound and overcorrect. This will repeat and cycle until the entirety of the impact energy has dispersed. Unfortunately, this means the eye may suffer significant damage during the entire process. The damage from compressive injury can affect every tissue in the eye, from the lids and ocular surface, to the muscles, soft tissue, and blood vessels of the eye. In this chapter, the various effects of blunt injury on the posterior segment will be discussed in detail in the corresponding tissue sections.

The vitreous body is in the core of the eye, providing structural support with its thick gel composition. This gel is called vitreous humor and is strongly attached to the surrounding retina. As people age, this gel begins to liquefy and creates pockets with decreased structural support. This is called syneresis and can start from an early age. Liquefied pockets in the vitreous can often cause the perception of floaters in the eye and is a benign condition. However, in the elderly, this vitreous liquefaction can result in detachment of the vitreous from the retina. In traumatic situations, tension forces on the vitreous can cause pulling and result in damage to the thin film of the retina. Pockets of liquefied vitreous can pull away and increase the risk of developing traumatic vitreous detachment with resulting hemorrhage.

Vitreous hemorrhage occurs when the blood vessels in the posterior eye rupture, often from the shearing forces of blunt trauma. These mechanical forces damage the vessels or capillaries in the retina, and the blood spreads into the vitreous gel. As with all bleeding, the likelihood of occurrence increases with more severe trauma. Injuries severe enough to penetrate the eye will also likely have bleeding in the vitreous space. With injuries causing vitreous hemorrhages, patients can present with a constellation of symptoms.

Patients with only vitreous hemorrhage and no anterior eye injuries will typically present with painless vision loss. As the posterior eye does not possess somatic pain fibers, the complaint of painless visual deficits should trigger the worry that there is damage anywhere from the posterior eye to the visual cortex in the brain. Severe unilateral vision loss usually emanates from an ocular cause. Vitreous hemorrhage is associated with a variety of visual changes. Patients may see floaters, cobwebs, shadows, or a red hue in their visual field. Patients who are not initially bothered by these symptoms can have worsening of the symptoms overnight and wake the next morning with severe vision loss. As the patient lays supine, the blood tends to settle within the visual axis where light focuses on the retina, blocking a person's vision. Therefore if the diagnosis of vitreous hemorrhage is made early, it is important to emphasize sleeping with the head elevated at least 30°, or even sleep sitting upright overnight. Due to the influence of gravity, this will allow pooling of blood toward the bottom of the eye, outside the visual axis. This will also allow for more efficacious followup examination by a retinal specialist.

In order to make the diagnosis of vitreous bleeding/hemorrhage, a fundus exam will reveal the presence of blood but will not connote implications or guide appropriate management. When examining the vitreous body, intravitreal-structures may impair the view. One common cause is asteroid hyalosis, caused by degenerative opacities that reflect light and look like asteroids in the night sky on exam seen in Fig. 10.27a, b. Old vitreous hemorrhage gives a similar appearance, called synchesis scintillans. This makes examining the fundus difficult and requires skill to look beyond the vitreous deposits and examine the underlying fundus (Fig. 10.28). However, the direct fundus exam does not include the peripheral retina and indirect ophthalmoscopy will be needed to detect peripheral tears. B-scan ultrasound of the eye can help supplement the initial exam. In contrast, if the patient has severe trauma with an open globe, the examination methods mentioned previously can probably be foregone in favor of an orbital and globe CT scan. Depending on the findings, patients can be managed outpatient, or require urgent surgical consultation.

For patients with severe injuries resulting in open globes, they should be placed on surgical protocol and ophthalmology should be urgently consulted for possible urgent surgical interventions. In patients with structurally intact globes and blood obscuring the view of the retina, a

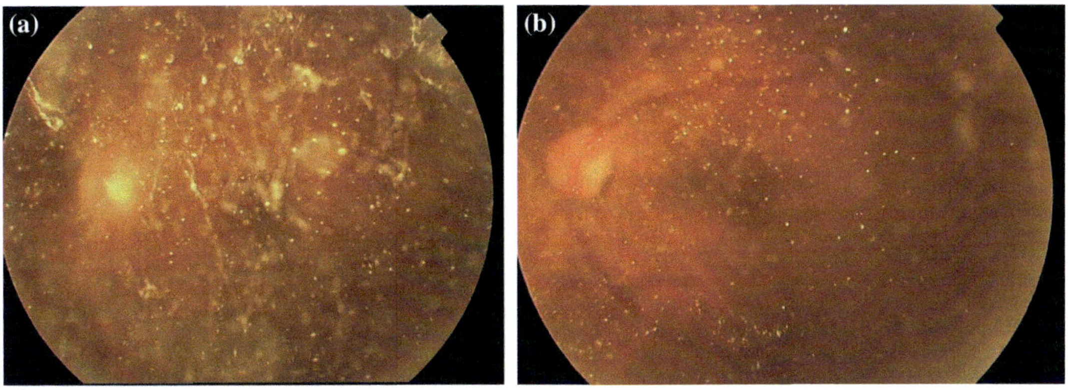

Fig. 10.27 **a** Asteroid hyalosis in the vitreous is depicted. **b** Asteroid hyalosis

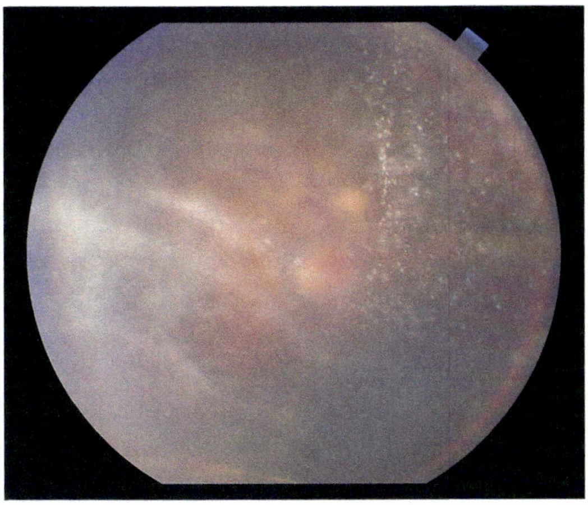

Fig. 10.28 Synchesis scintillans in the vitreous due to old vitreous hemorrhage

B-scan ultrasound may be used to help rule out retinal detachment and allow for timely (<24 h) referral to retinal specialists for evaluation. Patients with less severe vitreous bleeding and visible tears in the retina should be referred for urgent consultation for possible retinal surgery. Finally, patients with small vitreous bleeding and good retinal visibility in all 360° on scleral depressed examination with the absence of tears can be comfortably sent to retinal specialists for outpatient management.

With trauma to the eye, patients can occasionally develop **vitritis**, which is an inflammatory reaction in the vitreous body severe enough to cause uveo-scleral transudation or swelling. In this scenario, the inflammatory cells and proteins migrate into the vitreous and condense, decreasing translucency. The vitreous becomes hazy and triggers blurred vision or spotty vision in the areas of inflammatory protein aggregates. Inflammation in the eye can cause blood vessel dilation and a red eye with photophobia. Patients with these symptoms may have multiple underlying conditions, and therefore require examination of their fundus. Any more than a trace amount cells in the vitreous is an emergency, as it may represent acute infection [18]. On exam, there may be clumps or debris in the vitreous that are mobile. In addition, the anterior eye exam may reveal the presence of hypopyon. This would increase the suspicion of post-traumatic endophthalmitis

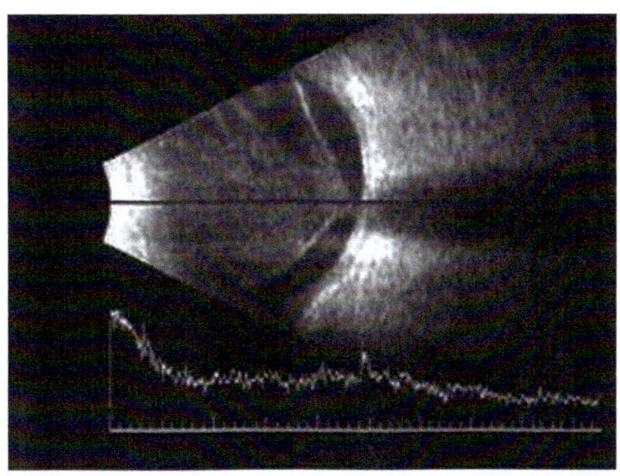

Fig. 10.29 B-scan ultrasound image of traumatic endophthalmitis with dense vitreous opacification and also retinal detachment. The retina remains attached at the optic disc in retinal detachments

(Fig. 10.29) and is an ocular emergency (see also Endophthalmitis Sect. 10.9.

There are a few other concerning traumatic conditions associated with the vitreous humor. However, they can be difficult to diagnose on exam. Both of these conditions require the ability to perform a scleral depressed fundus exam, which is much more difficult than the regular fundus exam. In addition, in order to perform a scleral depressed exam, there must be complete certainty that the globe is structurally intact. Otherwise, there is a risk that intraocular tissue will prolapse out with pressure. If there is certainty the globe is intact and the examiner is adept at performing the scleral depressed exam, it is important to examine the deep peripheral retina in all patients with ocular trauma. This type of definitive exam cannot be easily performed soon after trauma due to patient discomfort, but certainly must be repeated on subsequent examinations.

One rare traumatic condition is retinal/vitreous base dialysis (Fig. 10.30). The anterior edge of the tear occurs at the ora serrata, the junction of the peripheral retina with the ciliary body; the posterior edge of the tear occurs at the vitreous base [18]. As this region is located anteriorly and behind the iris, these tears can be easily missed. These tears can sometimes, but not always cause retinal detachments. Patients with retinal dialysis need evaluation by a retinal specialist though surgery is not always necessary. Isolated retinal dialyses with subretinal fluid are usually subtotal detachments and are usually treated best with cryotherapy and scleral buckling.

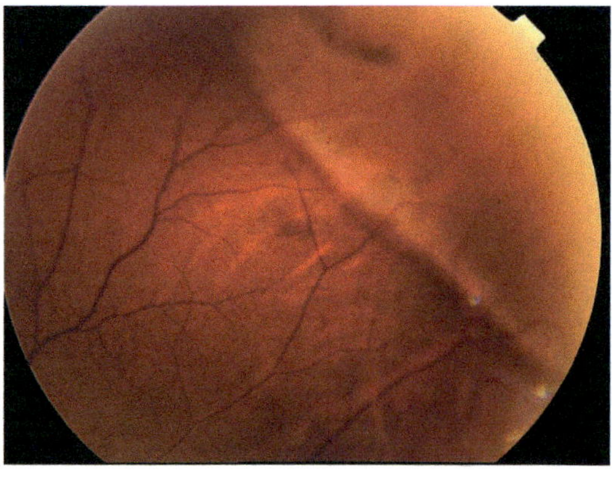

Fig. 10.30 A relatively posterior vitreous base dialysis is seen

Choroid

The choroid layer of the eye is the main vascular component in the eye as a whole and to the posterior pole. The vessels are the main source of nutrients and oxygen to the retina, and thus damage will impact retinal integrity and vision.

Direct trauma to the eye or low pressure within it (hypotony) can cause serous choroidal effusions and or bleeding into the supra-choroidal space and under the retina. They are generally termed "choroidals" or "choroidal detachments." They are believed to be caused by a transudation of serous fluid into the potential space or to tearing of the choroidal vessels. Depending upon the nature of the fluid collection, the appearance can differ from light in color (imparted by the overlying retina) and density to quite dark and dense. It can have an intermediate appearance if it has both components within the "choroidal." The B-scan ultrasound and radiographic image appearances will differ as expected along this fluid-blood spectrum based on their respective densities. The choroidals are usually multiple and concentric/ symmetrical (2–8 based on physical and anatomic geometry), limited to the periphery, concentric, and parallel to the ora serrata and dome-shaped. If they are large, they bow forward and can block vision and the view to the posterior pole. If they are very large, they can nearly touch each other or even meet in the mid-vitreous cavity from 180 degrees-apart locations. If they appear to touch, they are termed "kissing choroidals" (Fig. 10.31). Vision in this case is necessarily no better than HM or LP. Non-urgent surgical drainage by a retinal surgeon is usually indicated in this situation as direct contact in a previously non-vitrectomized eye can lead to retinal tears when the choroidals recede. In the event that the choroidals are caused by hypotony, they may recur after surgical drainage. A coincident choroidal rupture may allow choroidal blood to leak into the neurosensory retina which imparts a poor visual prognosis due to cellular oxidative damage from blood. On the

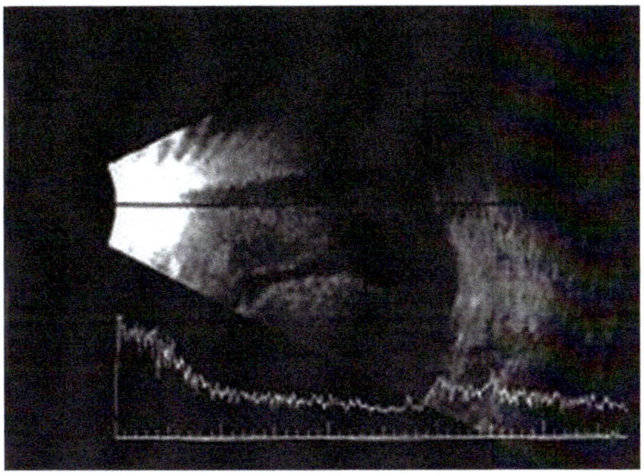

Fig. 10.31 B-scan image of large serous-hemorrhagic choroidals. They are nearly "Kissing"

bright side, large choroidals exert a "buckling effect" on the retina, and retinal detachment does not generally coexist except in cases of globe and retinal penetration.

Choroidal rupture (previously discussed) is caused by deformation after severe blunt injury. In blunt trauma, the surrounding sclera's collagen structure can compress and stretch. This finding is uncommon outside of the posterior pole.

Ciliary Body

The ciliary body is the anterior aspect of the choroid vascular layer. The ciliary body is the demarcation line that separates the anterior and posterior segments of the eye. It contains blood vessels, but also connective tissue and muscles that allow the lens to change shape. It is also the source of the aqueous humor that fills the anterior eye. Therefore, trauma to this structure can cause severe sequelae.

An important consequence is the cyclodialysis cleft, when the ciliary body separates from the underlying sclera. Patients usually present following blunt trauma with pain and photophobia. With significant disruptions in the ciliary body, there are usually notable deformities in the shape of the iris. There will usually be significant hypotony from disturbance of the uveo-scleral outflow (enhanced outflow by the cyclodialysis cleft) [19]. The cleft can spontaneously close later on, or as a result of surgical procedures, which will lead to very high intraocular pressure.

Anterior globe perforation will lead to an irregular pupil and is a helpful sign if present in the setting of high velocity injuries. Patients can develop corectopia, a displaced or abnormally shaped pupil. In other scenarios, the iris can be deformed causing more than one pupil to be present in the eye, called pseudopolycoria. In severe cases, the cyclodialysis can cause excess drainage of the aqueous humor called hypotony. This can cause retino-choroidal folds (Fig. 10.32).

Patients with less severe presentations of ciliary body rupture require more skill to diagnose. In mild cases of ciliary body rupture, patients can develop recession of the angle of the eye. This can contribute to late secondary glaucoma. The diagnosis can be made with a gonioscopy lens to observe the drainage network of the eye. However, this requires specialized training and is not easily performed, nor is it of upmost importance early on. Instead, imaging with ultrasound biomicroscopy (UBM) can be used for definitive diagnosis. UBM uses high frequency sound waves to create high resolution imaging of the ciliary body and anterior chamber [20]. It is by far the best tool to look for ruptures of the ciliary body and is more sensitive than gonioscopy. However, UBM is a very specialized tool and not usually available in the emergency hospital setting.

For management, patients can be treated with cycloplegic drops and topical steroids to decrease their pain and photophobia. Patients should also

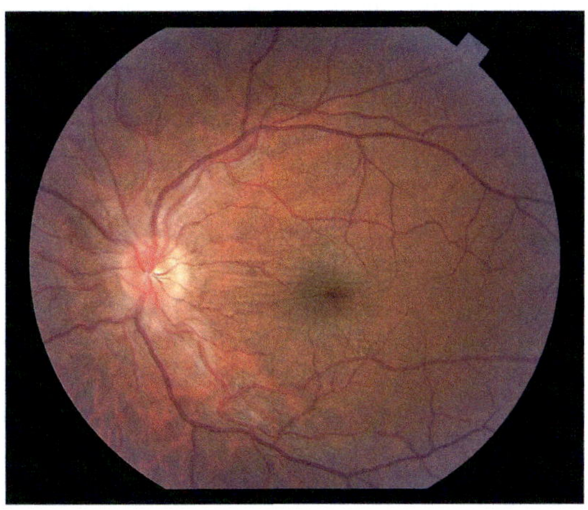

Fig. 10.32 Retino-choroidal folds are seen in an eye with hypotony

be placed on surgical protocol in the event they require more urgent intervention. Depending on the severity of their injury, they may be able to be monitored as an outpatient with retinal specialists as the eye heals. However, patients with an evident cyclodialysis sometimes require surgical closure and close followup to prevent secondary complications from the trauma.

Sclera

The sclera is the strong connective tissue casing that makes up the white of the eye. Therefore it can withstand a degree of punishment from blunt trauma. However, the sclera will tear or break with substantial trauma to the eye.

The most common trauma that can occur to the sclera is a laceration. Patients will typically present with eye pain and photophobia. Most will have significant conjunctival chemosis. Chemosis is the presence of swelling or edema of the conjunctiva. In most cases of scleral rupture, patients will have changes in pupil due to prolapse of intraocular contents at the laceration site with resultant pulling on the uvea.

Patients with suspected scleral lacerations should be examined under the slit lamp to look for the site of injury. However, patients should receive an immediate non-contrast CT of the orbits to identify areas with small lacerations to rule out the possibility of intraocular foreign bodies. Posterior ruptures are not always visible at the slit lamp, but do present with hypotony and corneal folds. These can be self-sealing, but are devastating injuries with a very poor prognosis for globe salvage. In addition, ophthalmologists can perform Seidel testing, using fluorescein strips on the wound at the slit lamp to identify fluid leaks from areas of scleral laceration. Leaking will signal that the globe is open and requires immediate repair. However, non-leaking lacerations require ruling out the possibility of prolapsed tissue sealing the wound as well. These injuries will also require urgent repair in the operating room.

When this type of injury is suspected, and especially if patients have been diagnosed with scleral lacerations on exam, immediate topical antibiotic therapy is imperative. Patients should be started on hourly topical broad-spectrum antibiotics with topical third- or fourth-generation fluoroquinolones like ciprofloxacin or moxifloxacin (Vigamox). Importantly, patients should also be given a dose of IV antibiotics (also third- or fourth-generation fluoroquinolones). PO versions may also be used with a sip of water, but this is not preferable. The presence of intraocular content extrusion shifts the severity from urgent to hyper-emergent. However, all patients should be placed on surgical protocol and started on anti-emetics. In addition, these patients' damaged eyes should be shielded for protection until ophthalmology can assess the stability of the eye and the need for the surgical intervention. Scleral lacerations are time sensitive and a delay in closure will impact the prognosis and final visual acuity [21]. Simple corneal lacerations, involving only the anterior segment, can usually be repaired by the general ophthalmologist. The retina begins approximately 5 mm posterior to the anatomic limbus, so lacerations and perforation posterior to this point will necessarily involve the retina (Figs. 10.33 and 10.34). Unfortunately, patients with lacerations involving the posterior part of the eye have a poorer prognoses and repair can be highly challenging and difficult. These very posterior lacerations may self-seal due to uveal and retinal tissue incarceration but it is important to inform the patient that the prognosis for useful vision in cases of this sort is very, very poor. Globe salvage is the intended benefit of surgery in these instances, with primary enucleation or evisceration often a reasonable and considered alternative especially with NLP vision (see Plastics Trauma chapter).

Patients with high-energy trauma can develop injuries severe enough to rupture the sclera. The transfer of energy into the eye through blunt injury can trigger full-thickness wounds of the eye wall. These patients will present with severe pain and should immediately be evaluated to rule out possible scleral ruptures. Patients should also receive urgent CT studies of the head to rule out intra-orbital, intracranial, or intraocular foreign bodies and evidence of penetrating trauma. Patients with confirmed scleral ruptures should not have any manipulation of their eye due to

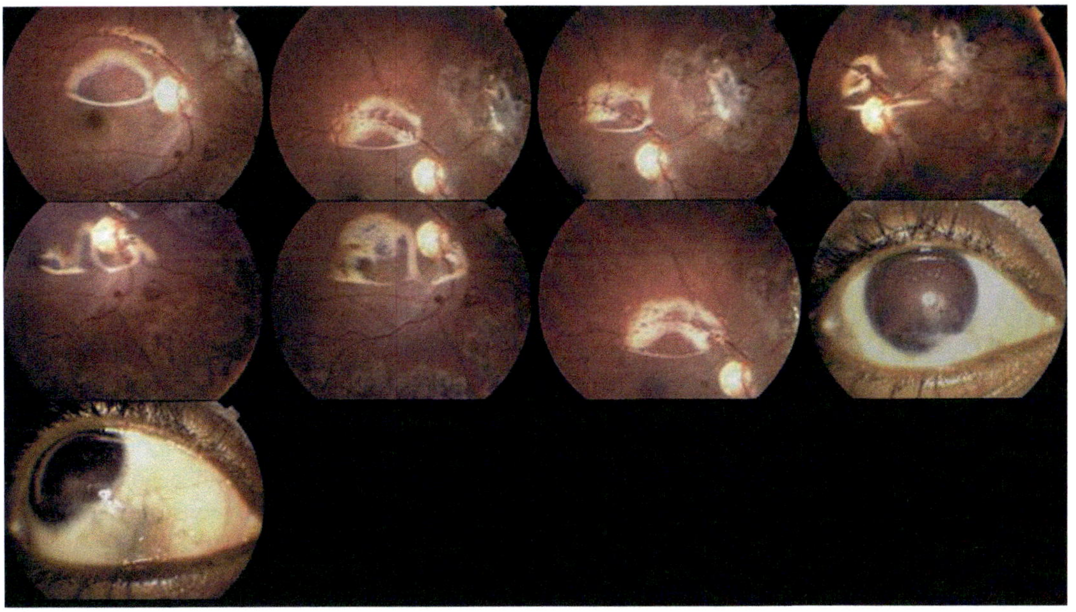

Fig. 10.33 Series of images of a right eye which sustained rupture with loss of some uvea. Cornea and scleral lacerations were closed primarily. Several days later, cataract extraction, PPV and retinal detachment repair were performed with endolaser and silicone oil injection (seen above)

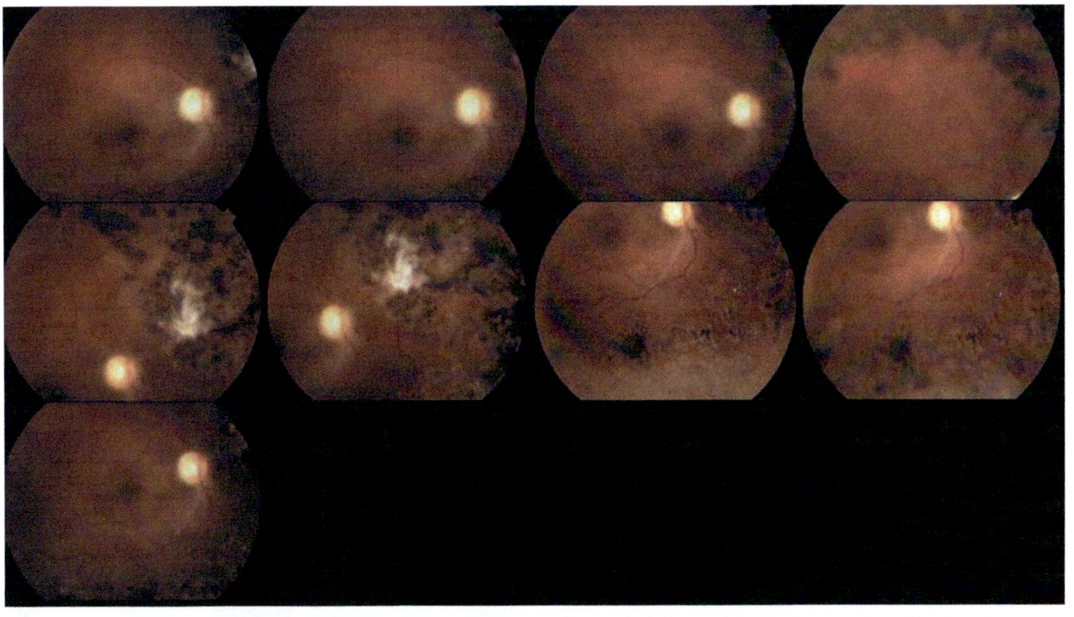

Fig. 10.34 Patient shown in 10.33 approximately ten years after the event. Silicone oil was removed 6 months after the trauma and she was left aphakic. The vision is 20/80 with contact-lens correction, which is an excellent outcome in a case of this sort

risk of further ocular content extrusion. Even gentle manipulation such as opening of the eyelids can create enough pressure to extrude ocular contents. These patients should immediately have eye shields placed and consulted for surgery. Patients should then be placed on surgical protocol, and kept relaxed in bed. In addition, Valsalva situations should be avoided and patients should be started on anti-emetics if they are nauseous or vomiting. The increased pressure of vomiting can place severe stress on the open wound and cause further prolapse and loss of important intraocular tissues. These injuries are incredibly serious and immediate intervention is the best possible option for saving the patient's eye.

Posterior Segment Foreign Body

When differentiating types of intraocular eye injuries, terminology becomes important. Injuries on the surface of the eye or the structural wall can be open or closed. Closed globe injuries mean that the wound did not extend to the full thickness of the eye wall. Open globe injuries refer to impacts that create an open wound exposing the inside of the eye to the outside environment. This differs from ruptured globe injuries, which is due to blunt force traumas. The impact from blunt force can sever the weakest structural link in the eye at the moment of impact and create an open wound. Finally, penetrating eye injuries refer to objects that have forced themselves into the eye. These injuries are usually sharp objects that were able to embed into the eye. This differs from perforating eye injuries wherein objects enter and exit the eye in one strike. These objects had enough force to penetrate the eye, continue on the ballistic path, and then exit the eye wall [22]. Properly describing the injuries can help multispecialty teams determine the further workup needed and how to properly coordinate the appropriate interventions for the patient.

Higher energy impact or a very sharp edge is necessary for foreign bodies to enter the posterior segment during trauma. This is commonly seen in war with combat, blast injuries. In the current era, the battles fought in the Middle East have increased the incidence of these injuries, as the use of improvised explosive devices have increased the incidence of blast injuries. In the civilian environment, foreign body penetration is typically associated with work related injuries often with the use of power tools [23]. In these scenarios with high-risk stray projectiles, the lack of eye protection is the major risk factor in developing intraocular foreign body injuries. Therefore, history becomes a crucial component in determining the extent, severity and outcomes in patients with foreign body injuries.

Patients who present with a possible ocular foreign body may have a very wide spectrum of presenting symptoms including absolutely none. On the contrary, they may have severe pain, photophobia, and severe vision loss acutely. However, with time, the symptoms may progress and the secondary complications from having a foreign body in the eye will sometimes rapidly develop. The mechanism of injury will be very important (i.e., use of power tools or a "weed-wacker" with no eye protection). Therefore, immediate evaluation with radiographic imaging is prudent to look for foreign bodies (Fig. 10.35). Slit lamp and fundus exams can also confirm the presence of a retained foreign body as seen in Fig. 10.36a, b. Patients who appear to have intact eyes on slit lamp can undergo a B-scan ultrasound of the eye.

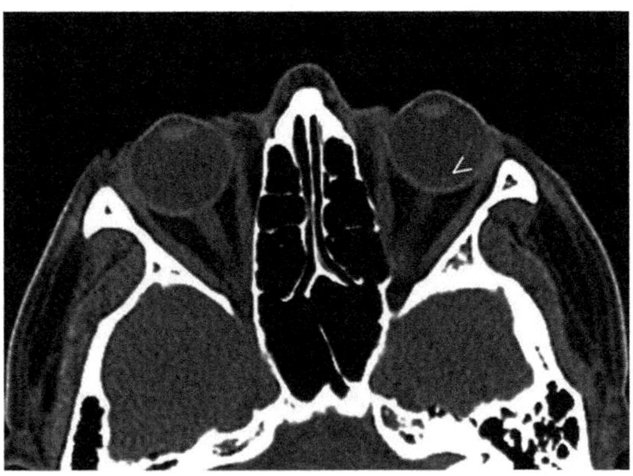

Fig. 10.35 CT scan of the globe and orbits showing area suspicious for globe rupture and retained intraocular foreign body in the left eye

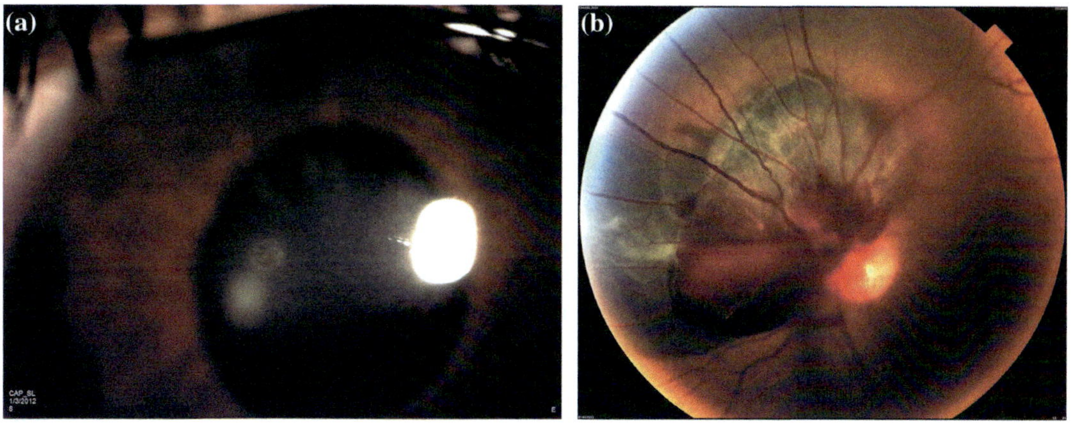

Fig. 10.36 **a** Slit lamp photo depicting corneal injury from foreign body penetration. **b** Fundus exam shows preretinal, subretinal and mild vitreous hemorrhaging due to foreign body penetration of the retina

However, any uncertainty for possible perforation or those with evidence of damage on or near the eye should get a CT of the orbits and globe. OCT examination can also confirm foreign bodies (Fig. 10.37) but it is not a first-line tool in diagnosis.

There is no greater potential danger than foreign bodies in the eye. Acutely, the injury caused by a foreign body is limited to the penetration into the eye and the tissues damaged. The initial symptoms of pain and vision changes depend on the damaged structures of the eye. Later, as the foreign body stays in the eye, there can be direct infectious or toxic risks to the eye tissues. Infectious organisms, or severe inflammation that develops can be very injurious [24]. Identifying the three main factors that influence the outcome may be important in management. These factors

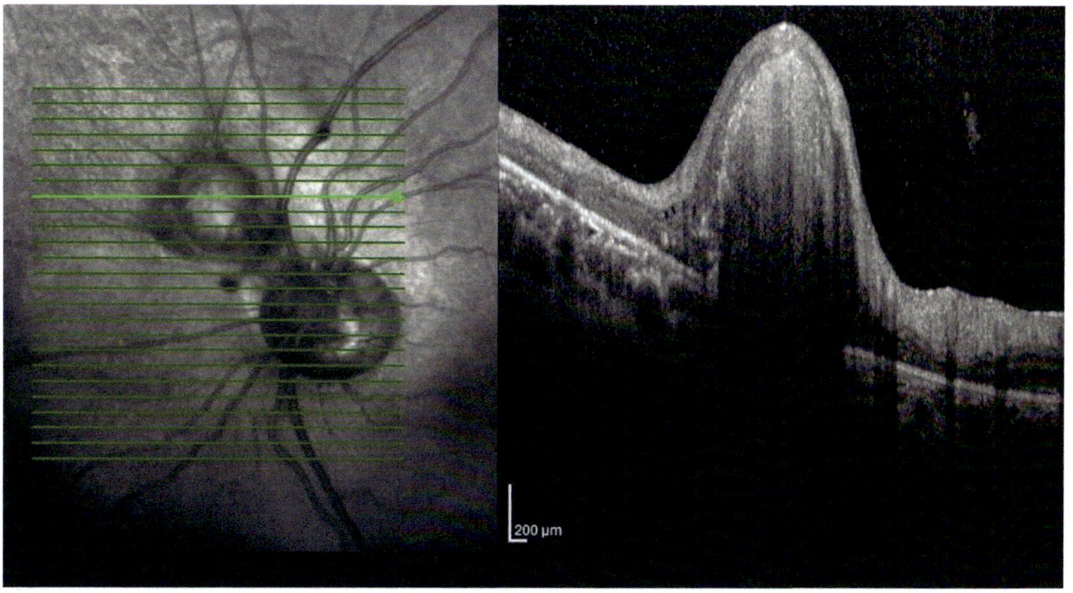

Fig. 10.37 OCT image through the area of the retained foreign body. History was presumptive for a fiberglass shard as the mechanism of injury

are the size, shape, velocity of projectile, and type of material of the foreign body.

Size is an important variable in intraocular foreign bodies. Larger sizes can be more easily identified yet will pose more damage in the path of injury due to the mass of the ballistic object. However, smaller sizes can be very dangerous due to the risk of missed diagnosis. Smaller foreign bodies may present with less acute damage, and thus history and exam is vital in finding the microscopic debris. As the length of time of the intraocular foreign body increases, the inflammation that develops will cause secondary damage to the eye, depending on the material, and make extraction more difficult [25].

Shape is a second important variable that is distinguished through the surface and structure of the foreign body. Smooth and more uniform-shaped structures have more linear and predictable ballistic paths. Irregular objects are less predictable in their motion and trajectories and may ricochet once in the eye. These objects have increased likelihoods of causing tissue tearing in addition to the initial penetrating injury. In addition, sharper objects can cause additional injury cutting tissue as the eye moves. Easily accessible items that can contribute to penetrating injuries range from knives, chisels, and glass materials in the workplace environment. Items such as pencils, thorns, or darts are common objects that can penetrate the eye and should be considered when obtaining the history [26]. Pressure placed on the eye after injury can deform and distort the eye triggering further damage and should be avoided.

Ball bearing (BB) guns have been popular in American culture for over a century. This means that BB-related eye injuries have also plagued children and young adults for equally long. The dangers of BBs lie in two main factors. They are often marketed as toys and thus are not as strictly regulated as are standard firearms [27]. However, these pellets can fire at speeds between 150 to 1000 feet per second. As approximately 250 feet per second is the threshold limit to penetrate the eye, many guns on the market should rather be labeled as weapons. However, once inside the eye, BBs present their own difficulties for retinal surgeons. Intraocular BBs are toxic to the eye as they are usually steel balls coated in a copper shell. (Copper toxicity will be discussed in a later section.) These small pellets, usually 4.5 mm in diameter, are difficult to remove via forceps [28]. In addition, as copper is not a strong magnetic metal, using magnetic tools do not aid in extraction either. This inability to obtain a firm grasp on the BB during extraction increases the risk of secondary damage from the surgical removal. Therefore, the best option is prevention by the use of protective eyewear and not using BB guns in the vicinity of other people.

The velocity of impact has a vital impact on whether the foreign body penetrates the eye. On average, objects need to reach a speed of 246 feet per second or 75 meters per second in order to penetrate the human eye [29]. At this speed, shape will play less of a role as the kinetic energy exceeds what the eye can endure. Therefore, suspicion of high velocity injuries in the home or workplace should be evaluated closely. Mechanized sanding or cutting tools used during woodwork, masonry, or plumbing may send off high velocity particulate matter, which may easily penetrate the eye. Hammering anything without adequate eye protection can also lead to eye penetration with foreign bodies. Counter intuitively, lower velocity foreign may cause more tissue damage because they drag tissue with them as they move through the eye; unlike high velocity foreign bodies that penetrate tissue more cleanly, but deeper.

Some metallic foreign bodies can remain in the eye for very long periods of time without inducing toxicity or inflammation (Fig. 10.38). Others lead to devastating organo-toxic or metallotoxic retinal injury and severe vision loss in short order (Fig. 10.39a–i). Electoretinography (ERG) can be performed at baseline during the recovery period and then serially examined for evidence of retinal toxicity. ERG however is not widely available as it rarely utilized, and requires both a skilled operator and expensive equipment. The electrical amplitudes of the ERG tracing will become reduced and ultimately extinguished with metallic toxicity such as with iron toxicity (siderosis).

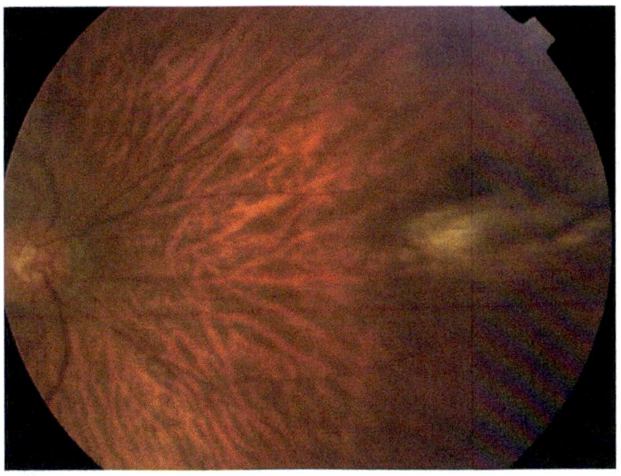

Fig. 10.38 This photo depicts a retained metallic intraocular foreign body in the nasal fundus that had occurred from injury in 1968. The vision is 20/25

Another form of damage from penetrating trauma is called sclopeteria (Fig. 10.40). Sclopetaria's root meaning is derived from old English and refers to a "claw," which can be seen on fundus exam [30]. This trauma differs, as it is not damage caused directly to the eye. Sclopetaria is secondary damage caused by objects that impact near the eye without penetrating the eye. The shockwave energy that transmits to the eye from the projectile causes the chorioretinal layer to rupture leaving the sclera exposed and visible. This can result in severe tears in the retina and vision loss in small areas with shallow retinal damage. The multiple forms of bleeding that occur in the retina and vitreous triggers fibrosis. Cryotherapy closely mimics the appearance (Fig. 10.14).

Again, diagnosis is confirmed with the acute appearance of the fundus showing claw-like tears and holes with white areas of sclera underneath. This shockwave damage presents problems with healing and interventions and is thus managed with outpatient observation. Luckily, the scarring of the tissue will often seal the retinal breaks and the risk of retinal detachment later on is very low [31]. Unfortunately for these patients, the final visual acuity will depend on the severity and location of the original injury.

Finally, the material composition of the foreign body presents an important factor in its management. The composition of the item that entered the eye and the object's sterility will all affect the severity of the damage [25]. Materials which are super-heated (from physical friction), such as during grinding of metals, may in fact be sterile due to heat treatment of the object immediately prior to entry into the eye or surrounding tissue. There are other objects with inert chemical properties such as plastics and glassware that do not trigger reactions in the eye or induce inflammation. It is due to this property that ophthalmologists are able to implant plastic and silicone lenses in the eye. There are other inert objects such as stone, sand, and other minerals that are also usually well tolerated. Infection may still occur from inoculation of flora from the ocular surface. Sometimes, these objects are harmless and increased damage can occur from the extraction itself. If the objects are not posing any risk to the integrity of the eye and not impeding vision, vitreo-retinal surgeons may recommend having the object remain in the eye with close monitoring.

However, this is not true for other organic vegetative materials. One commonly encountered injurious item such as wood is very dangerous to the eye. The cellular composition of wood products and plant materials often results in severe inflammatory reactions in the eye and can result in endophthalmitis. Live wood and vegetative material frequently harbor bacteria and/or fungal elements that can sequester within the eye allowing subsequent infection. These foreign bodies will need immediate attention and intervention. Identifying these wood and vegetative products may be highly difficult as they can be easily missed on radiographic imaging [31]. Wood products can range highly in density depending on the type of wood and the processing of the product. The variability in the density of the wood can mimic air bubbles, fat, or muscle in the eye [32]. Retention of vegetative or wood materials in the eye usually will result in loss of the eye.

Finally, metals that have oxidizing properties are at high risk of toxicity to the eye. Iron materials will oxidize in the eye and deposit into the cells of eye. This process is known as siderosis and can trigger many sequelae. Iron can

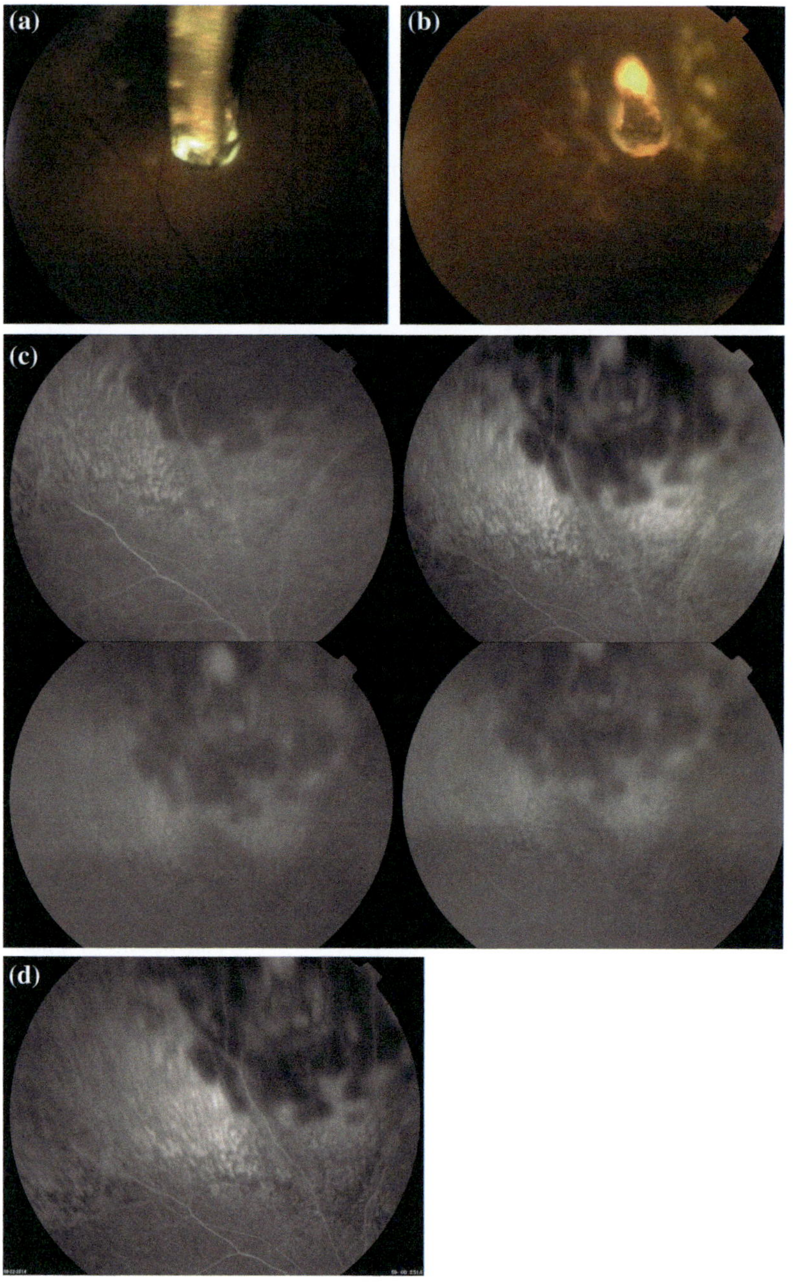

Fig. 10.39 This series of photos depicts a man who suffered a penetrating injury with a granite-like foreign body (**a**). He had initial primary closure (corneal repair), and then cataract extraction 7 days later (**b**–**d**). He refused PPV at that time for removal of embedded retinal IOFB, opting for observation instead. Three weeks later, he developed an APD. I month post-injury Macular OCT is shown 8/8/14–mild vitritis was then noted. SRF worsened 3 days later (**e**–**f**). Since retinal toxicity was detected, he opted for PPV and removal of IOFB. The retinal degeneration persisted despite complete IOFB removal (5 weeks post-injury)(SRF gone). 2 and 3 weeks after PPV, retinal appearance worsened (**g**–**i**). Vision is HM only

Fig. 10.39 (continued)

(e)

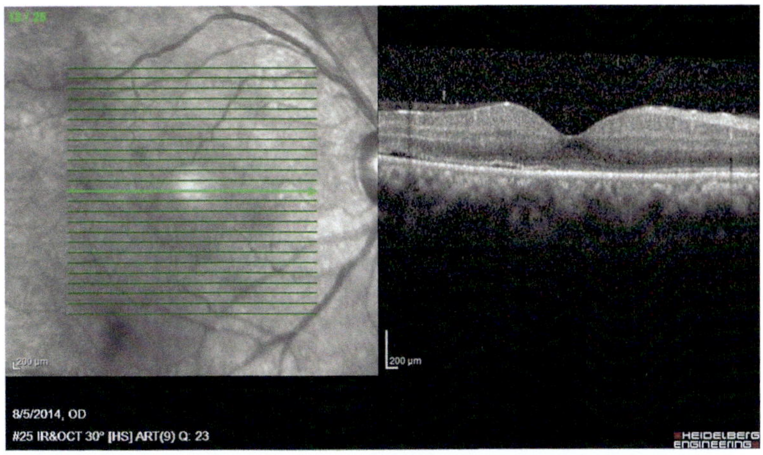

(f)

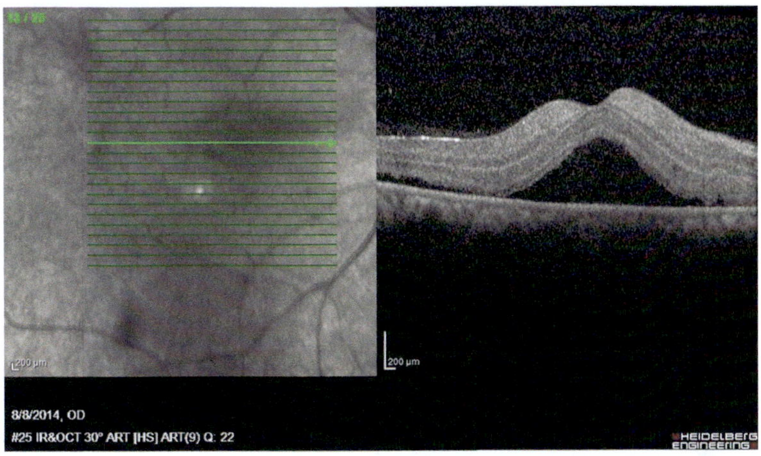

(g)

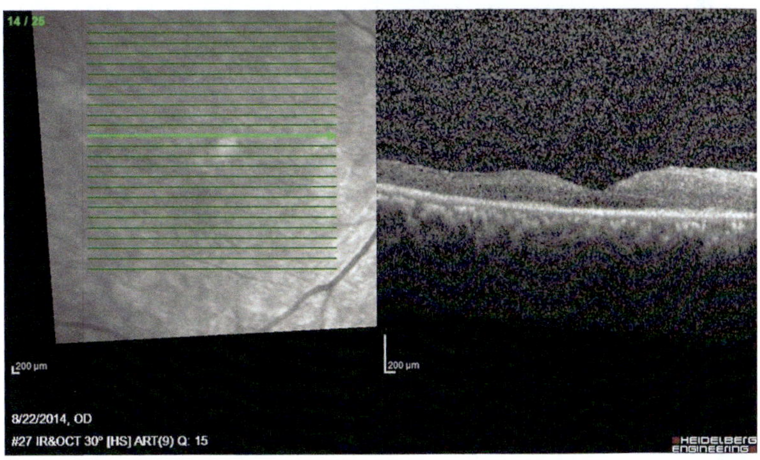

Fig. 10.39 (continued)

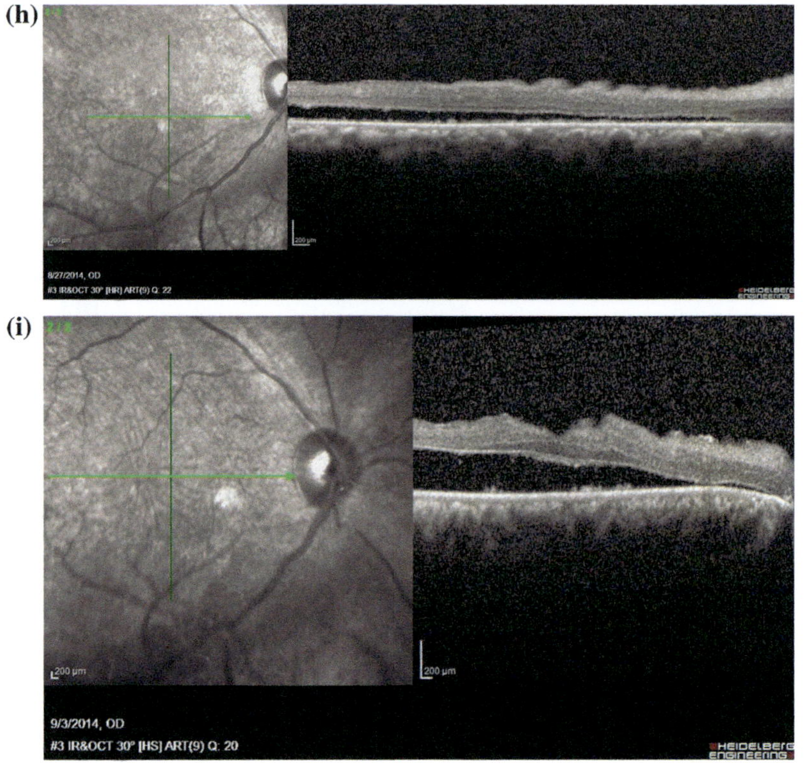

deposit into the iris pigment, triggering heterochromia or different colored irides, which in itself is not a problem. Iron deposition into lenses, however, can result in cataract formation and decreased visual acuity. More importantly, iron can also localize to the retinal pigment epithelium, causing toxicity to the cells, resulting in severe vision loss.

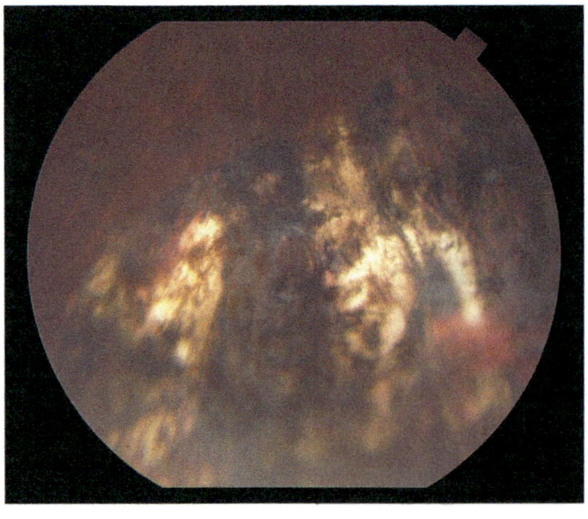

Fig. 10.40 Depicts the appearance of Retina sclopteria

Copper deposition in the eye is known as chalcosis and is extremely toxic to the eye. Copper triggers severe inflammation known as fulminant panophthalmitis and can result in the loss of the eye [33]. Copper in the eye can also disseminate and spread to neighboring tissues. Copper residues in the Descemet's membrane of the cornea can result in Kayser–Fleischer rings. Copper can also deposit into the lens forming unique cataracts with a sunflower like appearance. Copper may also deposit deeper in the vitreous and retina, discoloring the tissues and resulting in vision changes or loss.

An important variable in the decision to image for open globe injuries, and to delineate the presence of intraocular foreign bodies, is if the object is metallic and can be magnetized. This poses the primary concern in patients who are receiving imaging to map the extent of their trauma. If the metal is magnetic, then MRI will cause secondary tissue damage and is directly contraindicated. Therefore, if a foreign body is suspected, simply avoid MRI. However, when approaching surgery, specialized magnets can be used by the ophthalmologist to help extract the foreign object while performing surgery.

The therapy for a suspected intraocular foreign body is immediate administration of PO or intravenous antibiotics with third or fourth-generation topical fluoroquinolones preferred, and consultation for potentially urgent surgery [34]. Patients should be started on systemic and frequent instillation of topical broad-spectrum antibiotics immediately to reduce the risk of endophthalmitis. If deemed necessary, the intravitreal antibiotic therapy may very occasionally be used. The grace period before hyper-acute inflammation occurring in the eye is often 6–12 h. The prognosis worsens immensely [35]. Inflammation increases the difficulty of extraction and the risk of endophthalmitis increases concurrently. These sequelae, along with the possibility of secondary trauma from the surgical extraction of the foreign body, are significant concerns associated with any intraocular foreign body injury.

It is important to remember that trauma severe enough to have a foreign body enter the intraocular space will have consequences. When taking the history, if patients were near items with chemical or thermal properties, there may be additional damage in the eye. Dissipating heat can cause collateral thermal damage to nearby structures. Acid or alkali materials embedded within the eye will produce severe damage that cannot be easily neutralized. Blood vessels that tear in the eye will result in hemorrhage. If the trauma has penetrated through the globe, a retrobulbar hemorrhage is especially worrisome as the increased pressure can trigger a compartment syndrome, compress the optic nerve, and result in permanent vision loss [35]. Fundus examination may reveal disc swelling from the pressure exerted by the blood behind the eye. It is an important factor that should be kept in mind when reviewing the images of the orbit. Finally, over time, trauma may induce a severe diffuse, granulomatous uveitis called *sympathetic ophthalmia*, in the contralateral eye which can occur later on in life.

There are three main stages in the recovery of the posterior segment of the eye after an intraocular foreign body. The first stage is active healing, and may take up to 3 weeks. Poor vision in this stage is not an indication of the final visual acuity at full recovery. Over the next 4–12 weeks, the second stage of recovery addresses specific sequelae pertinent to the patient. This may involve close outpatient monitoring or even possible surgery of the eye. At this time, the vision is dependent on the amount of damage to the chorioretinal layer and the macula. These structures are very fragile and thus the vision at this stage is closely related to the final visual acuity at recovery. The final stage is delayed recovery when some improvement in the vision may occur, but this may be a minimal change over many years [36].

Solar/Thermal/Laser Trauma

Humans use light in the visible spectrum to see and interact with the world. However, it is important to remember that light in the extended spectrums are damaging to the eyes. Specifically, UV radiation from the sun can have a phototoxic effect in the eye. Patients with this type of trauma usually report prolonged staring directly into the sun, more frequently during a solar eclipse [37]. The vision loss is transient and will often improve over the course of months, with some permanent visual sequelae. Psychiatric patients have been known to stare at the sun, with resulting vision loss. These patients can be followed in the outpatient clinic.

Newer lasers on the market also use more focused beams that use shorter wavelengths with increased power. These can cause phototoxic effects in the eye, but can also transfer direct thermal energy into the sensitive structures in the retina. The laser light is absorbed by the melanin in the retinal-pigmented epithelium and can damage the retinal tissue. Depending on the severity of the retina damage, there may be temporary vision changes or permanent vision loss. The location of the laser damage on the retina is also important, as peripheral scarring may not impact vision. However, direct laser damage of the fovea will result in central visual changes that may be permanent. These traumatic occurrences are usually due to accidental trauma from laser pointers or workplace injuries seen in Fig. 10.41 [38]. Typically, low power lasers and commercially available laser pointers are safe due to their lower laser energy. However, as the unregulated market for higher power lasers have grown through Internet sales, so has the rate of accidental trauma to the eye [39]. Habitual laser-pointer damage causes serprentine-like atrophic linear tract marks in the retina and may also show coincident injuries to the iris stroma.

Infectious Endophthalmitis

Infection within the posterior eye, endophthalmitis is always devastating in the setting of trauma. This is due to the fact that direct inoculation has occurred in an immune-privileged area (the vitreous cavity). It usually results in loss of the eye. An exuberant immune-inflammatory reaction in itself is very damaging to the retina, as are the toxins expressed by the inoculum. As previously mentioned, organic material which is not super-heated is highly likely to lead to infectious endophthalmitis, whereas "hot" IOFBs will usually not harbor infectious organisms due to sterilization. Any IOFB should be presumed to have a potential for induction of infection, and to have caused endophthalmitis. If a decision is made to only observe, that should be done on a very frequent (hourly) basis, by a skilled eye-examiner for and assessed for interval change which can be very rapid.

Infectious endophthalmitis can be caused by any type of organism, but by far the most common are gram-positive bacteria (approximately 70%). This is due to the fact that skin flora is almost always gram positive, and has a chance to infect the eye indirectly as a result of any ocular perforation/penetration. This is the rationale for topical and systemic fourth-generation fluoroquinolones to be immediately administered post-trauma, as infection can occur at any time through an open wound. As with any infection, severity is directly related to virulence of the organism. Hyper-acute infections may be due to either an aggressive bacteria, or due to a large inoculum. Gram-negative infections are generally more severe than gram positive, due to the toxins that they express. Fungal infections are

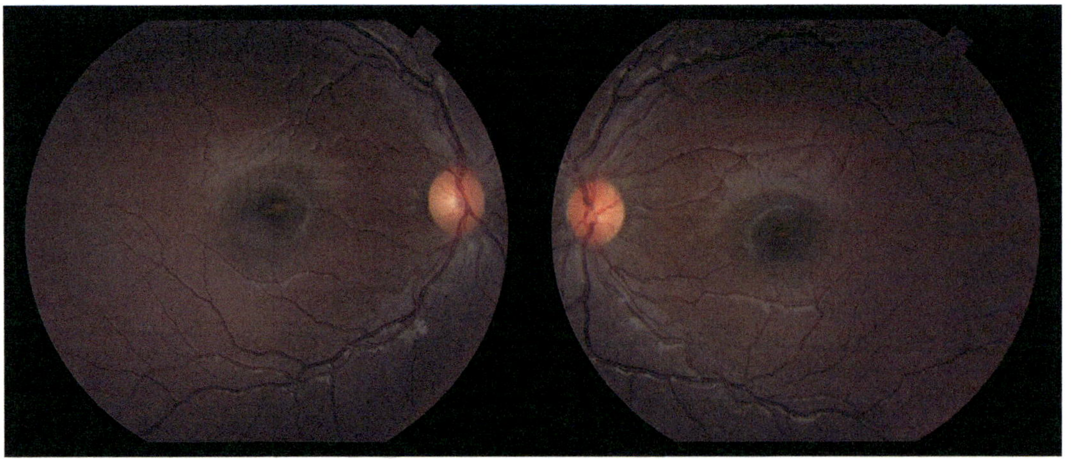

Fig. 10.41 Bilateral laser-induced maculopathy is shown. The 11-year old had purposely shined the laser beam into each eye consecutively for several seconds. The vision was approximately 20/30 o.u. at that time, and had improved to 20/20- o.u. at three-months followup

generally slower to declare themselves, so treatment can be specifically tailored to account for this if injury and inoculation with vegetative material is suspected.

Organic matter is sometimes associated with Bacillus infections (*B. cereus*), a highly prevalent, particularly virulent gram-positive rod.

Therefore, in cases of suspected endopthalmitis, a vitreous biopsy with anterior chamber aspirate or a pars plana vitectomy is needed to obtain gram stains and culture samples to identify underlying causes and to guide treatment [40]. Simultaneous injections of specially compounded intravitreal and subconjunctival antibiotics and/or anti-fungal medications are mandatory. An ophthalmologist who is vitreo-retina trained must perform these surgical procedures, and appropriate emergent consultation is necessarily required. Intraocular/ intravitreal injection cannot be performed with an open globe, as extrusion and loss of intraocular contents will surely occur.

The antiobiotics must be specially formulated for intravitreal injection in the pharmacy. This is owing to the fact that sterility and the concentrations are very critical. They can be given at the time of ruptured globe repair as well.

Vancomycin 0.5 mg/0.1 cc
Ceftazadime 2.25–2.5 mg/0.1 cc (range based on Pharmacist preference)
Amikacin 0.4 mg/0.1 cc

Vancomycin and Ceftazadime are the common choices, since they will cover all gram-positive organisms (most common) and most gram negatives. Amikacin is theoretically most toxic to the retina, so it would be reserved for suspected gram-negative infections. The choice ultimately should be left up to the vitreo-retinal specialist, but it would be acceptable to have all the aforementioned ordered and available as they take significant time to formulate (i.e., one hour). Anti-fungal medication (Voriconazole) can be given P.O. or I.V. in cases where vegetative material is retained in the eye, as it penetrates into the vitreous cavity to prophylax against the occurrence of fungal endophthalmitis. Anti-fungal intravitreal dosing is as follows:

Amphotericin B; 5 mg/0.1 cc
Voriconazole 50–100 mg/0.1 cc

Intravitreal injection must necessarily be accompanied by release of fluid from the eye, due to volume and pressure considerations. As mentioned, wounding leaking and loss of intraocular contents will occur is there is an open wound. Anterior chamber aspiration and/or needle vitreous biopsy is performed at the discretion of the treating physician and sent directly to the microbiology lab for gram staining and culture. Anterior chamber aspiration is safer than needle vitreous biopsy as it does not cause vitreous traction, which can lead to iatrogenic retinal tears.

Intravitreal injection is never a good considered option in cases with incidence of retained IOFB. The infection, if it occurs is caused by an inoculum that is simply too large to be cured by intravitreal injection alone. Furthermore, the chance of sub-acute severe inflammation and retinal degeneration is always a possibility. PPV, IOFB removal, and injection of intravitreal and subconjunctival antibiotics are indicated in virtually all cases of IOFB, let alone whether endophthalmitis is present. Prognosis is poor once endophthalmitis is recognized to have occurred.

Sympathetic Ophthalmia

See Sympathetic Ophthalmia chapter.

Posterior segment Surgery

There are several well-established surgical interventions and procedures that can be used to treat problems in the posterior segment of the eye. Most are very extensive and technical and need to be performed in the operating room, whereas others can be performed in the outpatient setting.

When trauma involves the posterior segment, one should consider how to expedite wound closure and to ultimately obtain adequate closure. When the scleral injury involves the area more than 5 mm posterior to the corneal limbus, the retina and vitreous are necessarily involved. One should have a good idea of the extent of the injury based on clinical acumen and imaging. Foreign bodies always need to be accounted for. The extent of the trauma will indicate whether posterior repair should be performed. Huge posterior ruptures with LP only or NLP vision will often neither be fixable nor result in ambulatory vision. However, exploration (versus primary enucleation) and closure with recognition of poor prognosis is usually indicated. As with any surgery, exposure is very critical. Yet, one tries at the same time to minimize extrusion of contents from the eye. A reasonable approach is to fully expose the sclera and sub-tenon's space near the site of injury in the 90–180° (1–2 quadrants) of involvement and extend to 270 or 360° if necessary depending upon the location of trauma and imaging results. After the eye is prepped and draped, conjunctival peritomy is made and the conjunctiva and Tenon's are separated from the limbus for the extent required. It is then very useful to identify and hook the rectus muscle insertions with 0-silk ties on fenestrated muscle hooks. The silk ties are used to help rotate the eye via the muscle insertions effectively during exposure and repair techniques. The sub-tenon's space is accessed by curved Steven's scissors. A Schepen's lid retractor is used for exposure of the scleral quadrants as an assistant helps with the inspection process. Foreign bodies and debris should be removed. The area can be irrigated with fluoroquinolone ophthalmic drops. Uveal tissue (or retina) should it be reposited prior to wound closure. As long as it is free of contaminants and foreign bodies, the wound should be closed with Nylon sutures (7–0). Exposed uvea should be excised from the wound. Very posterior ruptures are usually self-sealing, cannot be exposed or visualized and will be left. PPV surgery is sometimes then performed simultaneously in this setting, such as when an IOFB is present, but it is not mandatory. It can be planned in subsequent days, allowing for wound healing, multidisciplinary (Anterior segment and Plastics) involvement and planning of further surgery. Proper planning and informed consent is important in grave cases such as these.

The most commonly performed retinal and vitreous surgery is the three-port pars plana vitrectomy (PPV). The pars plana is the uveal tract structure near the junction of the sclera and the insertion of the iris. It is only structural in nature and does not function visually. It is virtually avascular, and is relatively elastic. These properties make the pars plana the ideal location to insert the tools used for vitreous and retinal surgery. In the vitrectomy, parts or nearly all of vitreous body will be removed permanently and replaced with aqueous fluid.

To perform a vitrectomy, retinal surgeons penetrate the conjunctiva and sclera with several (usually 3) small trocar-cannulas. They then use one of the cannulas to infuse balanced-salt solution, and the others to introduce a lighting device (light-pipe) and various cutting and aspiration instrumentation. The retinal surgeon then removes parts or the entire vitreous humor for the procedure via a vitrector hand-piece. Vitreous must be cut as it is aspirated, as suction alone induces pulling and traction damage to the retina. In trauma, this may be diagnostic in order to clear blood to visualize the retina when retinal tears are suspected. The vitrectomy procedure is also used to reattach the retina if detached (Figs. 10.42a–e). In penetrating injuries, retina and vitreous are usually incarcerated in the entry and exit sites, and this traction may be released with cutting maneuvers (retinectomy). It may also be used to prevent fibrovascular growth after traumatic inflammation, reducing the risk of retinal detachments in the future. This therapy, coupled with many more specific tools and techniques in the eye are the mainstay of retina repair.

Two-dimensional endoscopes are occasionally used along with vitrectomy instrumentation in cases of severe trauma with opacification of the cornea. If the lens capsule has been violated or the lens is subluxed (Fig. 10.43) or dislocated, it may represent an impediment to safe and effective PPV. Traumatic zonular damage may

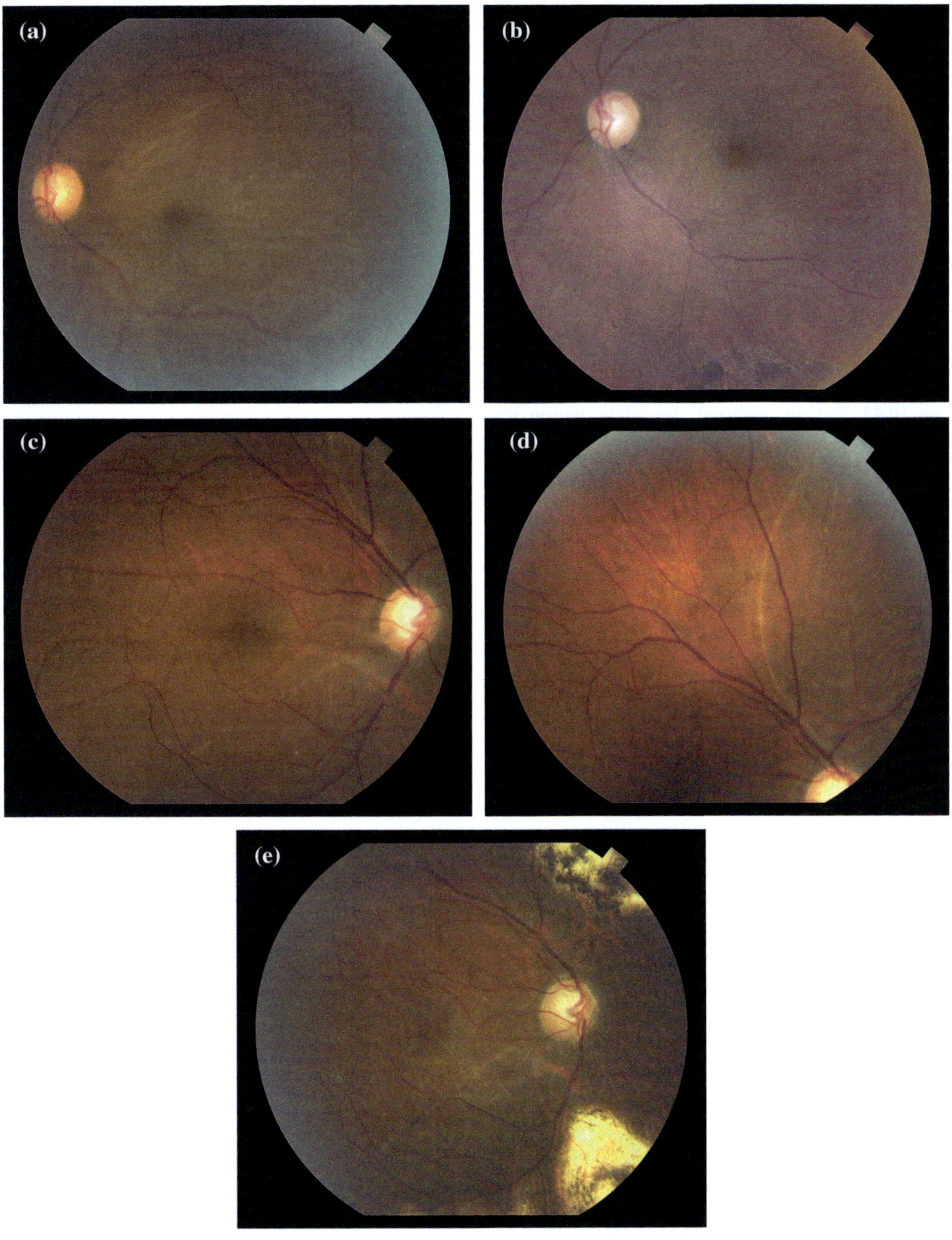

Fig. 10.42 a–e. Two cases of subtotal retinal detachment successfully treated via PPV, endolaser and SF6 gas injection

result in lens displacement in these cases. Lens extraction is then usually performed at the time of vitrectomy, when it is significantly opacified or subluxed/ dislocated. A vitrector is used to make a capsulotomy and remove the lens in younger patients, as the lens is softer in youth. In older individuals, a fragmentation hand-piece (fragmatome) is best utilized to remove the lens

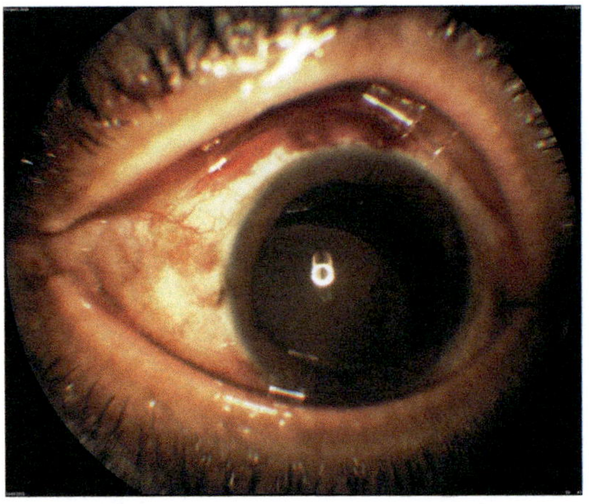

Fig. 10.43 Partially subluxed crysytalline human lens from acute blunt trauma

through a 20-gage pars plana incision. In less severe trauma, a conventional cataract operation using phacoemulsification instrumentation is inserted through a scleral tunnel or clear-corneal incisions and can be used to facilitate insertion of an intraocular lens if that is deemed appropriate. Coincident severe posterior segment trauma or retinal detachment usually contraindicates implantation of an intraocular lens at the time of primary repair as the lens complex will serve as a "scaffold" for the formation of most-undesirable anterior-loop proliferative vitreo-retinopathy (PVR).

Scleral buckling is another technique sometimes used to repair the retina after traumatic retinal detachments and retinal dialysis. Although it can be a standalone procedure in cases involving inferior-retinal detachments and significant retinal dialyses, this technique is also sometimes used in conjunction with pars plana vitrectomy in severe trauma cases. Scleral buckling elements vary in shape, contour and size. They are composed of silicone, either in the form of a dense porous sponge or as firm, but flexible elements. It is like a thin corset that wraps around the eye, placed under the four-rectus eye-muscles, keeping the retina attached properly through imbrication of the sclera (Fig. 10.14) as opposed to through external force. Retinal surgeons will begin by entering and then retracting the conjunctiva and Tenon's capsule and then isolating the four-rectus muscles. Once all four-rectus muscles have been marked with sutures, the buckle is passed underneath the muscles and secured with non-absorbable sutures. This additionally pushes the sclera onto the neurosensory retina and helps keep the cell layers intact during recovery. It also overcomes foreshortening of the retina when scarring is present and potentiates reattachment. The retinal pigment epithelium (RPE) forms a hypertrophic scar around tears and usually inhibits re-opening of holes and subsequent retinal re-detachment.

The use of thermal (cold/freezing) energy to seal the retina after breaks or tears is another common practice. This potentiates the RPE scarring at the injury sites. When subretinal fluid builds after retinal tears, the pressure and forces of the fluid can cause larger retinal detachments or recurrent detachments after surgery. Lasers or cryotherapy are the main tools to seal the tears and keep the retina structurally intact. When subretinal fluid is present, judicious use of cryotherapy is necessary. Lasers can be used in the outpatient setting for small tears or in the operating room in conjunction with larger tears that require additional surgery. It can also be used after the retina has flattened to prevent redetachment, either in the operating room or after scleral buckling or pneumatic retinopexy has flattened the retina.

However, use of laser is somewhat limited if the view of the retina is obstructed by blood. In this scenario, the blood can be cleared with vitrectomy surgery. On the other hand, if the tear is visible behind the blood, cryotherapy, or a red-colored laser can be expertly used to promote adherence of the retina to the pigmented epithelium. In this procedure, a cryotherapy probe is placed into the eye, and super cooled liquid nitrogen metallic probe is placed around the break to fix the retina back onto the posterior surface of the eye. Alternatively laser marks are placed around the break when there is very minimal, or no subretinal fluid. These treatments are typically performed in the outpatient setting with topical or local anesthesia (cryotherapy). In many patients with more extensive retinal detachments, the outcomes of surgery using lasers or cryotherapy as ancillary treatments are both successful [41].

Systemic Trauma Syndromes

Optic nerve avulsion is a rare occurrence when blunt trauma triggers a tear and detachment of the optic nerve from the globe. This is unique as the force of injury keeps the globe and sclera intact anteriorly and optic nerve sheath intact posteriorly [42]. The damage is very specific as blunt trauma can induce rotational forces on the eye, which avulses the optic nerve. It has been seen to occur in a numerous clinical settings. Orbital canal fractures can sever the optic nerve, but this is not a true avulsion. In other rare circumstances, penetrating trauma with foreign material in the medial orbit can directly sever the optic nerve near the insertion at the sclera [43].

Patients who suffer an optic nerve avulsion will present with sudden complete loss of vision. On examination, they will have no light perception in the eye, with a full second cranial nerve avulsion. As the nerve pathway is severed, they will also exhibit an afferent pupillary defect as the input for the reflex has been cut. A visible fundus exam may not be possible, secondary to the bleeding that occurs with such traumatic injuries to the eye. However, if the optic nerve is visible, there will be an excavation of the optic disc as the nerve has detached from the eye [44]. For patients without visible fundi, many imaging modalities can be used to assist in diagnosis.

Unfortunately, most of the current imaging modalities do not detect optic nerve avulsions well. However, confirming the presence of an avulsion injury is crucial, as it will change the treatment of the patient. CT scans of the orbit can be used but are limited in their ability to identify the abnormalities that reveal the injury [45]. MRI scans, with thin slices at the orbit, are similarly limited as they too can fail to identify the lesion. B-scan ultrasonography is another tool available to identify avulsion injuries, although the results may be inconclusive [44]. If available, OCT can help identify partial and full lesions at the optic nerve head. OCT can also be used to monitor the nerve fiber layer changes that occur after avulsion [42].

Treatment for optic nerve avulsions is limited, as the tissue cannot be functionally reconnected. However, confirming the diagnosis of optic nerve avulsion is crucial in deciding whether the patient will need surgical intervention. Therefore, it is important to determine the diagnosis from the history, clinical findings and the imaging study results. If the patient's presentation is simply due to traumatic optic neuropathy from the shock of the injury, their vision may improve with high-dose steroids or orbital decompression surgeries [46]. Unfortunately, these treatment modalities become moot if the nerve has been transected. These patients should be spared invasive treatments and therapies that will not change the final outcome, which is very poor (usually NLP vision).

Purtcher's syndrome is a rare retinopathy, with less than one case per million, which develops after systemic trauma, usually associated with impacts to the head or chest [47]. Patients may have a sudden loss of vision or may have a delayed period up to 48 h after the trauma before the vision changes occur [48]. These deficits can develop with visual field losses either unilaterally or bilaterally with intact peripheral vision. The current proposed theory is that head or chest trauma sends compressive vaso-occlusive forces that reach the eye and damages the endothelium. This damage is then believed to trigger a vasculitic process that contributes to the vision loss.

The diagnosis of Purtcher's retinopathy can be made with a fundus exam. The exam reveals patches of superficial retinal whitening with hemorrhage seen in Fig. 10.44. In addition, the optic nerve head can reveal pallor or edema. OCT imaging can demonstrate hyper-reflective inner layers of the retina. Fluorescein angiography can reveal choroidal vascular involvement with decreased capillary perfusion and late leakage from the injured capillaries of the retina. Acute pancreatitis, fat embolization from long bone fractures, hypertensive emergency, advanced AIDS and sepsis should be considered in the differential diagnosis.

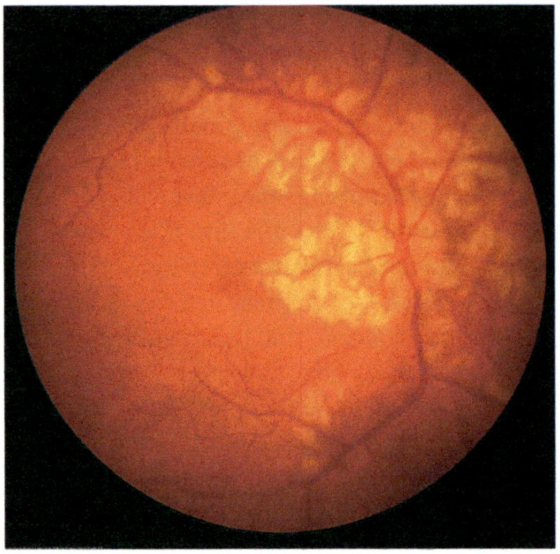

Fig. 10.44 Purtscher's retinopathy is shown. Image is courtesy of the ASRS image bank

Treatment of the underlying cause is the best initial step in the management of Purtcher's syndrome. High-dose IV corticosteroids were thought to be beneficial but have not been proven to be valuable in all patients [49]. In the end, observing patients in the outpatient setting and monitoring recovery is the best management for these patients.

Terson's syndrome is a rare scenario of vitreous hemorrhage associated with a subarachnoid hemorrhage. However, it is not caused by blood extending into the eye. These two hemorrhages are two separate bleeds linked by the increased intracranial pressure (ICP) related to the subarachnoid hemorrhage. This increased pressure acts on retinal venules, triggering the bleeding [50].

The treatment urgency of this ocular syndrome is second to the management of the subarachnoid hemorrhage. Therefore, performing a fundus exam may be delayed as pharmacologically dilated pupils, used to perform the full ocular fundus examination, will interfere with the ability to continue neurologic monitoring of the patient. However, if the need to examine the eye is urgent, B-scan ultrasound can be used to look for vitreous bleeding. An un-dilated fundus exam may also reveal the loss of the red reflex from the vitreous bleed obstructing the view to the retina.

Treatment for Terson's syndrome is conservative as the vitreous hemorrhage can resolve spontaneously. This is also prudent as monitoring the neurologic state of the patient takes precedence. Once the patient has stabilized, if the vitreous hemorrhage continues to affect the patient, pars plana vitrectomy is the curative procedure.

Shaken baby syndrome, otherwise known as "non-accidental trauma," is a consequence of child abuse. Every year, many children lose their lives and more suffer through life-long disabilities due to child abuse. In the USA alone, around 1400 children per year suffer from the complications of shaken baby syndrome [51]. These children can present with numerous nonspecific findings and the diagnosis can be frequently missed. The typical child presents in an obtunded state. Illness and dehydration is the default diagnosis. However, once non-accidental trauma is suspected, a detailed eye exam with documented pictures and findings are required.

The ocular findings associated with shaken-baby syndrome are usually bilateral retinal hemorrhages seen in Fig. 10.45 [52]. These hemorrhages can occur in all regions of the eye with subretinal, intraretinal, preretinal, and vitreous bleeding that can extend from the posterior

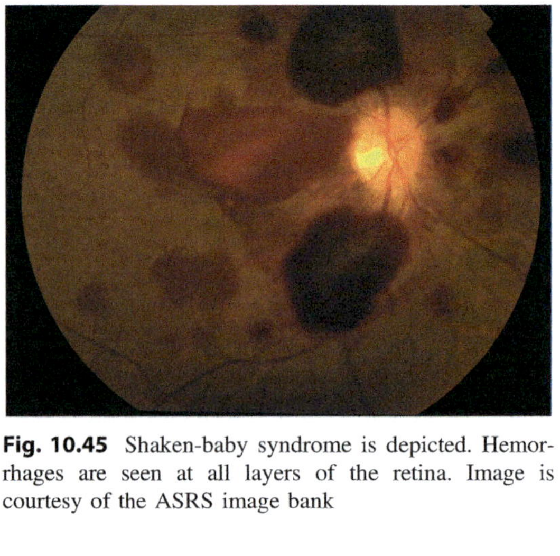

Fig. 10.45 Shaken-baby syndrome is depicted. Hemorrhages are seen at all layers of the retina. Image is courtesy of the ASRS image bank

pole of the eye to the far periphery. This is due to the recurrent acceleration-deceleration forces the child encounters during the shaking trauma. The shearing of the sensitive neuronal structures from the exerted forces results in the rupture of vessels and the retinal axons/nerve fiber layer. Children that present with evidence of bleeding in the eye from shaken baby syndrome are associated with poor visual and neurologic outcomes. This may also be secondary to the significant brain injury that is inflicted by the shaking trauma as well. Despite the very high sensitivity and specificity of bilateral retinal hemorrhages in diagnosing shaken baby syndrome, the diagnosis can only be made from the composite of multiple signs and symptoms.

Signs of ocular damage, systemic damage, with documented proof on imaging will help make the diagnosis of shaken baby syndrome. It is a difficult diagnosis to make for the clinician due to the severe consequences that occur. Failing to diagnose a child can result in their loss of life and future litigation. Making a diagnosis that proves to be incorrect may result in long legal battles to reunite parents with their children. However, making the diagnosis is necessary to protect the safety of the child. In addition, the high correlation of retinal hemorrhages in young children with abuse makes a good fundus exam a vital tool in the confirmation of the diagnosis of shaken baby syndrome. Retinal and vitreous bleeding in a baby is usually due to shaking, although acute myelogenous leukemia and X-linked juvenile retinoschisis can occasionally present with a similar appearance.

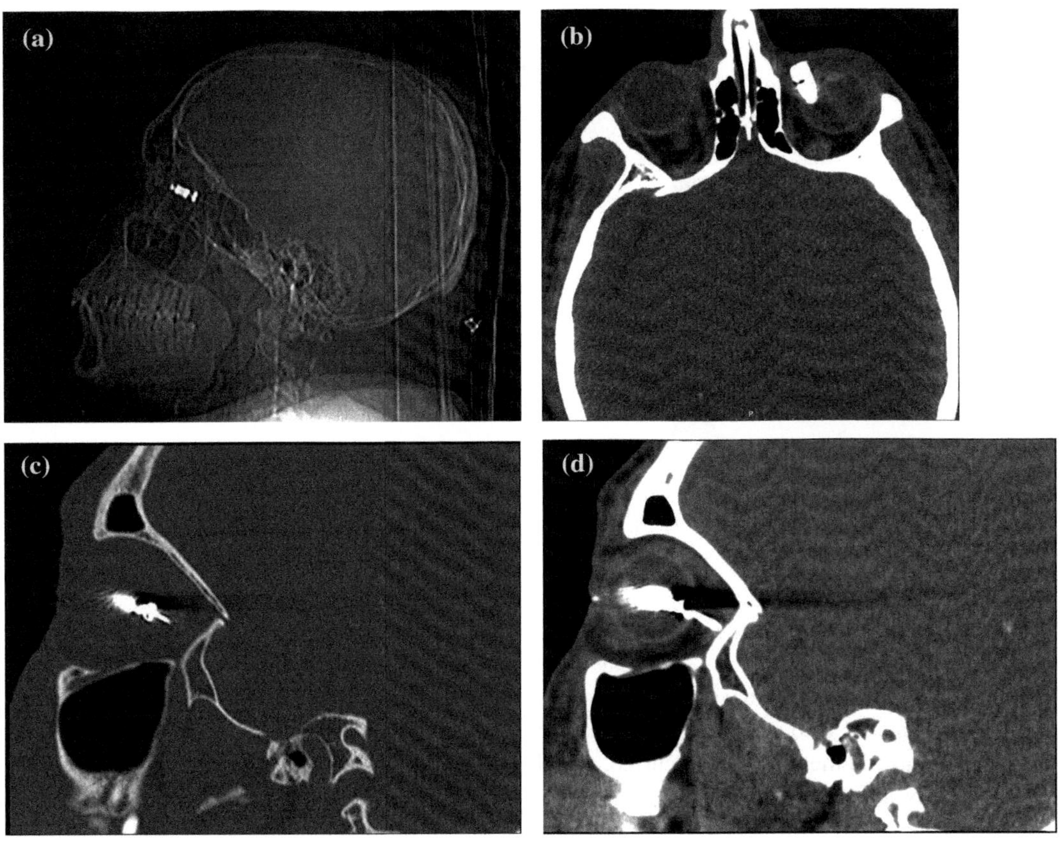

Fig. 10.46 **a–d** Case discussion 1: 20 year old male who sustained acute traumatic injury with a Taser dart to the left eye. Vision is light perception. What are the management considerations? (i.e. vitreo-retinal and removal or Plastics procedure or both.) Does neurosurgery need to involve?

(a)

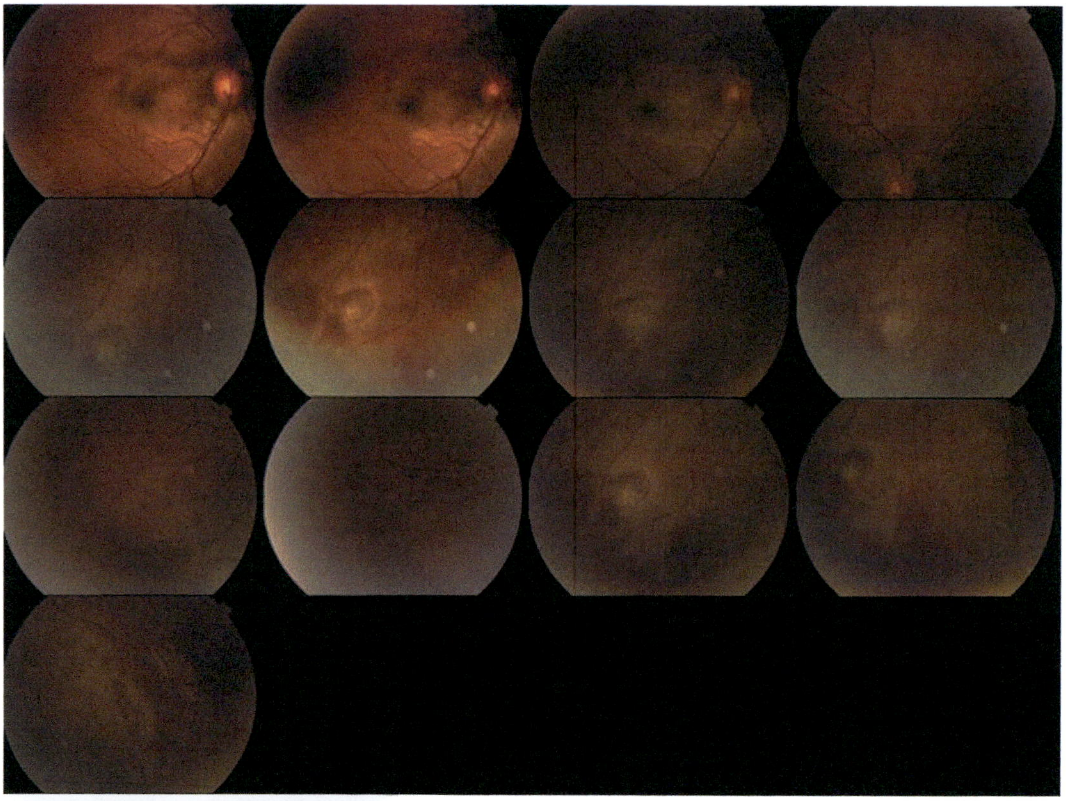

(b)

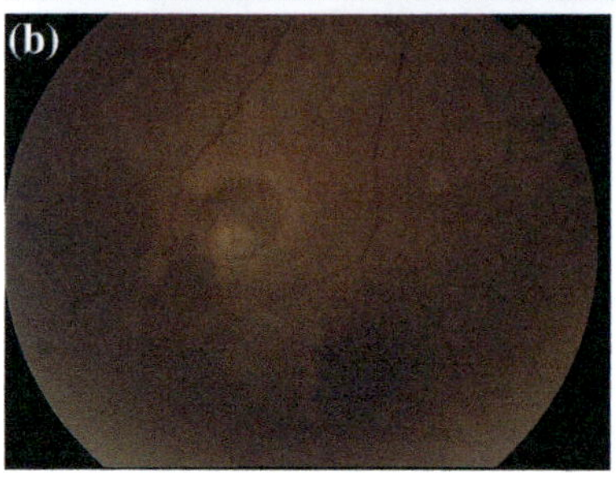

Fig. 10.47 **a**, **b** Case discussion: 2 28 year old male with acute trauma from a fist. The IOP is 18. Vision is 20/100 at near. There is severe photophobia and no conjunctival chemosis. What is the management? VH, commotio, white without pressure change. Urgency of retinal evaluation?

Unfortunately, the prognosis for good vision after shaken baby syndrome is very bleak. The shearing neuronal damage caused by the trauma is not repairable. It also indicates that shearing neuronal damage in the brain has occurred. Good final vision is associated with good initial neurological exam findings, visual responses and pupillary reactions. However, if these signs are poor, the odds of recovery are quite low. Documentation by a pediatric ophthalmologist or retinal specialist is mandatory to assist in criminal prosecution of perpetrators. Proactive education and prevention play important roles in parent education in order to prevent future children from having to suffer physical trauma. (Figs. 10.46, 10.47 and 10.48).

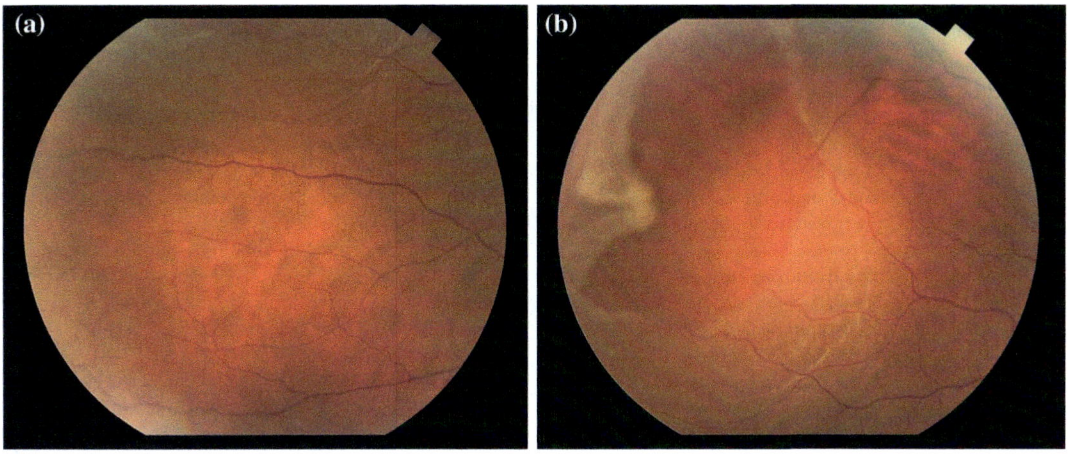

Fig. 10.48 **a**, **b** Case discussion: 3 48 year old male. Vision is 20/25. Uncertain if the eye was traumatized. Is this an RRD? It looks different from most RRD as the retinal vessels course over what is seen, at first glance, to be a large tear. This represents a case of senile retinoschisis full-thickness detachment that will need surgery as an inner layer break has occurred due to traumatic PVD

References

1. "Eye Safety." Centers for Disease Control and Prevention. Centers for Disease Control and Prevention, 25 Feb 2015. Web. Available at: http://www.cdc.gov/niosh/topics/eye.
2. McGwin G, Xie A, Owsley C. Rate of eye injury in the United States. Arch. Ophthalmol. 2005;123 (7):970–6.
3. Shiuey Y, Lucarelli MJ. Traumatic hyphema: outcomes of outpatient management. Ophthalmology. 1998;105(5):851–5.
4. Di Lauro S, Castrejón M, Fernández I, et al. Loss of visual acuity after successful surgery for macula-on rhegmatogenous retinal detachment in a prospective multicentre study. J. Ophthalmol. 2015;2015:821864.
5. Aironi V, Gandage S. Pictorial essay: B-scan ultrasonography in ocular abnormalities. Indian J. Radiol. Imaging. 2009;19(2):109–15.
6. Kubal WS. Imaging of orbital trauma. Radiographics. 2008;28(6):1729–39. doi:10.1148/rg.286085523 Review.
7. Smith MJ, Walline JJ. Controlling myopia progression in children and adolescents. Adolesc Health Med. Ther. 2015;13(6):133–40. doi:10.2147/AHMT.S55834 eCollection 2015. Review.
8. Wilkinson CP. Interventions for asymptomatic retinal breaks and lattice degeneration for preventing retinal detachment. Cochrane Database Syst. Rev. 2014;9: CD003170.
9. Diaz RI, Sigler EJ, Randolph JC, Rafieetary MR, Calzada JI. Spectral domain optical coherence tomography characteristics of white-without-pressure. Retina. 2014;34(5):1020–1.
10. Kubota M, Hayashi T, Arai K, Tsuneoka H. Choroidal neovascularization after blunt ocular trauma in angioid streaks. Clin. Ophthalmol. 2013;7:1347–51.
11. Doi S, Kimura S, Morizane Y, Shiode Y, Hosokawa M, Hirano M, Hosogi M, Fujiwara A, Miyamoto K, Shiraga F. Successful displacement of a traumatic submacular hemorrhage in a 13-year-old boy treated by vitrectomy, subretinal injection of tissue plasminogen activator and intravitreal air tamponade: a case report. BMC Ophthalmol. 2015;7(15):94.
12. Rishi E, Gopal L, Rishi P, Sengupta S, Sharma T. Submacular hemorrhage: a study amongst Indian eyes. Indian J. Ophthalmol. 2012;60(6):521–5.
13. Toth CA, Benner JD, Hjelmeland LM, Landers MB 3rd, Morse LS. Ultramicrosurgical removal of subretinal hemorrhage in cats. Am. J. Ophthalmol. 1992;113(2):175–82.
14. Gupta A, Mazumdar S, Choudhry S. Practical approach to ophthalmoscopic retinal diagnosis. New Delhi: Jaypee Brothers Pvt. Ltd.; 2009.
15. Miller JB, Yonekawa Y, Eliott D, Kim IK, Kim LA, Loewenstein JI, Sobrin L, Young LH, Mukai S, Vavvas DG. Long-term follow-up and outcomes in traumatic macular holes. Am. J. Ophthalmol. 2015;160(6):1255–1258.e1.
16. Ahn SJ, Woo SJ, Kim KE, Jo DH, Ahn J, Park KH. Optical coherence tomography morphologic grading of macular commotio retinae and its association with anatomic and visual outcomes. Am. J. Ophthalmol. 2013;156(5):994–1001.e1.
17. Kiel J, Chen S. Contusion injuries and their ocular effects. Clin. Exp. Optom. 2001;84(1):19–25.
18. Vote BJ, Casswell AG. Retinal dialysis: are we missing diagnostic opportunities? Eye (Lond). 2004;18(7):709–13.

19. Wang M, Hu S, Zhao Z, Xiao T. A novel method for the localization and management of traumatic cyclodialysis cleft. J. Ophthalmol. 2014;2014:761851.
20. Gentile R, Pavlin C, Liebmann J, Easterbrook M, Tello C, Foster F, et al. Diagnosis of traumatic cyclodialysis by ultrasound biomicroscopy. Ophthalmic Surg. Lasers. 1996;27(2):97.
21. George CW, Slack WJ. Corneal and scleral lacerations. A five-year review. Am. J. Ophthalmol. 1962;54:119–23.
22. Birmingham Eye Trauma Terminology System (BETTS); International Society of Ocular Trauma. Available at: http://isotonline.org/betts/.
23. Ehlers JP, Kunimoto DY, Ittoop S, Maguire JI, Ho AC, Regillo CD. Metallic intraocular foreign bodies: characteristics, interventions, and prognostic factors for visual outcome and globe survival. Am. J. Ophthalmol. 2008;146.3:427–433.
24. Napora KJ, Obuchowska I, Sidorowicz A, Mariak Z. Intraocular and intraorbital foreign bodies characteristics in patients with penetrating ocular injury. Kliniki Oczna 2009;111.10:307–312.
25. Babar TF, Khan MT, Marwat MZ, Shah SA, Murad Y, Khan MD. Patterns of ocular trauma. J. Coll. Physicians Surg. Pak. 2007;17(3):148–53.
26. Khaw PT, Shah P, Elkington AR. Injury to the eye. BMJ. 2004;328(7430):36–8 (Review).
27. Laraque D. American Academy of pediatrics committee on injury, violence, and poison prevention. Injury risk of nonpowder guns. Pediatrics. 2004;114 (5):1357–61.
28. Joseph DP, Meredith TA. A new BB forceps. Arch. Ophthalmol. 2000;118(11):1574–5.
29. Powley KD, Dahlstrom DB, Atkins VJ, Fackler ML. Velocity necessary for a BB to penetrate the eye: an experimental study using pig eyes. Am. J. Forensic Med. Pathol. 2004;25(4):273–5.
30. Ahmadabadi MN, Karkhaneh R, Roohipoor R, Tabatabai A, Alimardani A. Clinical presentation and outcome of chorioretinitis sclopetaria: a case series study. Injury. 2010;41(1):82–5.
31. Desai A, Parihar R, Mathews J, Akduman L. Occult wooden posterior segment intraocular foreign body. Ophthalmic Surg. Lasers Imaging Retina. 2014;45 (1):58–61.
32. John SS, Rehman TA, John D, Raju RS. Missed diagnosis of a wooden intra-orbital foreign body. Indian J. Ophthalmol. 2008;56(4):322–4.
33. Rathod R, Mieler W. An update on the management of intraocular foreign bodies. 2011. Available at: http://www.retinalphysician.com/articleviewer.aspx?articleid=105554.
34. Kernt M, Kampik A. Endophthalmitis: pathogenesis, clinical presentation, management, and perspectives. Clin. Ophthalmol. 2010;24(4):121–35.
35. Knox FA, Best RM, Kinsella F, et al. Management of endophthalmitis with retained intraocular foreign body. Eye (Lond). 2004;18:179–82.
36. Yeh S, Colyer MH, Weichel ED. Current trends in the management of intraocular foreign bodies. Curr. Opin. Ophthalmol. 2008;19(3):225–33. doi:10.1097/ICU.0b013e3282fa75f1 Review.
37. Gregory-Roberts E, Chen Y, Harper CA, Ong T, Maclean MA, Fagan XJ, Carden SM. Solar retinopathy in children. J. AAPOS. 2015;19(4):349–51.
38. Turaka K, Bryan JS, Gordon AJ, Reddy R, Kwong HM Jr, Sell CH. Laser pointer induced macular damage: case report and mini review. Int. Ophthalmol. 2012;32(3):293–7.
39. Consumer health information: illuminating the hazards of powerful laser products. Silver Spring, MD: Food and Drug Administration, 2009. Available at: http://www.fda.gov/downloads/ForConsumers/ConsumerUpdates/UCM167564.pdf.
40. Ahmed Y, Schimel AM, Pathengay A, Colyer MH, Flynn HW Jr. Endophthalmitis following open-globe injuries. Eye (Lond). 2012;26(2):212–7.
41. Lira RP, Takasaka I, Arieta CE, Nascimento MA, Caldato R, Panetta H. Cryotherapy vs laser photocoagulation in scleral buckle surgery: a randomized clinical trial. Arch. Ophthalmol. 2010;128(12):1519–22.
42. Chaudhry IA, Shamsi FA, Al-Sharif A, Elzaridi E, Al-Rashed W. Optic nerve avulsion from door-handle trauma in children. Br. J. Ophthalmol. 2006;90(7):844–6.
43. Mumcuoglu T, Durukan HA, Erdurman C, Hurmeric V, Gundogan FC. Functional and structural analysis of partial optic nerve avulsion due to blunt trauma: case report. Indian J. Ophthalmol. 2010;58 (6):524–6.
44. Sawhney R, Kochhar S, Gupta R, Sood S. Traumatic optic nerve avulsion: role of ultrasonography. Eye (2003). (n.d.);17:667–670. doi:10.1038/sj.eye.6700411.
45. Foster BS, March GA, Lucarelli MJ, Samiy N, Lessell S. Optic nerve avulsion. Arch. Ophthalmol. 1997;115(5):623–630. Erratum in: Arch. Ophthalmol. 1997;115(8):1070.
46. Sosin M, De La Cruz C, Mundinger GS, Saadat SY, Nam AJ, Manson PN, Christy MR, Bojovic B, Rodriguez ED. Treatment outcomes following traumatic optic neuropathy. Plast. Reconstr. Surg. 2016;137(1):231–8.
47. Agrawal A, McKibbin M. Purtscher's retinopathy: epidemiology, clinical features and outcome. Br. J. Ophthalmol. 2007;91(11):1456–9.
48. Behrens-Baumann W, Scheurer G, Schroer H. Pathogenesis of Purtscher's retinopathy. Graefes Arch. Clin. Exp. Ophthalmol. 1992;230(3):286–91.
49. Gil P, Pires J, Costa E, Matos R, Cardoso MS, Mariano M. Purtscher retinopathy: to treat or not to treat? Eur. J. Ophthalmol. 2015;25(6):e112–5.
50. Mazurek M, Krzystolik K, Lachowicz E, Kubasik-Kladna K, Czepita D. [Terson syndrome–a literature review]. Klin Oczna. 2014;116(1):59–63 (Review).
51. All About SBS/AHT. The National Center on Shaken Baby Syndrome. Available at: http://www.dontshake.org/sbs.php?topnavid=3&subnavid=27.
52. Kivlin JD, Simons KB, Lazoritz S, Ruttum MS. Shaken baby syndrome. Ophthalmology. 2000;107 (7):1246–54.

11 Sympathetic Ophthalmia

E. Clifford Lazzaro

Sympathetic ophthalmia (SO) is an uncommon, devastating disease which is difficult to treat once started. Ophthalmic surgeons, whether they have repaired a perforated globe or performed a pars plana vitrectomy, consider the development of this autoimmune uveitis a most serious sight threatening event. This is a disease in which a patient's good eye became diseased because the patient's other eye was penetrated or perforated and suffered uveal damage. SO is a bilateral disease. Its name was coined by Sir. William Mackenzie [1], a nineteenth century ophthalmologist who used history taking and keen powers of observation, aided by contact lenses in his examination of the eye. He did not use the Von Helmholtz ophthalmoscope which had just been invented. The pathology was described by Dalen in 1904 and Fuchs in 1905 [2]. Despite mankind's march toward civilization, accidents, assaults and war are agents involved in the etiology of SO. However, intraocular surgery has replaced globe trauma as the number one cause of this disease, although this is debated in the literature.

A 5-year old boy presented to the ER of Brooklyn Eye and Ear Hospital in 1970 with complaints of pain, decreased vision, and light hurting his red left eye. As a second year ophthalmology resident, I was about to examine my first patient who had developed SO. The young boy exhibited all the findings of a granulomatous panuveitis. His right eye had been enucleated the year earlier, following a repair of a perforated globe secondary to a pencil injury. The right eye pathology slip in his chart stated perforated globe with heme and disruption of intraocular contents post-surgical repair. Our pathologist reviewed the slides and reversed the diagnosis to SO. We sent the slides to Dr. Lorenz Zimmerman at the AFIP who confirmed the diagnosis. Corticosteroids used locally and systemically brought the uveitis in his remaining eye to quiescence over several months [3]. We then tapered the steroid slowly over several more months. Our patient did quite well despite occasional flare-ups treated by reinstitution of steroid therapy. Additionally, no evidence of sarcoid, TB, toxoplasmosis, Vogt Koyanagi Harada (VKH) syndrome, herpetic disease, or syphilis was found.

Tempus fugit and the year is now 2015. I had become a 75-year old Jurassic park ophthalmologist about to retire from an academic position at The State University of New York—(SUNY) Downstate Medical Center. A 40-year old male from the Caribbean presented to our eye clinic at Kings County Hospital Center in Brooklyn, NY. Ocular exam revealed a bilateral granulomatous panuveitis. Our patient had been punched in his left eye (injured eye) some 4 weeks earlier, and had not sought medical attention until arriving in Brooklyn when his symptoms began. The exam of his OS revealed prolapsed uveal tissue under the conjunctiva anterior to the insertion of the superior rectus tendon. The anterior chamber was

E.C. Lazzaro (✉)
Department of Ophthalmology, The State University of New York (SUNY) Downstate Medical Center, Brooklyn, USA
e-mail: niccliff@aol.com

S.C. Kaufman and D.R. Lazzaro (eds.), *Textbook of Ocular Trauma*,
DOI 10.1007/978-3-319-47633-9_11

slightly deeper OS than OD. No hyphema was present. Phacodonesis was present. No cataract or lens capsule injury was apparent. A granulomatous panuveitis was present OU, more intense in the OD (the sympathizing eye) than in the OS (the injured inciting eye) [4]. No confirmatory findings of Vogt–Koyanagi–Harada (VKH), sarcoid, TB, herpes, toxoplasmosis, or syphilis were found. A diagnosis of SO was made and steroid treatment commenced.

The ophthalmologist must be fastidious in evaluating the proptotic ecchymotic patient with subconjunctival heme. In addition to orbital fracture, occult rupture of the globe must be ruled out. Careful globe exploration surgery should be done when there is a suspicion of globe rupture, especially in the presence of low intraocular pressure, lid laceration and/or intraocular heme on the injured side.

The question of who should repair an orbital fracture is important. While ENT and oral maxillary surgeons [5] may know how to repair an orbital fracture, are they able to identify a globe penetration or perforation? If this surgery is done by other than an oculoplastic surgeon, should careful ophthalmic evaluation be done before our colleagues in another specialty perform the repair?

Sympathetic ophthalmia SO is a bilateral granulomatous panuveitis secondary to traumatic or surgically induced uveal damage. The disease may present as early as 5 days or as late as 66 years post injury [6]. An autoimmune etiology is suggested by the lymphocyte, macrophage, and giant cell response in the uveal tract [7]. Genetic makeup [8] (i.e. HLA-DR4, HLA-DQw3, and HLA-DRw53) may increase the susceptibility to developing SO.

The clinical exam of the SO patient may reveal mutton fat keratic precipitates (KPT), anterior chamber flare and cells, posterior synechiae, cyclitis with decreased accommodation, vitritis, choroiditis with various degrees of choroidal thickening, Dalen-Fuchs Nodules, papillitis, serous detachments of the retina, occasional areas of choroidal and retinal vasculitis, cataracts, and glaucoma. The Dalen-Fuchs Nodules can be found in some 25% of SO patients. The nodule is not specific for SO, as it can be found in VKH and sarcoid patients as well. The Dalen-Fuchs Nodules [9] appear as yellow white spots 60–70 um in diameter. They are located near the equator mostly. Histologically, these nodules are made up of histiocytes and pigment epithelial cells. While inflammation of the choriocapillaris is not the usual finding, it is sometimes found. Several other panuveitis diseases must be considered in the differential diagnosis of SO including VKH, sarcoid, tuberculosis, toxoplasmosis, syphilis, herpes simplex and zoster, Behcet's disease, and intraocular lymphoma. The history of no accidental or surgical trauma antecedent to the "uveitis" developing is usually the case in these entities.

The VKH patient may have headache, meningismus, and dysacousia accompanying or preceding the uveitis. Such is not usually the case in SO. As time goes on, the VKH patient may develop poliosis, alopecia, and vitiligo. Asian, Middle Eastern, Native American, and Hispanic people are the patient populations mostly involved. The VKH patient is more likely to have bilateral exudative retinal detachments than is the SO patient. The VKH patient is more likely to demonstrate involvement of the choriocapillaris than is the SO patient.

The sarcoid patent may present with enlarged lacrimal, parotid and/or salivary glands. A fever may be present. Enlarged parotid glands and fever is known as Heerfordt's syndrome. Erythema nodosum is sometimes present as is lupus pernio on occasion. Hilar lymphadenopathy on chest X-ray and other pulmonary findings are often seen. Noncaseating granulomas of the conjunctiva can appear as chalazia. The sarcoid granuloma may even be present in the bundle of His and cause bradycardia. An elevated angiotensin-converting enzyme level is sometimes found. The ocular exam will sometimes reveal granulomatous panuveitis with a multifocal choroiditis. Candle wax drippings near the veins will outline periphlebitis.

The patient with tuberculosis may have active tuberculosis or TB in the past. A PPD test would be positive (usually) and might even have incited the uveitis. An interferon gold test would be positive. Evidence of pulmonary infiltration, and scarring, particularly in the upper lobes, might be present. Acid fast bacilli may be present in the sputum. A solitary choroidal granuloma or a multifocal choroiditis can be present. Periphlebitis of the retinal veins is another feature.

The toxoplasmosis patient may have a history of exposure to cats. The mother of the patient may have been exposed to cats as well. The eating of undercooked meats and unclean vegetables are also etiological factors. The chorioretinitis is sometimes bilateral as can be an anterior uveitis. An old pigmented chorioretinal scar may be near a new yellow chorioretinal lesion seen hazily through the dense fog of a vitritis (headlight in the fog).

Syphilis, the great masquerader can present with nongranulomatous as well as granulomatous uveitis. Ocular disease is usually seen during the secondary stage, but it can be seen in all three stages. When the diagnosis of ocular syphilis is made, HIV should be ruled out and vice versa as there may be overlapping risk factors. The patient with secondary syphilis presents with a generalized maculopapular rash that involves the palms and soles. A positive VDRL (earlier) and a positive FTA-ABS test (later) will be present. Many diseases including Lyme can give false positive tests for syphilis. If one performs an anterior chamber tap on a patient with iritis who has secondary syphilis, one may demonstrate by dark field microscopy the presence of Treponema pallidum. A neuroretinitis might accompany the anterior uveitis. Retinal artery and vein occlusions are sometimes seen. The treatment must be treatment for neurosyphilis.

The patient with herpes zoster (HZV) involving the eye will demonstrate the typical painful vesicular rash, usually unilateral. A panuveitis might accompany the dermatologic findings. An optic neuritis and/or an extraocular muscle problem can be present. The cornea may show dendrites (without the terminal bulbs). There is hyposensitivity of the cornea and an acute retinal necrosis occasionally can be present. The patient usually develops HZV only once. Herpes simplex types one and two can cause an iridocyclitis. The latter can be accompanied by a panuveitis occasionally. If the uveitis has not been preceded by a keratitis, the correct diagnosis of the recurrent herpetic uveitis might not be made until much later in the course of the disease. Typically, the herpes simplex patient presents with a dendritic keratitis (dendrite with terminal bulbs) and the corneal sensitivity is diminished. The anterior uveitis may be accompanied by elevated intraocular pressure. A panuveitis is occasionally accompanied by acute retinal necrosis. Viral studies of corneal scraping smears, culture, and even polymerase chain reaction testing can be confirmatory.

The Behcet's disease patient will have an HLAB51 genetic predisposition. This rare disease of mostly younger patients is thought to be caused by a generalized vasculitis. Pulmonary artery aneurysm, GI, cardiac and neurological problems may be present. An anterior chamber hypopyon may be seen. Retinal artery and vein occlusion may develop. Oral ulcers are frequently present, and genital ulcers and erythema nodosum can occur as well. The disease is more common in Middle Eastern, Mediterranean, and Asian populations.

Intraocular lymphoma can present with what looks like bilateral posterior (and anterior) uveitis. Glaucoma, uveitis, and neuro-ophthalmic signs are sometimes part of the diagnostic picture. While steroids are helpful in the beginning, they do not help for long. A vitreous biopsy [10] (with appropriate cell studies, cytokine analysis, and PCR demonstrating neoplastic B cells) should be done. An MRI of the brain will reveal an intraocular lymphoma. Primary intraocular lymphoma is less common than extension from brain parenchymal primary CNS lymphoma. This disease is not only sight threatening but life threatening .

Previous data indicates that young males (more prone to accidental injuries than females) and the elderly (more prone to falls) presented with SO in higher numbers than did patients who had undergone intraocular surgery. Present data indicates less SO patients among young males as our societies have adopted more accident precautions. Obviously, if our societies engage in more wars, our young men and women might experience injuries to their eyes which could result in a higher SO incidence. Surgery on the elderly now is the major etiological component behind SO statistics today [11]. Vitreoretinal operations including pars plana vitrectomy, multiple ocular procedures on the same eye, cataract and glaucoma operations (the cyclodestruction operations) contribute to the number of patients who develop SO. Thus, while 0.2–0.5% of traumatic injuries result in SO, and only 0.01% of planned surgical cases develop SO, the total number of patients who develop SO after scheduled intraocular procedures exceeds the total number of patients who develop SO following traumatic injuries. More people receive planned intraocular procedures than people who sustain traumatic globe injuries.

The histological findings in SO reveal lymphocyte, macrophage [11], and giant cells infiltrating the entire uveal tract. This is a bilateral disease. CD4 T cells are present in the early stages of the disease, followed by CD8 T cells in the later stages (an attempt at downregulation). B cells are seen in 5–15% of choroidal infiltrates. Patient with HIV may not develop SO until their immune status is restored after HAART. [12] S. antigen [13], photopsin [14] interphotoreceptor retinoid binding antigen [15], recoverin [16], and melanin antigens [17] are possible stimuli that may play a role in the development of the delayed cellular SO response, a class 4 immune response. In the intact eye, these and other antigens are sequestered in the privileged inside compartment of the eye [18]. These antigens may travel via the bloodstream to the spleen and blocking antibodies may form, but all is quiet. However, when uveal (and or retinal) tissue antigens exit the eye secondary to ocular injury, and when these antigens get to conjunctival lymphatics, they are transported to regional lymph modes where an immune response is launched. The latter has been studied in the laboratory by Chan et al. who injected melanin [19] subconjunctivally into experimental animals and produced experimental autoimmune uveitis OU.

Gelatinase B [20] and metalloproteinases are involved in leukocyte recruitment and in T and B cell activation. Tumor necrosis factor [21] upregulation (along with its receptor, nitric oxide synthase) in SO may result in nitration of mitochondrial cell products such as cytochrome C which is located on the inner segments of the photoreceptor, leading to photoreceptor apoptosis. M1 Macrophages and their cytokines make up the lava of SO and add to the destruction caused by this bilateral disease. These three areas of research may result in new avenues of SO treatment.

It has been reported that most cases of SO develop in the first 2–3 months after eye injury. Ninety percent were alleged to have occurred by 1 year. Many more cases are being reported in patients 1 year post injury. Classically, enucleation of the totally blind eye injured with no visual potential was advised to be done between 10 days to two weeks post injury. But sympathetic ophthalmia has developed as early as 5 days and as late as 66 years post injury [22]. Is there a grace period that fits one and all? Different genetic makeups, different quantities of uveitis antigens spilling onto the conjunctiva, different times of primary repair after injury are all factors affecting that answer.

Classical teaching advises that SO is less frequently associated with enucleation, compared with evisceration. There is even debate as to whether enucleation can prevent SO's development. After all, SO has developed in a patient who underwent enucleation as early as 5 days post injury [23]. Is 5 days too long a grace period? One report cites no cases of SO developing after over 500 eviscerations [24]. While there are certainly reports of SO following enucleation to prevent SO development, we still would recommend enucleation over evisceration as the surgeon's ability to completely eliminate all the uveal tissues and retinal tissue from inside the scleral shell may not always be possible in evisceration procedures. Many oculoplastic surgeons do, however, favor evisceration over enucleation for cosmetic reasons. At present, there is a shift toward evisceration over enucleation in terms of prevention, as the superiority of enucleation over evisceration as a method of prevention is debatable. If SO develops in a patient who has undergone early and meticulous repair of a ruptured globe, enucleation and evisceration have not been shown to ameliorate the SO or to result in a better outcome. Lubins reported in 1980 that enucleation done within 2 weeks of SO development resulted in better visual outcome. Chic and Foster, in 2002 [25] found no improvement in outcome when enucleation was preformed after SO developed. Bilyk [26] found no benefit in terms of visual outcome when enucleation was performed after SO developed. In fact, the inciting eye might end up with better vision.

The pharmacologic management of SO includes corticosteroids; cytotoxic agents such as chlorambucil [27], cyclosporine [28], a T-cell inhibitor with renal and hepatic toxicity, and biological agents such as anti-interleukin 2 therapy [29]. Steroids can be combined with cytotoxic agents or cyclosporine, allowing for steroid sparing. As steroids can cause hypertension, diabetes, osteoporosis, necrosis of the femoral head, and susceptibility to infection, the ophthalmologist will need the rheumatologist, internist or oncologist to monitor the patient with SO. The use of the intravitreal steroid implant [30] can help control the uveitis for up to 2.5 years and thus lessen the amount of steroid and other systemic medicines needed to control the SO.

In evaluating how well our SO patients are doing on the pharmacologic agents employed, we rely on the slit lamp exam, contact lens and indirect ophthalmoscopic exam of the retina, and ancillary studies. The B scan [31] will aid in the study of choroidal thickening. The OCT [32] can be used to follow the resolution of exudative retinal detachment. ICG and FA studies can delineate areas of retinal staining and pooling of fluid in areas of retinal detachment. Pharmacologic agents can be increased or supplemented with different agents based on the clinical conclusion reached by the above comprehensive approach to treatment response.

In conclusion we believe the ophthalmologist should:

(1) Perform early and meticulous repair of the rupture globe to lessen the amount of uveal tissue (and or retinal) antigen that might be taken by the lymphatics to the regional lymph nodes.
(2) Perform early enucleation or evisceration only in cases of no vision or useful visual potential as an attempt to prevent the development of SO.
(3) Perform no enucleation or evisceration once SO has developed.
(4) Use local and systemic corticosteroids in high doses. Add cytotoxic agents, cyclosporine and/or biologicals when needed. This should be done in conjunction with internal medicine, oncology, or rheumatology.
(5) Co-manage with retinal service who may wish to use an intravitreal implant.

References

1. Serpell G. Sir William Mackenzie: sympathetic ophthalmia and glaucoma before ophthalmoscopy. ANZ J Surg. 2009;79:926–9 (Royal Australian College of Surgeons, Monash Medical Center Melbourne, Victoria, Australian).
2. Chin C, Whitcups S, Nussenblatt R. Sympathetic Ophthalmia and Vogt-Koyanagi-Harada Syndrome Chapter 51 in Duane's textbook of ophthalmology. 2010.
3. Chin C, Whitcups S, Nussenblatt R. Thirty two cases of sympathetic ophthalmia retrospective study at notional eye institute from 1982–1992. Arch Ophthalmol. 1995;113(5):579–600.
4. Albert DM, Diaz-Rohena R. A historical review of sympathetic ophthalmia and its epidemiology. Surv Ophthalmol. 1989;34:1–14.
5. Chaithanyaa N, Devireddy S, Kumar K, Gali R, Aneja V. Sympathetic ophthalmia: a review of the literation. Oral Surg Oral Med Oral Pathol Oral Radiol. 2012;113(2):172–6.
6. O'Keefe S, Leng T. Sympathetic ophthalmia. American Academy Ophthalmology. 2014 Eye Wiki.
7. Chan CC, Benezra D, Rodriguez M, Hsu M, Palestine A, Murphee A, Nussenblatt R. Immunohistochemistry and microscopy of choroidal infiltration and Dalen-Fuchs nodules in sympathetic Ophthalmia. Ophthalmology. 1985;92(4):580–90.
8. Davis J, Mittal K, Freidlin V, Mellow S, Optican D, Palestine A, Nussenblatt R. HLA association and ancestry in VKH disease and sympathetic ophthalmia. Ophthalmology. 1990;97(9):1137–42.
9. Reynard M, Riffenburgh R, Minkler D. Morphologic variations of Dalen-Fuchs nodules in sympathetic ophthalmia. Br J Ophthalmol. 1985;69(3):197–201.

10. Gonzalez J, Chan C. Biopsy techniques ad yields in diagnosing primary intraocular lymphoma. Int Ophthalmol. 2007;27(4):241–50.
11. Chin C, Nussenblatt RB, Fujikawa LS, Palestine A, Stevens G, Parver LM, Luckenbach M. Immunohistochemistry and election microscopy of choroidal infiltration and Dalen Fuchs nodules in sympathetic ophthalmia. Ophthalmology. 1985;92(4):580–90.
12. De La Fuente MA, Alejandra N, Ferner P, Fernandez G, Sarasa J, Sanchez O. Sympathetic ophthalmia in HIV injection, a clinicopathologic case report. J Ophthalmia Inflammation Injection. 2012;2 (3):161–4.
13. Kozak Y, Sakai J, Thillaye B, Faure JP. S antigen—induced experimental autoimmune neuro-retinitis in rats. Current Eye Res. 1981;1(6):327–37.
14. Schalkenm J, Winkens H, VanVugt H, DeGrip W, Broekhuyse R. Rhodopsin induced experimental autoimmune uveoretinitis in monkeys. Br J Ophthalmol. 1989;73(3):168–72.
15. Grey I, Wiggert B, Redmond TM, Kuwabara, T. Uveoretinitis and pinealitis induced by immunization with interphotoreceptor retinoid-binding protein. Invest Ophthalmol Vis Sci. 1986;27(8):1296–300.
16. Chu X, Chan C. Sympathetic ophthalmia: to the twenty first century and beyond. J Inflammation Infections. 2013;3(1):49.
17. Chan CC, Hikita N, Dastgheib K. Experimental melanin—protein-induced uveitis in the Lewis rat. Immunologic Process Ophthalmol. 1994;101 (7):1275–1280.
18. Barker C, Billinghanic RE. Immunoloically privileged sites. Adv Immunol. 1977;25:1.
19. Chan C, Hakiti N, Dastgheib K, Whitcups S, Gray J, Nussenblatt R. Experimental melanin—protein induced uveitis in the Lewis Rat. Ophthalmology. 1994;101:1275–80.
20. Struyf S, Van Den Broeck C, Van Damme J, Opdenakker G, Geboes K, Kestelyn P. Expression of chemokines and gelatinase in sympathetic ophthalmia. Eye. 2007;3(5):649–57.
21. Parikh J, Saraswathy S, Rao N. Photoreceptor oxidative damage in sympathetic ophthalmia. Am J Ophthalmol. 2008;140(6):866–75.
22. Furusato E, Shine D, Cao X, Furusato B, Nussenblatt RB, Rushing E, Chan C. Inflammatory cytokine and chemokine expression in SO: pathology study. Histopathology. 2011;3(9):1145–51.
23. Arevalo J, Garcia R, Al-Dhibi H, Sanchez J. Update on sympathetic ophthalmia. Middle East Afr J Ophthalmol. 2012;19(1):13.
24. Phan L, Hwang T, McCulley T. Evisceration in the modern age. Middles East Afr J Ophthalmol. 2012;19(1):24.
25. Lubins J, Albert D, Weinstein M. Sixty five years of SO: a clinicopathologic rev. Ophthalmology. 1980;87:109–21.
26. Chu D, Foster C. Sympathetic ophthalmia. Int Ophthalmol Clin. 2002;42(3):179–185.
27. Bilyk J. Enucleation, evisceration, and sympathetic ophthalmia. Curr Opin Ophthalmol. 2000;11(5):372–86.
28. Yang C, Liu J. Chlorambucil therapy in sympathetic ophthalmia. Am J Ophthalmol. 1995;119(4):482–8.
29. Demico F, Kiss S, Young, L. Seminars in ophthalmology. 2005;20:191–197.
30. Pasadhika S, Rosenbaum J. Update on the use of systemic biological agents in the treatment of non-infectious uveitis. Biologics. 2014;8:67–81.
31. Myoung J, Asker G, Kiss S. Treatment of noninfectious positive uveitis with dexamethasone—intraocular implant. Clin Ophthalmol. 2010;4:1423–1426.
32. Castiblanco C, Adelman R. Imaging for SO: impact on diagnosis and management. Int Ophthalmol Clin. 2012;52(4):173–181.

Optic Nerve, Visual Pathways, Oculomotor System, and Consequences of Intracranial Injury

12

Valerie I. Elmalem, Laura Palazzolo and Marib Akanda

Introduction

The spectrum of neuro-ophthalmic injury is wide, involving decreased visual acuity, oculomotor injury, visual field deficits, and/or blindness [1]. The neuro-ophthalmic status of a trauma patient should be carefully reviewed following high impact trauma, especially in cases of head injury [2]. Signs of neuro-ophthalmic involvement may be difficult to assess if the patient is obtunded or comatose, yet early management is often critical to prevent severe morbidity or mortality.

This chapter describes traumatic damage to the optic nerve, visual pathways, and oculomotor system. The material will enable the practitioner to recognize neuro-ophthalmic manifestations of eye and head trauma, promptly diagnose, and efficiently manage these patients.

V.I. Elmalem (✉) · L. Palazzolo · M. Akanda
Department of Ophthalmology, The State University of New York (SUNY) Downstate Medical Center, 450 Clarkson Avenue, Box 58, Brooklyn, NY 11203, USA
e-mail: valerie.elmalem@downstate.edu

L. Palazzolo
e-mail: laura.palazzolo@downstate.edu

M. Akanda
e-mail: marib.akanda@downstate.edu

Imaging in Orbital and Head Trauma

CT Imaging of the Orbit

CT scanners acquire multiple X-rays from various angles to produce cross-sectional images. Tissues are assigned radiodensity based on an attenuation scale measured in Hounsfield units (HU). Water is assigned an attenuation of 0 HU, air is -1000 HU, soft tissue is usually in the range of +10 to +60, bone is +700 to around +1000 depending on the density, and metal is usually well above +1000. Since we are unable to distinguish over 1000 shades of grey in a single image, CT images are usually acquired in a specified narrow range, also called windowing (e.g. - soft tissue or bone window). Coronal, sagittal and axial slices of the same region are obtained using multiplanar reconstruction (MPR) and maximum intensity projection (MIP) to allow visualization of surrounding structures in different image planes.

CT scans can be used to visualize the bony structure of the orbit as well as the soft tissues including the extraocular muscles and nerves. In Fig. 12.1, the four rectus muscles and superior oblique muscles are visible as grey regions arranged around each optic nerve, which is grey and labeled "o." The bony orbit itself is white.

As evidenced in Fig. 12.1, the orbital and paraorbital bony anatomy is easily visualized in CT imaging and can help determine if bony pathology such as fractures are present. Although MRI has significant advantages to CT as described below, CT may be the only option

S.C. Kaufman and D.R. Lazzaro (eds.), *Textbook of Ocular Trauma*,
DOI 10.1007/978-3-319-47633-9_12

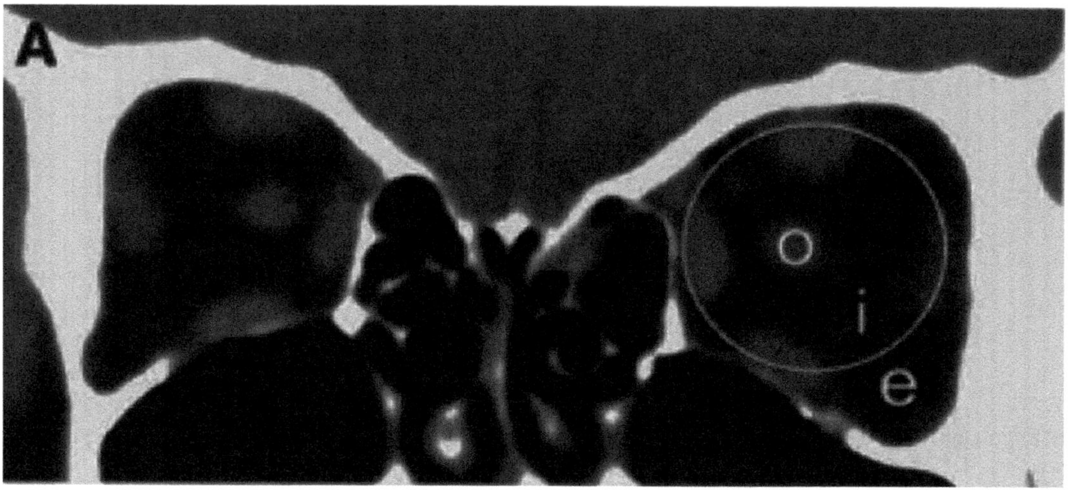

Fig. 12.1 Coronal CT image (soft tissue window) demonstrating bony anatomy and extraocular muscles of the orbit: *o* optic nerve, *i* intraconal space, *e* extraconal space, *circle* border between intraconal and extraconal spaces formed by connecting the extraocular muscles. *Source* Fig. 1 from van der Pol C, Chakraborty S, Nguyen T, Torres C, Glikstein R, Gao J. Imaging Anatomy and Pathology of Extraocular Muscles in Adults. Canadian Association of Radiologists Journal [serial online]. November 2014;65(4):366–371 6p. Reprinted with permission from Elsevier

Table 12.1 Appearance of various tissue types in unenhanced T1 and T2 weighted MRI images

Tissue	T1	T2
Air	Very dark	Very dark
Blood, acute	Dark to intermediate	Dark
Blood, chronic	Dark rim with variable center	Dark rim with variable center
Blood, hyperacute	Intermediate	Intermediate
Blood, subacute	Bright rim	Bright
Bone, cortical	Very dark	Very dark
Bone, marrow	Bright	Intermediate
Cortical gray matter	Dark	Bright
Cerebrospinal fluid	Very dark	Very bright
Fat	Very bright	Intermediate to dark
Muscle	Dark	Dark
Optic nerve	Dark to intermediate	Intermediate
Proteinaceous fluid	Intermediate to bright	Intermediate
Sclera	Dark to intermediate	Intermediate
Vitreous	Dark	Bright
Water	Very dark	Very bright
White matter	Bright	Dark

Adapted from Table 2.1 of Dutton [5]
Available from: Discovery eBooks, Ipswich, MA. Accessed January 30, 2016. Permission received from Clinical Key.

in cases with ferromagnetic metallic foreign bodies. The low cost of CT and ability for rapid acquisition of images make it preferable in the immediate evaluation of trauma, as its resolution still allows for adequate visualization of key structures such as the ophthalmic artery and ocular motor nerves [3].

MR Imaging of the Orbit

MRI provides the advantage over CT of improved visualization of the soft tissues without obscuration by surrounding bony structures, and additionally avoids exposing the patient to ionizing radiation. Weighting of the MRI changes how structures appear [brighter (hyperintense) or darker (hypointense)] based on time for longitudinal and horizontal relaxation of the magnetic moments. In T1 weighted images, tissues with shorter times for longitudinal relaxation will appear brighter, while those with longer times for longitudinal relaxation will appear darker. In T2 weighted images, the same concept applies but for horizontal relaxation times. Table 12.1 elaborates on which particular tissues appear bright or dark on T1 versus T2 imaging.

(a) (b) (c) (d)

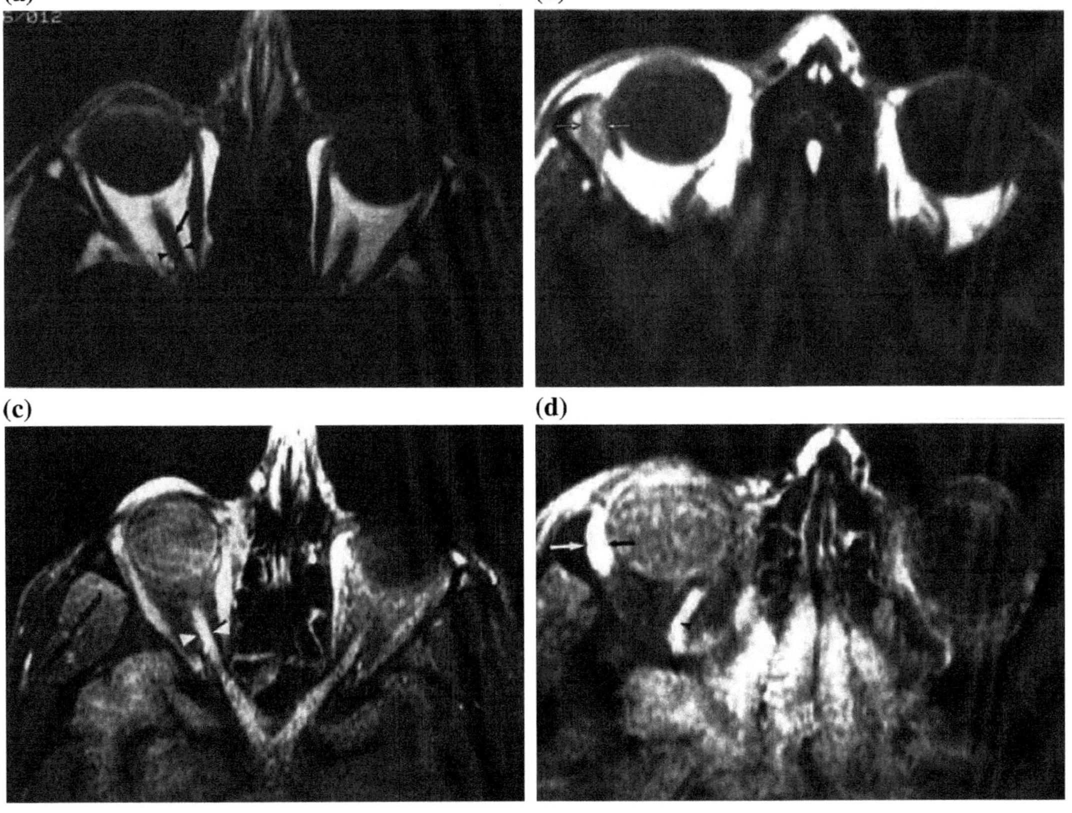

Fig. 12.2 The effects of fat suppression in imaging of normal orbital anatomy demonstrated by axial T1 weighted MRI (**a**, **b**) and axial T1-weighted MRI with fat suppression (**c**, **d**). **a** Hyperintense fat around normal structures produces an artifact (*arrow*) that causes the optic nerve to appear enlarged (*arrowheads*). **b** Hyperintense fat obscures visualization of the lacrimal gland (*between arrows*). **c** Fat suppression better reveals the optic nerve (*arrowheads*) against low-intensity CSF. **d** Fat suppression also increases the contrast between the lacrimal gland (between *arrows*) and surrounding structures, and allows for visualization of the superior ophthalmic vein (*arrowhead*), which is now hyperintense compared to the suppressed fat. From J Simon, J Szumowski, S Totterman, D Kido, S Ekholm, A Wicks, and D Plewes. Fat suppression MR imaging of the orbit. AMNR 1988 9:961–8. Reprinted with permission from American Journal of Neuroradiology

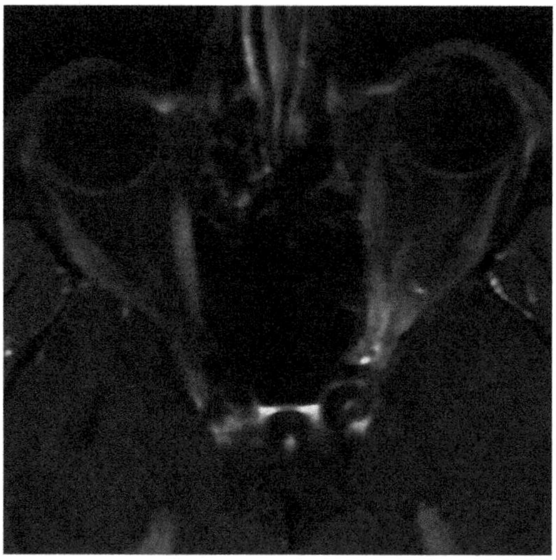

Fig. 12.3 Axial T1 image with gadolinium and fat saturation of the orbits showing enhancement of the soft tissue structures in the left orbital apex. This patient presented with painful ophthalmoplegia and proptosis. *Source* From Ferreira et al. [262]. Reprinted with permission from Science Direct

The preferred imaging in ocular trauma is currently high-resolution T1 MRI of the brain and orbits with contrast and fat suppression sequences [4]. The fat suppression prevents intraconal and extraconal fat from obscuring other enhancing lesions with its own bright signal and can be performed by using chemical shift imaging or short T1 inversion recovery sequences (STIR) [5]. The benefit of fat suppression is illustrated in Fig. 12.2 for normal anatomy.

As seen in Fig. 12.2, axial images can be used to evaluate many of the structures of the orbit, such as the optic nerve and superior ophthalmic vein. The level of the axial slice can demonstrate some structures together in one image, such as the lateral and medial rectus muscles if the slice is taken at the level of the optic nerve. Axial images can also be used to identify important structures before and during their passage through the orbital apex, as in Fig. 12.3, where inflammatory changes at the left orbital apex can be visualized.

Mid-sagittal MR images of the orbit are able to demonstrate the globe, extraocular muscles, optic nerve, and surrounding fat and bony structure. In the sagittal image in Fig. 12.4, the superior and inferior rectus muscles as well as the inferior rectus and orbicularis oculi muscles are dark grey structures shown along their course to the globe. Sagittal images taken more lateral or medial would demonstrate more of the extraocular muscle anatomy and omit the optic nerve (not shown). T2-weighted gradient refocused-echo (GRE) imaging appeared to improve the evaluation of diffuse axonal injury (DAI) in TBI [6]. In the comparison study between T2 and T2-GRE imaging, more focal traumatic hemorrhages were seen on the GRE imaging as depicted in Fig. 12.5.

Optic Nerve Trauma

Traumatic Optic Neuropathy (Basic Definitions)

Cranial nerve II, the optic nerve, transmits afferent visual inputs from the retina that eventually reach higher cortical processing centers in the occipital lobe. In traumatic optic neuropathy (TON), complete or partial impairment of visual function follows orbital or head trauma due to damage of optic nerve fibers [7, 8].

Direct or indirect forces may damage the optic nerve. Blunt trauma to the head or orbit is the more common cause of TON, termed indirect TON [9]. The force of closed head trauma is transmitted through the surrounding soft tissue and bony optic canal to the optic nerve, disrupting optic nerve fibers [10, 11]. In direct TON, penetrating injury causes direct stress to the optic nerve with resultant anatomical disruption [9, 10, 12]. Direct TON is less common than indirect TON and has a worse prognosis for long-term visual potential [7].

Optic Nerve Anatomy

There are four anatomical divisions of the optic nerve: intraocular (1 mm), intraorbital (24–28 mm), intracanalicular (9 mm), and intracranial (16 mm) (see Fig. 12.6) [11].

Intraocular The intraocular ON is comprised of the optic disc, prelaminar area (anterior to lamina

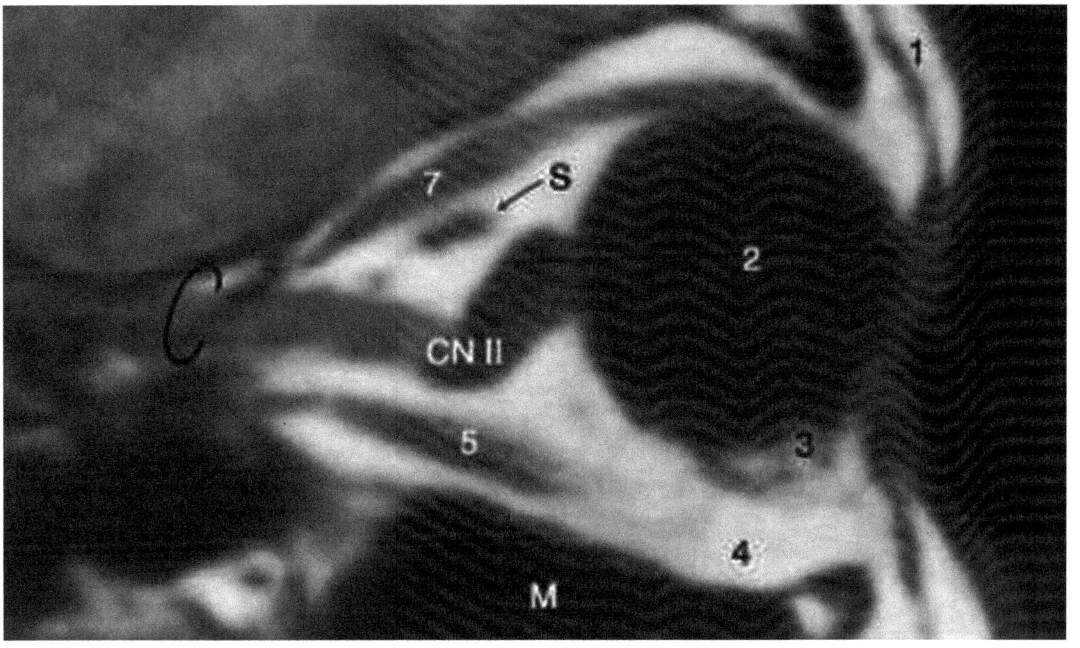

Fig. 12.4 Mid-sagittal T1 MRI, lateral view of the orbit. Orbital contents: *1* orbicularis oculi muscle, *2* globe, *3* inferior oblique muscle, *4* retrobulbar (extraconal) fat, *5* inferior rectus muscle, *7* superior rectus muscle, *S* superior ophthalmic vein, *M* maxillary sinus, *CN II* optic nerve. From Moore K, Dalley A, Agur A. Clinically Oriented Anatomy [e-book]. Philadelphia: Wolters Kluwer Health/Lippincott Williams and Wilkins, 2010; 2010. Available from: SUNY Downstate Brooklyn—Catalog, Ipswich, MA. Reprinted with permission from LWW

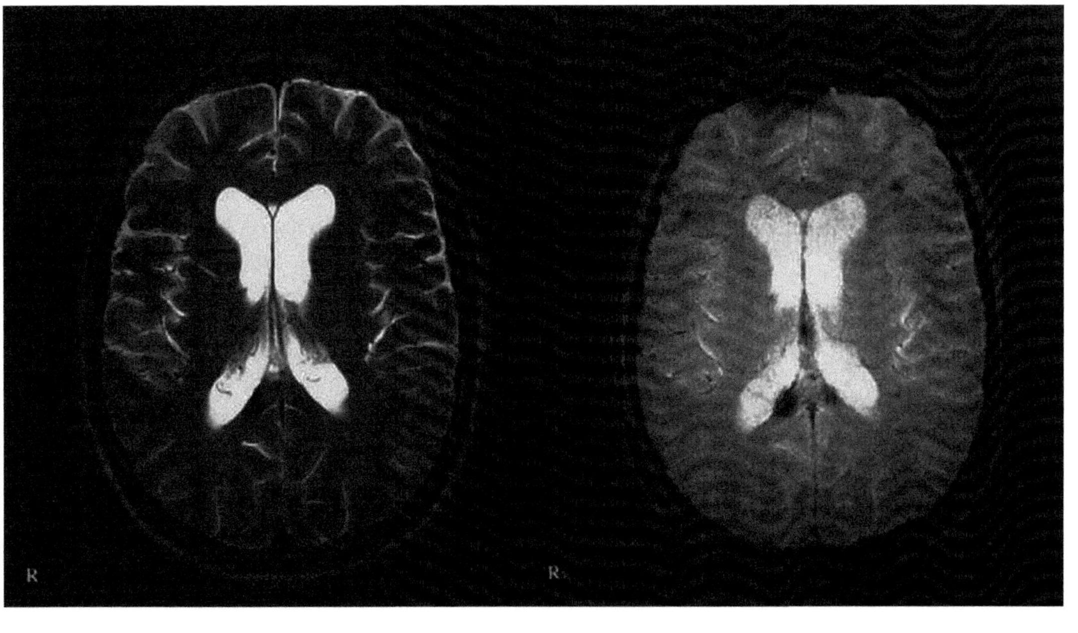

Fig. 12.5 *Left* T2-weighted image of a 42M in a MVA suffering traumatic microbleeds evident in the posterior corpus callosum; *Right* T2-GRE image revealing additional traumatic microbleeds in the left side of the splenium and the gray–white matter junction of the frontal lobes. From Scheid et al. [6]. Reprinted with permission from American Journal of Neuroradiology

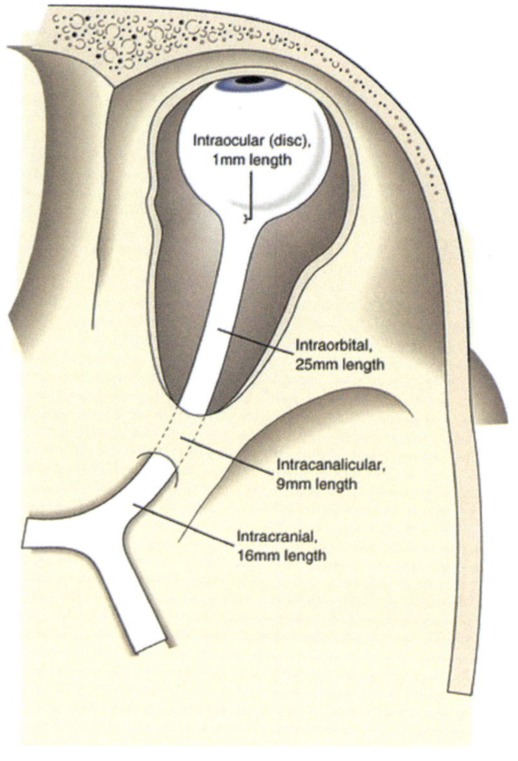

Fig. 12.6 Optic nerve segments. From Yanoff M, Duker JS (eds) Ophthalmology, 2nd edn. St Louis, Mosby, 2004. Reprinted with permission from Elsevier

cribrosa), and laminar area. Beginning at the optic disc, 1.2 million retinal ganglion cell (RGC) axons exit the globe through the scleral canal to form the optic nerve. The RGC axons are physically supported by the lamina cribrosa and metabolically supported by interweaving astrocytes [9]. The lamina cribrosa is a system of 10 connective tissue plates integrated with the sclera, and axon bundles are transmitted through openings in the lamina cribrosa.

Intraorbital Posterior to the lamina cribrosa, the optic nerve fibers are myelinated by oligodendrocytes and surrounded by a meningeal sheath (pia mater, arachnoid mater, and dura mater). At this point, the optic nerve is within the muscle cone of the eye. The intraorbital part of the optic nerve is longer than the distance between the posterior globe and optic canal. This length difference allows for optic nerve laxity in the orbit and facilitates unrestricted globe rotation. Before entering the optic canal, the optic nerve passes through the annulus of Zinn.

Intracanalicular The optic canal travels through the lesser wing of the sphenoid bone. In the optic canal, the dural sheath surrounding the optic nerve fuses with the periosteum and immobilizes the nerve.

Intracranial At the transition from intracanalicular to intracranial segments, the optic nerve passes under a dural fold called the falciform ligament. The final intracranial portion of the optic nerve does not have a dural sheath. The optic nerve terminates at the optic chiasm where the neural fibers continue posteriorly as the optic tracts.

Vascular Supply (see Fig. 12.7). The short posterior ciliary arteries, branches from the ophthalmic artery, provide vascular supply to the optic nerve head. The short posterior ciliary artery distribution has few anastomoses, so the optic nerve head is susceptible to ischemia in cases of poor perfusion [13]. The primary blood supply along the length of the optic nerve is from pial branches of the surrounding meninges. The branches are supplied by the posterior ciliary arteries, which are small branches from the ophthalmic artery. Although the central retinal artery and vein travel within the anterior 10–12 mm of the optic nerve, only a small portion of optic nerve vascular supply is from the central retinal artery (see Table 12.2 and Fig. 12.7).

Optic Nerve Anatomy—Clinical Application to Trauma

The clinical picture of TON varies based on the anatomical site of injury. In posterior optic nerve injury, the most common injury, the optic nerve is damaged posterior to the entry point of the central retinal vessels [12]. In anterior optic nerve injury, a less common presentation, damage is anterior to where the central retinal artery enters the optic nerve. In this injury, visual loss is often

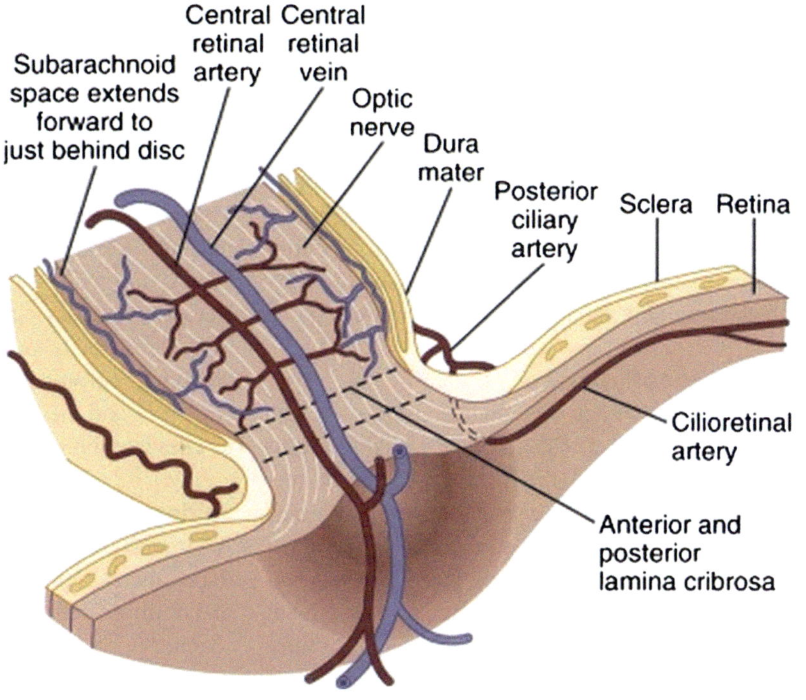

Fig. 12.7 From Balcer LJ and Prasad S, "Abnormalities of the Optic Nerve and Retina". Reprinted with permission from Springer Publishing Company

associated with abnormalities in the retinal circulation [8].

The most common site of optic nerve injury is intracanalicular. In a study of 42 patients with TON, 71.4% of injuries occurred at this location [11, 14]. The dural sheath of the optic nerve is adherent to the periosteum in the optic canal, and such areas of dural sheath attachment are highly susceptible to trauma [14, 15]. Coup and contrecoup forces in blunt head trauma cause the greatest degree of injury at transition sites between mobile and fixed segments of the nerve [16]. Traumatic stress disrupts the pial vessels within the optic canal, and neuropathy may result from decreased vascular supply to the optic nerve [16]. In addition, the majority of blunt forces from frontal head injury are transmitted to the optic foramen [14, 17]. With the direct trajectory of force and the closed, inflexible space of the optic canal, there is higher risk of compression, shearing, contusion, and stretching injuries to the intracanalicular optic nerve [17].

The optic nerve is also susceptible to traumatic forces in the intracranial segment where the optic nerve passes under the falciform dural fold [8]. The falciform dural fold may impinge on the optic nerve and produce shearing forces during blunt trauma [18]. Still, the intracranial

Table 12.2 Regional differences in vascular supply to the optic nerve

Segment	Blood supply
Intraocular Optic disc Prelaminar Laminar	Retinal arterioles Branches of posterior ciliary arteries
Intraorbital	Intraneural branches of central retinal artery; pial branches from CRA and choroid
Intracanalicular	Ophthalmic artery
Intracranial	Branches of internal carotid and ophthalmic arteries

optic nerve is relatively shielded from injury by the surrounding soft tissue and bone. Shearing forces are first absorbed by the intracanalicular optic nerve and often do not reach the intracranial segment [17].

Comparatively, injury of the intraocular optic nerve segment is rare. The intraorbital segment of the optic nerve is usually spared from injury due to its laxity within the orbit and shielding by the surrounding fat and extraocular muscles [17].

TON Pathophysiology

There is an evolving understanding of the pathophysiology of TON, which is likely multifactorial [19, 20]. One perception of indirect TON describes primary and secondary injuries. With primary injury, the immediate outcome of trauma is contusion necrosis [8]. There is irreversible shearing of RGC axons and subsequent RGC degeneration [8, 12, 21]. Secondary injury is caused by optic nerve edema within the rigid optic canal, which produces a compartment syndrome [9]. Edema may be driven by the initial trauma or the resultant ischemia. The optic nerve is highly susceptible to edema from ischemia, inflammation, or compressive forces because its axonal transport system has a high-energy requirement and is easily disrupted. The compartment syndrome exacerbates ischemia by further limiting blood supply to the RGCs, and many RGCs undergo apoptosis [12]. Because primary injury is irreversible, TON treatments focus on limiting secondary injury. Evolving protocols include neuroprotection strategies and medical or surgical decompression to alleviate the edema [21–23].

Epidemiology and Mechanism

A large 2009 survey of patients in the UK estimates the minimum incidence of TON as 1 per one million people per year [24]. TON occurs secondary to head injuries (see Table 12.3). In prospective studies, the incidence of TON following head trauma varies between 0.5 and 5%

Table 12.3 Reports on common mechanisms of TON

Author/References	Cases	MVA/bicycle accident	Fall	Assault	Other
Pirouzmand [27]	50	32 (64%)	12 (24%)	5 (10%)	1 (2%)
Urolagin [32]	8	7 (88%)	–	–	1 (12%)
Roccia [37]	14	5 (36%)	4 (28%)	1	4 (28%)
Lee [24]	121	26 (22%)	31 (26%)	26 (20%)	38 (31%)
Lubben [40]	65	30 (46%)	–	7 (11%)	33 (51%)
Kountakis [41]	34	19 (54%)	9 (26%)	5 (15%)	–
Levin (IONTS) [28]	133	58 (46%)	27 (21%)	18 (14%)	24 (19%)
Joseph [42]	14	5 (35%)	4 (29%)	3 (21.4%)	2 (14%)
Seiff [43]	36	15 (42%)	13 (36%)	4 (11%)	4 (11%)
Spoor [44]	21	10 (48%)	3 (14%)	8 (38%)	0 (0%)
Lessell [29]	33	22 (67%)	8 (24%)	2 (6%)	1 (3%)
Millesi [45]	29	18 (62%)	6 (21%)	5 (17%)	–
Nau et al. [39]	18	9 (50%)	5 (28%)	1 (6%)	–
Anderson [14]	7	4 (57%)	2 (12%)	–	–
Matsuzaki [46]	33	20 (60%)	7 (21%)	4 (12%)	2 (6%)
Bodian [47]	6	4 (67%)	2 (33%)	–	–
Total	622	284 (46%)	133 (21%)	89 (14%)	110 (18%)

Adapted and updated from Walsh and Hoyt's Clinical Neuro-ophthalmology with permission from Dr. N.R. Miller. "Other" includes injuries from falling objects, iatrogenic (after FESS), gardening accidents, explosive accidents, and sport accidents [24, 37, 40] of closed head injuries [8, 19, 20]. In adult patients, the predominant mechanisms of TON include falls, assault, and motor vehicle accidents (MVAs; see Table 12.3). In pediatric populations, mechanisms for TON are similar and primarily include falls from a height, MVAs, and sports injuries [25, 26]. TON is more frequently diagnosed in men and younger patients, averaging around 30 years old [7, 24, 27–29]

In patients with mid-facial fractures, 2.5% develop TON [30]. The likelihood of TON increases with more severe head trauma. There is 6–10% rate for patients with zygomaticomaxillary complex fractures [19, 31, 32], and patients with nasoethmoid complex fracture have 1.6 times greater chance of developing TON [27].

Less common causes of TON in adults are secondary to recreation-associated trauma during sports or iatrogenic [24]. Iatrogenic TON has been identified secondary to orbital surgery [33], osteotomies [34, 35], facial fracture repair [36, 37], and endoscopic sinus surgery [32, 38].

Other serious injuries often coexist, including orbital wall fractures, closed globe injuries (both anterior and posterior segment), ocular adnexal injuries to eyelid, extraocular muscles, orbital foreign body, skull fractures, and intracranial bleeding [24, 29]. However, it is difficult to predict the likelihood of TON solely based on the severity of the trauma [39].

Diagnostic Work-Up

History The diagnosis of TON is primarily clinical [9, 10]. There are often delays to diagnosis if the patient presents with impaired consciousness or unstable condition secondary to multisystem trauma [10, 19, 48]. The history frequently reveals a mechanism of head trauma, as stated above, followed by subjective decrease in visual acuity. Detailed questions should be asked about the mechanism of trauma, including the potential for ocular foreign bodies with penetrating injury. Determine the time course for visual change and time when the injury occurred [11]. Also investigate the patient's past ocular history, including any previous trauma or surgery to the involved eye.

Physical Examination If there is suspicion for TON, assess pupillary reactivity, visual acuity (VA), visual fields, and color vision, perform a funduscopic examination on all patients. Examination may be limited due to lid ecchymosis, edema, or other extensive facial trauma [49].

Pupillary Examination The most reliable early sign of optic nerve dysfunction is the presence of a relative afferent pupillary defect (RAPD) [20]. A RAPD will be present with the exception of bilateral and symmetric TON [10, 11]. This can be examined regardless of a patient's level of consciousness, so it is an invaluable measure for the diagnosis of TON in unconscious patients [39].

Visual Acuity Testing Patients with TON often have an acute decrease in VA following trauma. Occasionally, decrease in VA is delayed over weeks secondary to inflammation and edema or development of an optic nerve sheath hematoma [8, 20]. Visual acuity is often 20/400 or less in the affected eye [10]. In studies, 40–60% of patients initially present with light perception or worse [24, 32, 44].

Visual Field Testing Variable visual field defects are observed following TON. Commonly observed visual field defects following TBI are scattered visual field loss (58%) and homonymous visual field defects (22%) measured by confrontation method [50, 51]. If there is partial optic nerve avulsion, visual field loss will correspond to the location of injury [15].

Color Vision Testing Color vision is often decreased in TON. In one report, 76% of patients with TON visualized 12/17 or fewer Ishihara color plates [24].

Fundus Examination Findings of a RAPD and a normal fundus examination increase the likelihood of TON. In posterior optic nerve injury, the fundus appears normal during the early clinical stage [12, 24]. With an anterior optic nerve injury, there may be optic disc swelling, dilated and tortuous retinal veins, or retinal hemorrhages

[11, 15, 24]. Optic atrophy develops over the following weeks, and becomes evident 4–6 weeks after injury [9, 11, 19]. Therefore, it is useful to monitor patients with repeated dilated fundus examinations following closed head trauma. Of note, the fundus examination may initially be difficult to complete if there is coexisting intraocular hemorrhage (IOH), thus a repeat fundus examination should be performed at a later date in these instances.

Additional Physical Examination Assess ocular adnexa for other effects of trauma, including crepitus or step-off from orbital fractures [10]. Evaluate for oculomotor dysfunction, including ability to perform extraocular movements, strabismus, and accommodative and vergence defects [52]. Identify proptosis, which may be associated with intraorbital hemorrhage and can be difficult to diagnose if there is also periorbital swelling. Complete a full ophthalmic examination to identify additional ocular consequences of head trauma, such as corneal abrasion, traumatic cataract, and vitreous prolapse [53].

Imaging Imaging has uncertain clinical value. There is no consistent correlation between the finding of an optic canal fracture, the severity of visual loss, and the prognosis for visual recovery [17].

Computerized Tomography (CT) CT is the best imaging tool to identify optic canal fracture, intracranial mass lesion, such as a hematoma, subluxated lenses, or other specific pathology compromising the optic nerve [11, 19]. There is no clear protocol for imaging studies in the diagnosis of TON. Some clinicians use CT scan for all cases, while others reserve imaging based on clinical severity or when contemplating the need for therapeutic interventions [20]. For example, CT imaging is part of surgical planning for optic nerve decompression [10, 49].

Magnetic Resonance Imaging (MRI) MRI is an alternate imaging modality to assess intracranial mass lesions. It is used for patients with a clear history of trauma and no likelihood of metallic foreign bodies. However, MRI may be difficult to perform in critically injured patients [19].

Ultrasound B-scan ultrasonography is an inexpensive imaging modality that can be used in closed orbit injury [11]. It has demonstrated utility for early diagnosis of traumatic optic nerve avulsion. Optic nerve avulsion is often associated with concomitant vitreous hemorrhage that obstructs visualization of the fundus, and B-scan allows visualization despite intraocular bleeding [54].

Visual Evoked Potentials (VEP) Flash visual evoked potential (FVEP) is a useful form of VEP because it can be performed in patients despite level of consciousness, lid hematomas, or refraction abnormalities [39]. VEP should be measured in both eyes, with the uninjured eye as a control [11]. The presence and amplitude of VEP predicts visual outcome in TON [55]. Deformed evoked potentials correlate with morphological changes of the optic nerve and measurements of reduced pupillary reactivity [39].

Fluorescein Angiography (FA) FA is used in the evaluation of anterior optic nerve injury, such as understanding the degree of retinal vessel involvement in optic nerve avulsion [56, 57].

Prognosis

In patients with indirect TON, there is a correlation between initial and final visual acuity. Patients who are NLP on presentation have little or no visual acuity improvement regardless of medical, surgical, or conservative management [7, 43, 58]. If there is no visual recovery after 48 h, the prognosis for final visual improvement is poor [20, 59]. Furthermore, younger patients have greater likelihood of visual recovery [60].

Measurements of the RAPD with neutral density filters indicate that patients with an initial RAPD of 2.1 log units or less can have visual acuity improve to 20/30 or better, while patients with an initial RAPD of 2.1 log units or greater have little visual improvement [17, 61].

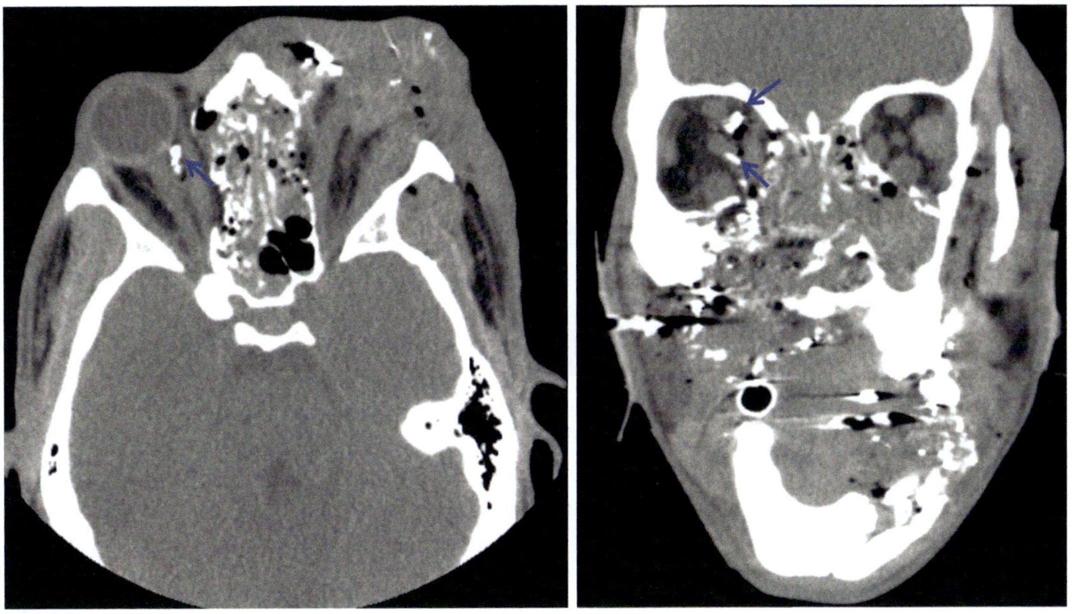

Fig. 12.8 Case study. This patient is status post gunshot wound to the face. On presentation, VA NLP OU. Bone fragments identified in the right orbit (*arrows*) causing direct trauma to the anterior medial intraorbital segment of the optic nerve. Severely traumatized left ruptured globe required primary enucleation with implant

Loss of consciousness following trauma is associated with a poor visual prognosis [20]. This finding may be related to a higher impact injury. Similarly, the presence of an orbital fracture is associated with smaller improvements from initial to final visual acuity due to a greater force of traumatic impact and greater severity of optic nerve trauma [7, 62]. Patients with anterior orbital fractures have more visual acuity recovery than patients with posterior orbital fractures [62]. Patients with optic canal fractures have varied success with visual recovery [19, 20].

VEP can also predict patient prognosis for visual function. FVEP amplitudes that are 50% of normal greater predict a good visual outcome of 20/30 or better (compared to the uninjured eye) [20]. Initial absence of visual evoked responses is associated with minimal, if any, visual recovery and final visual acuity of 20/300 or less [19, 55].

Compared to indirect TON, direct TON has a poor prognosis in all cases. There is acute, severe visual loss and to date no clinical interventions have demonstrated significant benefit for vision recovery [7, 20].

Examples of Direct TON

Direct trauma to the optic nerve may result from fractures of the optic canal, injury, or compression by bony fragments (Fig. 12.8), penetrating foreign bodies, or mass effect such as an expanding hematoma [63]. The causes of direct optic nerve injury can be distinguished with physical examination and imaging techniques. Generally, the diagnosis of direct TON is best detected radiographically with CT [63].

Treatment strategies are often limited. However, patients have been documented to regain vision [64]. A direct optic nerve injury may irreversibly damage one section of the involved nerve, but leave other areas with the potential for visual recovery [15, 64].

Traumatic optic nerve avulsion

Optic nerve avulsion is a rarely reported form of anterior optic nerve injury [54]. Due to the

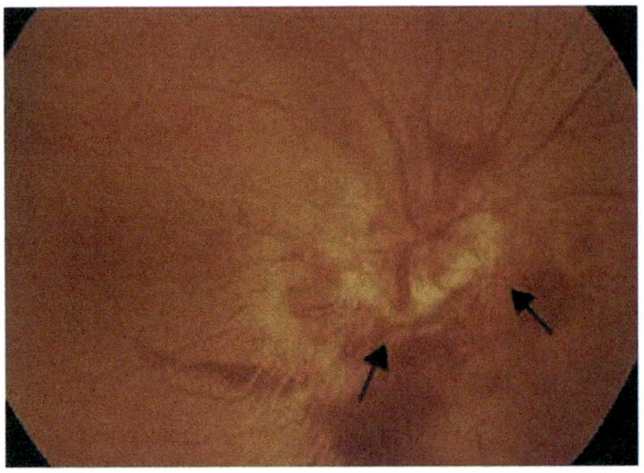

Fig. 12.9 Fundus photography demonstrating traumatic optic nerve avulsion. From Corrales and Curreri [66]. Reprinted with permission from Elsevier

difficulty with diagnosis, it is likely that the incidence of traumatic optic nerve avulsion is underreported. During trauma, the intraorbital optic nerve is forcibly separated from the globe at the lamina cribrosa, while the optic nerve sheath and adjacent sclera remain intact [54, 56, 65]. Avulsion may be partial or complete. In partial avulsion, there is segmental detachment of the optic nerve. In complete avulsion, there is full separation of the optic nerve from the retina, choroid, and vitreous and retraction of the lamina cribrosa from the scleral rim [56].

Mechanism Optic nerve avulsion may follow a wide variety of injuries, including severe facial trauma, blunt injury of the orbit, and globe concussion [54, 65]. A frequent mechanism of optic nerve avulsion is direct trauma to the globe in which a small foreign body enters the space between the orbital rim and the globe to displace the eye [56, 66, 67]. For example, this can occur from a strike in the eye by a finger during contact sports such as basketball or boxing [66, 68].

Pathophysiology Optic nerve fibers at the disc are susceptible to shearing forces as they pass through the lamina cribrosa because there is little supportive connective tissue in this location [69]. Suggested reasons for optic nerve tears at the lamina cribrosa refer to the traumatic forced rotation of the globe and resultant shearing forces, sudden increase in intraocular pressure driving the nerve posteriorly out of the scleral canal, or displacement of the globe concurrent with retropulsion of the nerve [9, 57, 69].

Clinical Presentation Acute, severe vision loss immediately follows orbital trauma [9]. Patients are often NLP on presentation with a RAPD. Because the anterior ciliary vasculature is maintained, the globe will have a normal appearance.

Diagnosis Fundus examination: The most specific means for diagnosis is fundoscopy (see Fig. 12.9). There is often a ring of hemorrhage encircling the visibly disrupted optic nerve head [8, 9, 15]. In the case of a partial avulsion, there are segmental depressions or excavation of the optic nerve head [56]. In complete avulsions, there is absence of the optic nerve head with a remaining "cavity" in its place [9, 54, 56]. There

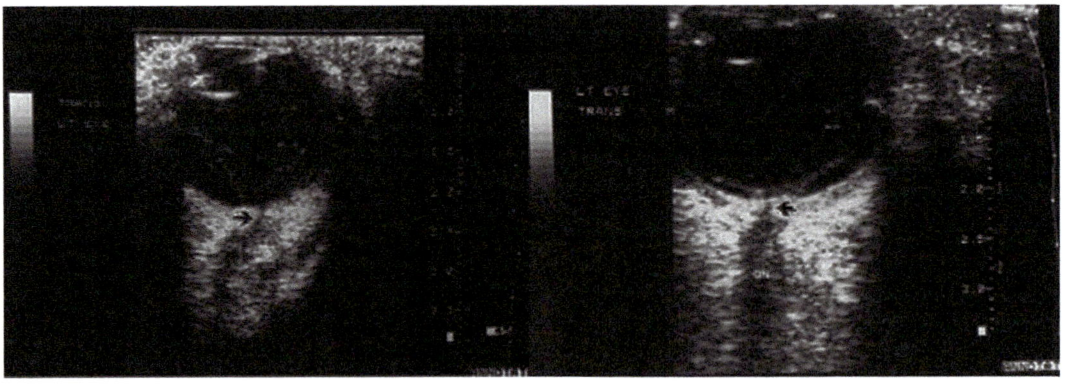

Fig. 12.10 B-scans demonstrating hypolucencies posterior to optic nerve head (*arrows*). From Sawhney et al. [54]. Reproduced with permission from Nature Publishing Group

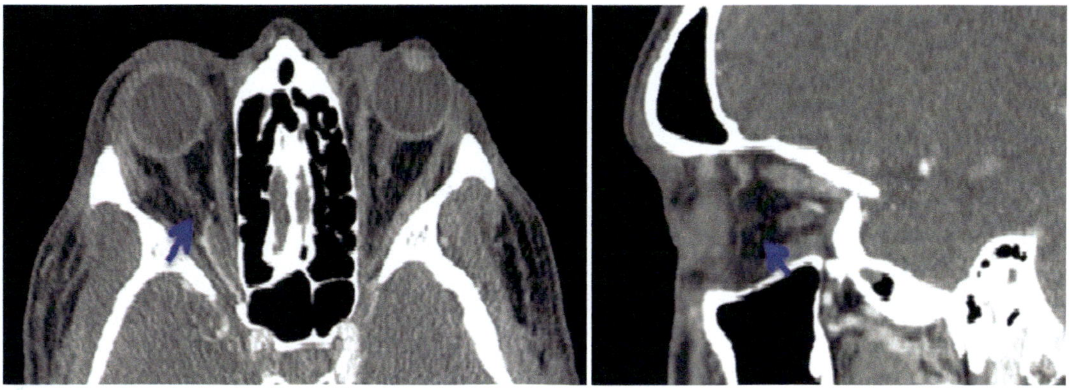

Fig. 12.11 Optic nerve transection *(arrow)*

are often limitations to the fundus examination. The clinical diagnosis may be delayed in its earlier stages by extensive vitreous hemorrhage, hyphema, or retinal hemorrhage that obstruct a clear view of the fundus [56, 57, 68].

Ultrasonography: Positive findings with B-scan include visualizing that the optic nerve does not reach the optic disc, hyperlucency anterior to optic nerve, and posterior ocular wall defects in the region of the optic nerve head (see Fig. 12.10) [54, 65]. At 4–6 weeks after injury, optic nerve head defects and ingrowth of glial scar tissue have been identified [70]. B-scan is especially useful in cases of vitreous hemorrhage or other obscuration of fundoscopy. However, B-scan has demonstrated variable success in the diagnosis of optic nerve avulsion [67].

Fluorescein Angiography: The retinal vasculature may be intact or have varying degrees of interruption following either partial or complete optic nerve avulsion. There may be a spectrum of normal filling, delayed filling, partial filling, or complete absence of retinal circulation [56].

CT/MRI: CT or MRI is not the preferred imaging modality. Results are inconsistent for the diagnosis of ON avulsion [54, 65, 67].

Treatment No medical or surgical treatments have proven helpful in cases of optic nerve avulsion [9, 67].

Optic Nerve Transection

Mechanism Optic nerve transection follows direct penetrating injury to the optic nerve. Transection may be complete or partial.

In cases of mid-facial blunt trauma, compressive forces directed on the superior orbital rim are transmitted to the orbital roof and optic canal [8, 14]. The forces can fracture the optic canal or orbital bones. Bony fragments are at risk of transecting the optic nerve (see Fig. 12.11) [9, 57]. Optic nerve transection may also follow injury from a penetrating foreign body.

In a review of the mechanisms of penetrating ocular trauma, optic nerve injury was most frequently caused by intentional self-inflicted injury. Common mechanisms of intentional penetrating eye injury included projectiles and blunt trauma (38%), projectiles (31%), and sharp objects (25%). Overall, penetrating eye injury is most frequently associated with projectiles (47%) [71].

Clinical Presentation Patients will have acute visual acuity loss and a RAPD. Early funduscopic examination is often normal, and optic nerve atrophy may be observed days following trauma (Fig. 12.12).

Diagnosis Diagnosis is largely based on clinical history of trauma, RAPD and acute vision loss with NLP visual acuity. CT scan may show a foreign body or bone fragment transecting the

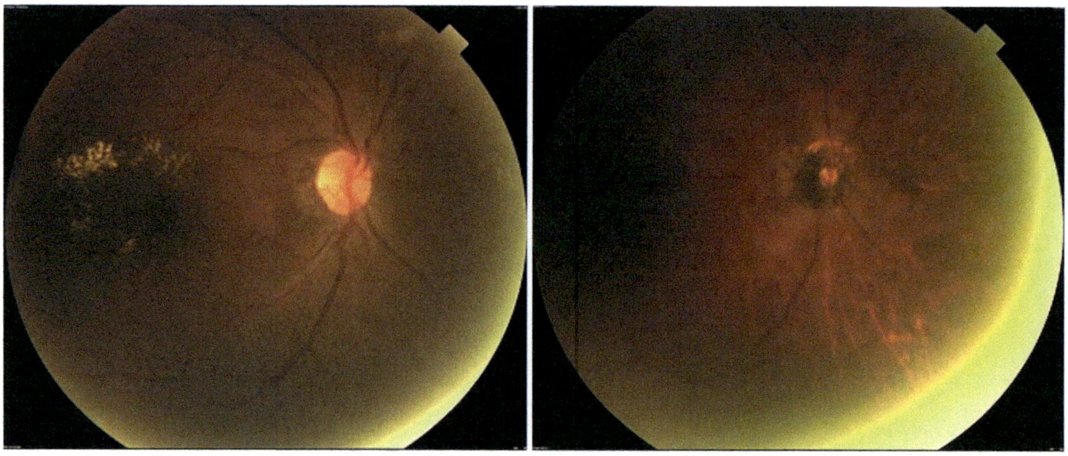

Fig. 12.12 Optic nerve transection (*arrows* in Fig. 12.11). Fundus photograph prior to the trauma (*left*) shows normal appearing optic disc. Fundus photograph several weeks after injury (*right*) reveals optic atrophy with peripapillary pigmentary changes

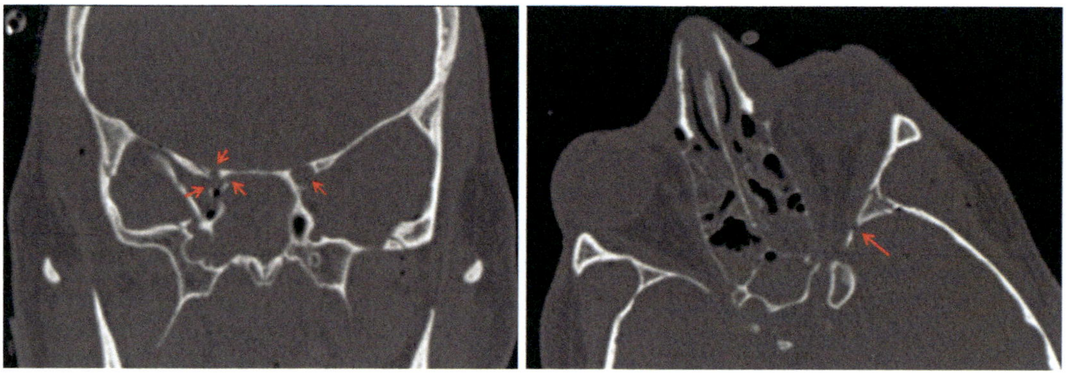

Fig. 12.13 23-year-old-male collided with an SUV while riding a motorcycle. He had a fixed, dilated left pupil. Fractures to the medial orbit, sphenoid sinus roof, and bilateral optic canal fractures involving all 4 walls of the optic canal. On *left*, bilateral optic canal fractures (*arrows*). On *right*, fracture involving superior orbital fissure (*arrow*)

optic nerve (Figs. 12.13, 12.14 and 12.15) and VEP amplitudes are decreased [9].

Management There is currently no effective management for optic nerve transection [9]. If there is extensive fracture, surgical repair can be pursued; however the damage to the optic nerve is irreversible [72].

Hemorrhage and Hematoma

Hemorrhage with the potential to cause direct TON may involve the optic nerve sheath, the optic nerve, or the potential space between the optic nerve and optic nerve sheath. In an autopsy series following patients with closed head trauma conducted by Crompton et al., 83% of autopsies had evidence of optic nerve sheath hemorrhage and 36% had hemorrhage involving the interstitium of the optic nerve [18].

Pathophysiology The hematoma or hemorrhage has a compressive effect on the vessels supplying the optic nerve and the optic nerve axons [15]. If blood is not evacuated promptly, there is risk of irreversible damage to the compressed optic nerve axons [73].

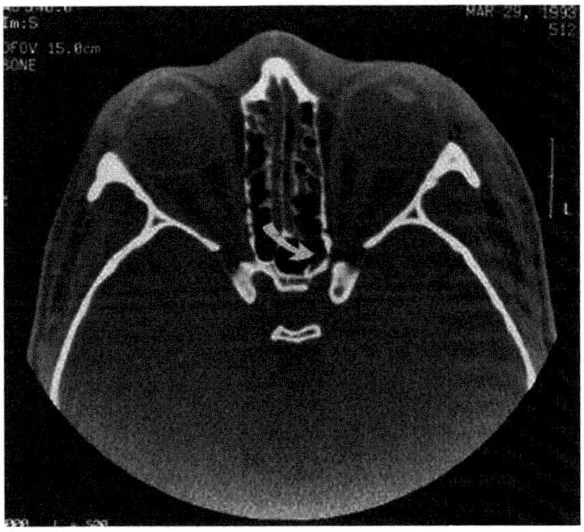

Fig. 12.14 CT scan of the head at the level of the optic canal with optic canal fracture in the left lateral sphenoid wall (*arrow*). From Walsh and Hoyt's Clinical Neuro-Ophthalmology, Chapter 9, pg. 436. Reproduced with permission from Robert Alan Goldberg, MD, University of California Los Angeles

Clinical Presentations Patients may present with proptosis, RAPD, and a sudden onset monocular decrease in visual acuity [9, 74, 75]. The optic disc may appear healthy in early stages, or optic disc edema can be present [75, 76].

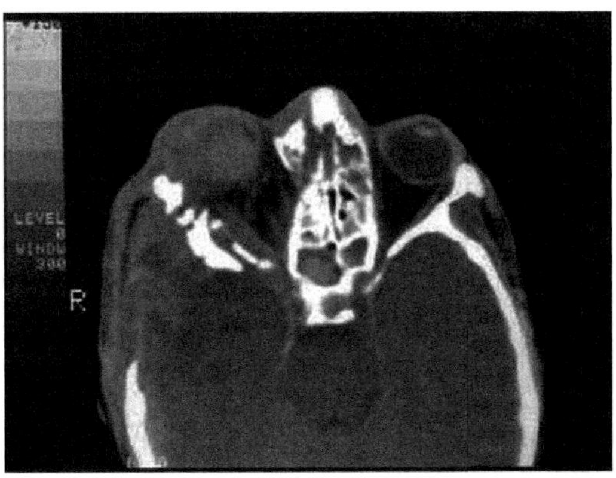

Fig. 12.15 CT scan of orbit with right optic nerve transection following penetrating trauma. From Sarkies 2004. NJC. Neuro-ophthalmological aspects of head injury. From Macfarlane R and Hardy D (eds) Outcome after head neck and spinal trauma. Butterworth Heinemann: Oxford, 1977 pp 163–177. Reproduced with permission from Elsevier

Diagnosis A CT scan can identify an optic nerve sheath hematoma (Fig 12.16). The affected optic nerve sheath will be expanded and hyperdense, and its increased size and density can be visualized [9, 74]. MRI is more specific than CT scan in detecting and localizing optic nerve hemorrhage [76].

Management Optic nerve sheath or intrasheath hemorrhage benefits from surgical drainage [15]. In optic nerve sheath hematoma, early nerve sheath fenestration to evacuate the clot is associated with greater recovery of visual acuity [9, 74, 77]. Megadose steroids have been used to treat optic nerve sheath hematoma, but their utility is unclear (See: Indirect TON Treatment section for discussion about corticosteroid use in TON) [75].

Orbital Compartment Syndrome

Orbital compartment syndrome describes an acute increase of intraorbital pressure. It may arise secondary to orbital hemorrhage or orbital emphysema. Because a fascial sheath and rigid bony walls enclose the orbital contents, small increases in intraorbital volume from blood or air can elevate the intraorbital pressure [37]. Arterial supply to the optic nerve can be compromised and lead to optic neuropathy [9, 15].

Mechanism Orbital hemorrhage can follow facial injury or surgery. Injection of retrobulbar anesthesia is a well-documented iatrogenic cause of orbital hemorrhage, occurring in 0.44–3% of cases [15].

Orbital emphysema is a common complication of orbital fracture, occurring in 50% of cases [78]. Nose blowing, coughing, sneezing, vomiting, or straining while lifting heavy objects by a patient with a blowout fracture can force air from the sinuses into the orbital space [78, 79]. Orbital emphysema is largely a benign process. However, air may become trapped in the orbit if a small fracture creates a one-way ball-valve mechanism [9, 15]. The trapped air increases intraorbital pressure and has a compressive, mass effect on the optic nerve [78, 80].

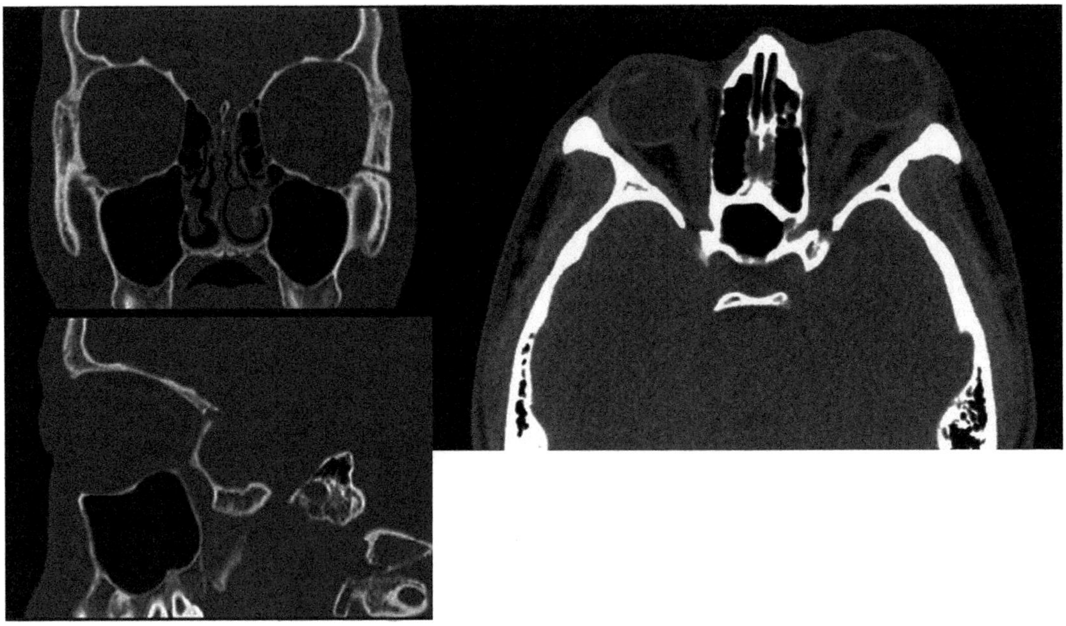

Fig. 12.16 Case study. Left optic nerve sheath hemorrhage following a forceful poke to the left eye while playing basketball. On presentation, he was NLP OS, pupils were 4 mm OD and 5 mm OS with a left RAPD, and he was unable to supraduct the left eye. **a** Coronal CT scan of the orbit with increased size of the left optic nerve, from hematoma. **b** Axial CT scan of orbit shows enlarged left optic nerve and left proptosis. He underwent emergent optic nerve sheath decompression without subsequent improvement of vision

Clinical Presentation Patients will experience acute onset proptosis, orbital pain, decreased visual acuity, RAPD, restricted extraocular muscle motility, and raised intraocular pressure [9, 15, 78, 80]. In ocular emphysema, palpation of the upper and lower eyelids may reveal tense underlying tissue [78].

Diagnosis Diagnosis is primarily clinical, in association with a history of facial trauma or recent orbital surgery. CT scan is useful to evaluate the fracture, identify presence of orbital emphysema or hemorrhage, and localize air pockets [80]. Facial radiographs may also reveal air within the orbit, but it is best confirmed with CT scan [80].

Management The goal of management is to rapidly decrease orbital pressure. Emergency surgical decompression by lateral canthotomy or cantholysis is essential [73, 78, 80]. The maximum potential for visual recovery follows surgical decompression within 2 h of injury [81]. In traumatic orbital compartment syndrome from retrobulbar hemorrhage, successful orbital decompression is achieved with lateral canthotomy and inferior cantholysis. When performed promptly, the patient may recover full visual function [82].

Examples of Indirect TON

Indirect TON is the most common form of optic nerve injury following blunt closed head trauma [9, 14, 28]. It involves the damaging effect of shearing forces on optic nerve RGCs (see section: TON Pathophysiology).

Treatment of Indirect TON

The treatment of indirect TON is currently debated. Before any treatment is initiated for TON, other treatable causes of visual loss should be ruled out [10, 83]. Approaches to indirect TON include conservative management, corticosteroids, optic canal decompression, and combined surgical and steroid treatment. In addition, research for neuroprotection strategies designed to repair damaged RGCs is ongoing.

Conservative Management

With conservative management for indirect TON, patients are observed for visual recovery. Interventions such as steroids or surgery are withheld [19]. Reports of spontaneous visual recovery following indirect TON are encouraging for conservative management, with a recovery rate of 30–60% [12, 20, 43, 83, 84]. The prognosis for spontaneous recovery is positively related to the patient's presenting visual acuity [12, 20]. A prospective study is needed to more clearly define the natural course of indirect TON [8, 83].

Corticosteroids

There is mixed evidence regarding the use of corticosteroids to treat indirect TON. High-dose corticosteroids administered soon after trauma may relieve optic nerve edema within the optic canal and decrease risk of damage to RGCs [14]. However, research outcomes have shown unclear benefits with corticosteroid treatment. There is debate on the best dose and time course of treatment. In addition, the risks of long-term disability and mortality from high-dose steroid regimens must be carefully considered.

In 1990, the multicenter, randomized, double-blind controlled National Acute Spinal Cord Injury Study (NASCIS 2) examined the use of "megadose" methylprednisolone following acute spinal cord injury [85]. An experimental group of patients with acute spinal cord injury was administered a bolus methylprednisolone dose of 30 mg/kg followed by infusion at 5.4 mg/kg/h for 23 h, while a control group received a placebo. Neurologic recovery was assessed with measurements of motor function, sensation to pinprick, and sensation to touch. Patients were followed up to 6 months after injury. The researchers found that patients who received methylprednisolone within 8 h of their injury had significant neurologic recovery, and this recovery remained stable when assessed 6 months following injury. Neurologic recovery was not observed in the placebo group or patients who received methylprednisolone greater than 8 h following trauma [85].

In a subsequent multicenter, randomized, double-blind clinical trial, NASCIS 3, researchers examined the outcome of extending the duration of megadose methylprednisolone treatment. Patients were treated within 3–8 h of acute spinal injury, and the study maintained the bolus dose of 30 mg/kg that was used in NASCIS 2 [86]. However, half of the participants received the 5.4 mg/kg/h methylprednisolone infusion for a total of 24 h and half of the participants received the infusion for 48 h. Neurologic recovery was measured and patients were followed for 6 months. The study results confirmed the neurologic benefit of early megadose corticosteroids following acute spinal injury. The study concluded that 48 h treatment benefits patients, if treatment is initiated 3–8 h after injury. This group had improved motor recovery and self-reported functional independence with 48 h steroid therapy. However, there was also an increased likelihood of severe sepsis and severe pneumonia in the 48 hour steroid infusion group. For patients who were treated within 3 h of injury, there was no significant difference between 24 and 48 h treatment regimens, and it was advised to continue using 24 h therapy for this group to reduce the complications of steroids [86].

Following the NASCIS 2 and 3 reports of neurologic recovery with megadose corticosteroids, researchers have sought to apply the results to patients with indirect TON [8]. An increasing number of patients with TON were managed with high-dose corticosteroids [10]. The results of research studies have varied widely. Several studies found a positive relationship between high-dose corticosteroids and recovery from TON [14, 44]. However, some studies comparing corticosteroid managed and conservatively managed patients with TON did not yield significantly different visual outcomes [29, 43]. There were also studies comparing corticosteroid management with surgical management that did not find a difference in treatment approach [62].

The research regarding indirect TON treatment has been limited by several factors. Many

Table 12.4 Classification of corticosteroid dosing and distribution in IONTS[a] [28]

	Corticosteroid dose (mg/day)	Percentage patients in IONTS
Megadose	≥5400	40
Very high dose	2000–5399	18
High dose	500–1999	19
Moderate dose	100–499	9
Low dose	<100	6

[a]8% of patients in IONTS had an unknown dose of corticosteroids

studies had small sample sizes or a lack of control group. Ability to compare studies has been greatly limited [10, 43]. Studies differed on multiple factors including differences in the timeline of treatment, corticosteroid dosing, baseline visual acuities, follow-up frequency, inclusion criteria, and exclusion criteria. Furthermore, in several studies, patients received combined corticosteroid and surgical treatment, which made it difficult to study the efficacy of each individual treatment [42, 73].

In 1999, the International Optic Nerve Trauma Study (IONTS) was established to address the limitations of indirect TON treatment research in evaluating the effect of corticosteroid treatment [28]. The study was designed as a randomized controlled trial, but was later modified to an observational nonrandomized study due to difficulties with patient recruitment. The study followed three types of treatment groups: corticosteroid only, surgical decompression only, and conservative management. In the corticosteroid treatment group, 40% received megadose steroids consistent with the NASCIS trials, while 60% received lower doses (see Table 12.4). For all treatment groups, the initial visual exam was conducted within 3 days of injury and treatment was initiated within 7 days of injury. Visual outcomes were assessed by change in VA. After adjustment for baseline visual acuity, the researchers concluded that there was no difference in visual outcome between the treatment groups [28].

In addition, the researchers did not find that timing or dose of treatment had an effect on the visual outcome. The researchers concluded that the the type of treatment should be made on a case-by-case basis, and there is no clear evidence to recommend one treatment over another [28].

The IONTS has merit as the first prospective study to evaluate the treatment of indirect TON. The researchers used a standardized method of defining and comparing visual improvement between the treatment groups [28]. The IONTS was a large patient study, and patient enrollment was great enough to detect statistical differences between the corticosteroid and surgical treatment groups [9]. However, there were study limitations. There were fewer patients in the conservative management group, and the conclusions regarding this group do not have as much power. Furthermore, the study design was not randomized, controlled, or masked. Because it became an observational study, there may have been selection bias regarding choice of treatment, and some patients were treated with both corticosteroids and surgery [8]. There were differences in corticosteroid dose, timing of treatment, and criteria for optic canal decompression between the patients [11].

Since the IONTS, corticosteroid research for indirect TON remains limited. The 2013 Cochrane Eyes and Vision Group review of steroids for TON identified only one randomized double-blind controlled trial to address the use of high-dose corticosteroids for indirect TON [20]. The research, by Entezari et al. in 2007, randomized patients with indirect TON to either a high-dose corticosteroid group (1000 mg methylprednisolone/day over 72 h) or a placebo group [58]. Patients were diagnosed with indirect TON within 7 days of injury based on clinical presentation of RAPD and decreased visual acuity. On average, they were treated within 52 h of injury. The patients were followed for 3 months and visual improvement was measured by visual acuity. At 3 months, there was no significant difference in visual recovery between the treatment and control groups. This conclusion supports the results of IONTS.

In addition to questions about corticosteroid efficacy, there have been concerns about treatment risks [63]. NASCIS 2 identified more frequent gastrointestinal bleeds in the steroid-treated group, and NASCIS 3 identified more severe sepsis and pneumonia in the 48-hour steroid-treated group [85, 86]. In addition, wound infections, pancreatitis, and acute psychosis have been reported following high doses of methylprednisolone [11].

In 2004, the Corticosteroid Randomization After Significant Head Injury (CRASH) trial investigated the safety of megadose corticosteroids administered for head injury [87]. The CRASH study was an international, multicenter, double-blind randomized placebo-controlled trial that enrolled 10,008 patients with head trauma. The patients were randomized within 8 h of injury. One group received a 2 g methylprednisolone over 1 hour in a 100 mL infusion, followed by a maintenance dose of 0.4 g/h for 48 h in a 20 mL/h infusion and the other group received a placebo. The doses were set to correspond with the NASCIS 3 trial. The study recruitment was stopped early when unmasked results indicated higher mortality rates in the steroid-treated group. At 2-week follow-up, there was a significantly greater risk of death from all causes for the patients in the corticosteroid group [87]. At 6-month follow-up, the researchers found a significantly higher risk of mortality and severe disability in the steroid-treated group [88]. This effect did not change based on injury severity or time from injury. The researchers concluded that corticosteroids are not recommended for cases of head trauma. The study results can extrapolate to the treatment of indirect TON because many of these patients also experienced head trauma [8].

Concerns about corticosteroid risk have been substantiated by animal studies. Steinsapir and coworkers examined the effect of very high-dose corticosteroids on injured optic nerves in rats [89]. Following crush injuries to the optic nerve, rats either received very high-dose methylprednisolone or saline placebo. When the optic nerves were examined six weeks after crush injury, the rats that underwent steroid treatment lost more axons than the placebo group. The study indicates that methylprednisolone may be directly toxic to a damaged optic nerve.

Further research with double-blind RCTs is needed to elucidate how steroids should be used in the treatment of indirect TON. Based on the IONTS and the study by Entezari et al., there is no clear evidence that steroids provide an additional benefit in the treatment of indirect TON. Future research regarding other doses and time-frames of corticosteroid treatment may alter these conclusions. Given the CRASH trial results, steroids should not be given to patients with head injuries. Other patients should be carefully evaluated on a case-by-case basis.

Surgical management

Surgical management of indirect TON is focused on reducing secondary injury to the optic nerve (See: Pathophysiology section). Optic nerve edema primarily affects the intracanalicular segment of the optic nerve. Optic canal decompression relieves the secondary intracanalicular compartment syndrome by providing more space for the edematous optic nerve and limiting post-injury ischemia [8, 11, 29, 90]. Early surgical intervention is believed to augment the potential for visual recovery [19, 91].

Surgical indications for TON are limited by research studies, which are primarily small and retrospective [19, 23]. The criteria are well defined for optic nerve hematoma, but surgical indications are less clear with optic canal fracture or indirect TON.

There is strong evidence to support surgical management in cases of hematoma (See: Direct TON-hematoma section). With retrobulbar hematoma or optic nerve sheath hematoma, urgent surgical decompression and evacuation of the hematoma is indicated [11, 58, 63]. Surgical evacuation of hematoma with optic nerve sheath fenestration for intrasheath hemorrhage quickly relieves optic nerve compression [24]. In case reports of patients with radiological evidence of enlarged optic nerve sheaths and gradual visual loss, there is a positive response to optic nerve sheath decompression with a high potential for visual recovery [8].

With optic canal fracture, surgical management with optic nerve decompression has been recommended. In particular, surgery has been recommended for comminuted canal fracture or radiologic evidence that the fractured optic canal segment impinges on the optic nerve [11, 19, 24, 28, 45, 58]. However, optic canal fracture has been identified as a poor prognostic factor, regardless of intervention, and researchers question if surgery is beneficial in all cases of optic canal fracture [20]. Poor outcome is related to optic nerve transection. If the bone fragments transected the optic nerve, the injury to RGCs is irreversible and optic canal decompression would not have an effect on visual function [19]. As a result, case studies indicate that surgical decompression for patients with optic canal fractures has low potential for significant visual improvement [92].

The considerations for indirect TON are not as well defined. Given the pathophysiology of indirect TON, optic nerve swelling is a commonly identified reason for optic canal decompression [8]. Intraneural edema, diagnosed radiologically and suggestive of indirect TON, has been cited as an indication for surgical management [11].

Surgical candidates are identified based on the likehood of visual recovery. Indirect TON patients with gradual visual decline and VA better than NLP are considered the best candidates for surgical decompression [49, 93]. Gradual visual change following injury is considered to indicate a reversible cause of vision loss, whereas sudden onset, acute and complete vision loss is more likely to indicate a nonreversible process such as optic nerve transection [14]. Given their poor prognosis, it is unclear if there is a benefit to treating patients with total, sudden vision loss following trauma [42, 94]. In retrospective studies, few patients (0–17%) with sudden vision loss who were NLP at presentation regained vision after surgical decompression [14, 95]. In comparison, the same retrospective studies indicated that the majority of patients with vision better than NLP experienced some degree of visual recovery either after surgical decompression or conservative management [95].

Because the guidelines for optic canal decompression are unclear, the surgery should only be considered for conscious patients [15, 83]. These patients are able to undergo a full ophthalmic exam to first rule out other causes of visual loss [42]. They can also be counseled regarding the risks and benefits of surgery, and actively participate in the decision-making process [10, 90].

It is widely understood that earlier management of indirect TON yields better visual outcomes. Several reports define effective surgical management as occurring within 1 week of trauma [15, 49, 60, 96].

High-resolution CT scans of the intraorbital and intracanalicular optic nerve are helpful to visualize optic nerve pathology and evaluate the need for surgical management [49]. CT findings that indicate a need for surgical management include an enlarged optic nerve sheath suggestive of hemorrhage, optic nerve edema, or optic canal fracture [42, 49]. After surgical need is identified, CT scans are further utilized in surgical planning [42]. For example, imaging the orbital apex identifies the relationship of the optic nerve and the carotid artery, which is critical to reduce intraoperative complications [90].

There are a variety of surgical techniques for optic nerve decompression. In all approaches, a wall of the optic canal is removed to provide room for the edematous optic nerve [45]. The earliest technique for optic canal decompression, developed in the 1960s, takes an intracranial approach to reach the optic canal [15, 92, 97]. With a craniotomy, surgeons are able to directly visualize a large area of the brain and potentially discover coexistent areas of brain damage following trauma [45]. However, the intracranial approach has significant risks to the patient and outcomes are overall poor [14, 49]. It is an invasive procedure and requires an external incision. Possible consequences of intracranial optic nerve decompression include frontal lobe edema due to the need to retract the frontal lobe, and the loss of olfaction [91, 94, 96].

Extracranial approaches to reach the optic canal were developed as a less invasive way to achieve optic canal decompression [49]. There are a variety of extracranial approaches, and all surgical techniques have the same final step of removing a wall of the optic canal to achieve decompression. The extracranial transethmoidal approach is most frequently used [10, 42]. Approaches that have been reported include transconjunctival [73, 98], transantral [92], transethmoidal [60, 92, 99, 100], transnasal [10], and lateral facial [101]. Combined techniques include transethmoidal/transorbital [90], transethmoidal/transsphenoidal [91], endonasal transsphenoidal [96, 102–104] and transconjunctival/intranasal endoscopic approaches [94].

Extracranial approaches offer several advantages over intracranial optic canal decompression. Because the approach is less invasive, it can be completed under general anesthesia [45, 92]. There is no external incision, no risk of frontal lobe edema or decreased olfaction, a faster recovery time, and decreased morbidity compared to intracranial techniques [91, 94, 96].

Although safer than intracranial surgery, extracranial optic canal decompression has several reported complications. All of the extracranial approaches risk cerebrospinal fluid leak, meningitis, intraorbital infections, and accidental dural exposure [11, 23, 91]. For example, in the IONTS, 3 out of 33 patients treated with extracranial decompression experienced CSF leak, and one developed meningitis postoperatively [28]. Enophthalmos may result from expansion of orbital volume [90, 94].

There is risk of damage to the surrounding anatomy in the orbit and the sellar region [9]. Direct, thermal, or ischemic injury to the optic nerve can occur intra-operatively [14, 90, 105]. There may be injury to the lacrimal apparatus, ophthalmic artery, or surrounding brain tissue [11, 91, 92, 94]. With a transconjunctival approach, there is risk for medial rectus entrapment and injury to the globe [94]. All approaches to optic canal decompression carry the serious risk of injury to the carotid artery because the optic nerve travels close to the carotid artery near the sphenoid sinus [10]. There is high mortality associated with damage to the carotid artery due to difficulty controlling hemorrhage, subsequent intracerebral hypoperfusion, and extravascular dissection of the expanding hematoma [90]. If carotid artery laceration occurs, immediate management should include sinus pressure packing tamponade, carotid artery ligation, and possible endovascular tamponade [90].

Ultimately, selection of surgical method should be individualized. Surgeon experience, location of pathology, and patient anatomy should all be considered. The intracranial approach still has use if intracranial pathology secondary to trauma also needs to be addressed [90]. When pathology is localized to the optic nerve, an extracranial approach is safer for the patient.

As with corticosteroid treatment, the decision to manage indirect TON with surgical decompression has not been standardized and the choice to perform surgery should also be made on an individual basis. Several studies have reported success with optic nerve decompression; however, these are frequently uncontrolled, small, retrospective case studies so it is difficult to make clear conclusions about surgical indications or timing [49, 60]. Furthermore, it is not possible to compare published studies because a variety of intracranial and extracranial surgical decompression techniques are employed, and frequently corticosteroid treatment is given to surgical patients in non-standardized regimens [11, 91]. There is also a recruitment bias prevalent in the literature, with selection of patients who have worse baseline visual acuities or have already failed corticosteroid treatment [11, 12]. Based on a Cochrane Review examining Optic Nerve Decompression for TON, there are no randomized controlled trials in which any form of surgical intervention for TON, either on its own or in combination with steroids, was compared to steroids alone or no treatment [23]. The IONTS (see: Corticosteroid Treatment section) could not find a reason to recommend surgical management for indirect TON over corticosteroids or conservative management [62].

Without clear evidence that surgical decompression benefits patients with TON, and given the well-known risk factors of the surgery, the decision to perform optic nerve decompression will remain controversial until further research is conducted [23].

Other Treatment Strategies

The goal of experimental treatment studies for TON is neuroprotection. Following trauma, irreversibly damaged RGCs release neurotransmitters and inflammatory factors that induce apoptosis of nearby, undamaged RGCs. New treatment strategies aim to prevent the receptive secondary apoptosis and minimize total damage to the ON [11, 19, 83]. For example, glutamate inhibitors prevent apoptosis in animal models [106]. Neurotrophic factors including fibroblast growth factor [2, 107], brain-derived neurotrophic factor [108, 109], and ciliary neurotrophic factor [110, 111] combat growth factor deficiencies following TON and promote survival of remaining RGCs. Additional neuroprotective research includes the anti-inflammatory small heat-shock protein crystalline [112], nitric oxide synthase inhibitors [113], tumor necrosis factor-alpha inhibitors [114], calcium channel blockers [115], the immunosuppressant FK50 [6, 116], and erythropoietin [117]. These interventions are promising, but still in early stages of investigation.

Traumatic Pupillary Abnormalities

Two significant types of traumatic pupillary abnormalities are Adie's tonic pupil, a dysfunction of the ciliary ganglion, and Horner syndrome, which involves dysfunction of sympathetic pathways of the nervous system. Both disorders produce characteristic changes in the pupil that are described below.

Adie's Tonic Pupil

Adie's tonic pupil results when postganglionic parasympathetic nerves to the iris sphincter and ciliary muscle are lost. The loss of this innervation results in a fixed dilated pupil that reacts poorly to light, but will constrict to near stimuli. When the near stimuli are removed, the characteristic tonicity becomes apparent as the pupil slowly relaxes. Additionally, Adie's tonic pupil is known to be supersensitive to weak miotic agents such as pilocarpine due to cholinergic denervation [118]. Adie's pupil can be associated with findings such as decreased deep tendon reflexes and the presence of anhidrosis. This triad of findings is known as Ross syndrome [119].

Adie's tonic pupil is often idiopathic. Women are more often affected with a mean age of 32 years [120]. The tonic pupil initially presents unilaterally in 80% of cases, and the chance of second pupil involvement is 4% per year [120]. Underlying causes that may be responsible for the parasympathetic denervation include traumatic, iatrogenic, viral, and neoplastic etiologies.

Horner Syndrome

Horner syndrome involves disruption of the sympathetic efferent fibers that normally cause the pupil to dilate, assist the lid in retraction, and enable perspiration of the forehead. The sympathetic pathway involved begins in the hypothalamus and, over the course of three neuron synapses, descends down the cervical cord, exits through the ventral rami of C8, T1, and T2, and joins the paraverterbral sympathetic chain to ascend some levels before continuing along the wall of the carotid artery and exiting the carotid wall to innervate its targets [121]. Dysfunction along the pathway, as depicted in Fig. 12.17, results in the typical findings of Horner syndrome: ptosis, miosis, and anhidrosis.

Epidemiology

Spontaneous internal carotid artery dissection has been reported to present as Horner syndrome in approximately 28–41% of cases [122]. Internal carotid artery dissection occurs with an incidence of 2.6–3.0 in 100,000, and with equal occurrence rates in males and females, most often of young and middle-ages [123].

In one study of combat-associated ocular trauma, Horner syndrome due to upper chest and neck injury represented approximately 1% of the

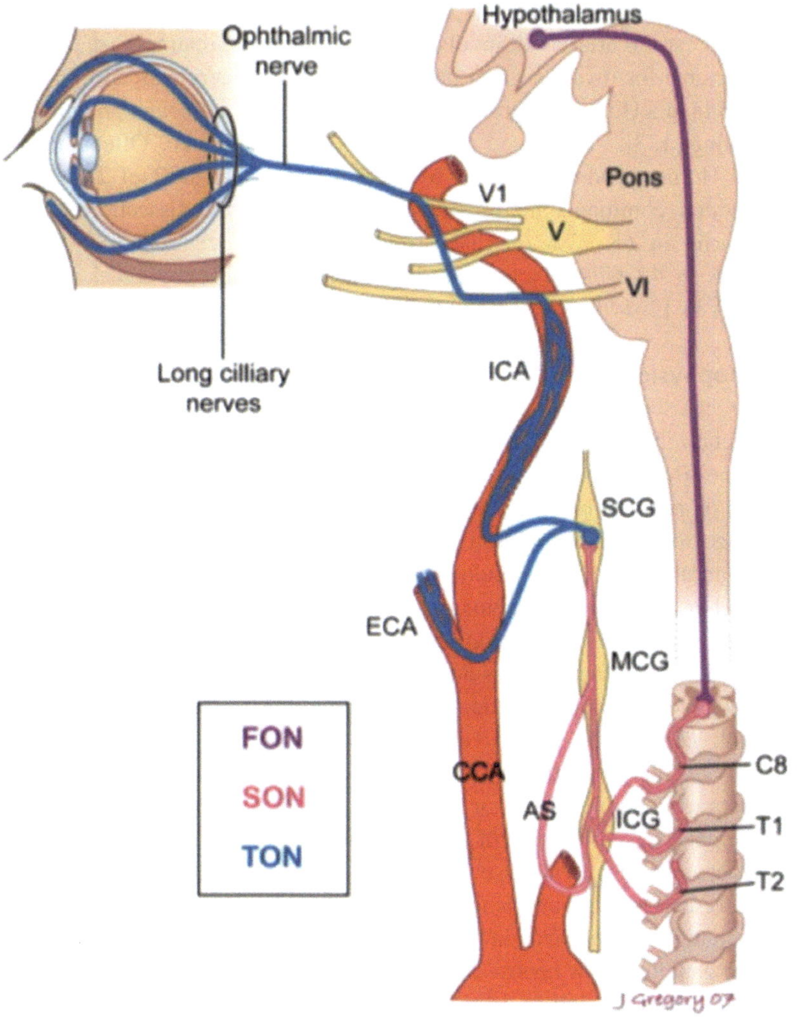

Fig. 12.17 Three-neuron sympathetic innervation of the eye. *AS* ansa subclavia; *ECA* external carotid artery; *ICA* internal carotid artery; *ICG* inferior cervical ganglion; *MCG* middle cervical ganglion; *SCG* superior cervical ganglion; *FON* first-order neuron; *SON* second-order neuron; *TON* third-order neuron. From Reede D, Garcon E, Smoker W, Kardon R. Horner's Syndrome: Clinical and Radiographic Evaluation. Neuroimaging Clinics of North America [serial online]. January 1, 2008;18(Cranial Nerves):369–385. Available from: ScienceDirect, Ipswich, MA. Reproduced with permission from Science Direct

total cases. Similarly, a series of TBI patients demonstrated Horner syndrome in 0.9% of cases [124]. In one rare case, Horner syndrome was reported as a direct consequence of first rib fracture, itself a rare occurrence, suffered in a motor vehicle accident without carotid dissection [125].

Iatrogenic Horner syndrome can be a rare complication of different surgical procedures involving the head and neck, as described below. Even with closely associated procedures, such as conventional thyroidectomy, the occurrence of Horner syndrome has been reported to be as low as 18 cases between 1993 and 2015 [126].

Pediatric Horner syndrome, although rare, can be acquired or congenital. One study determined the pediatric incidence to be 1.42 per 100,000 patients younger than 19 years, and congenital syndrome to occur in 1 in 6250 births [127]. In a series of 73 pediatric patients with Horner syndrome, 42% were considered congenital or caused by birth trauma, 15% were acquired without surgical intervention such as by neoplasm or trauma, and 42% were acquired with surgical intervention as the cause [128].

Presentation

Horner syndrome consists of the three classic findings of ptosis, miosis, and anhidrosis. Though these three findings make up the syndrome, dysfunction along the third-order, postganglionic neuronal fibers that run along the internal carotid artery will involve only the fibers responsible for mydriasis and lid retraction, thus resulting in a Horner syndrome with spared facial sweating [123].

In Horner syndrome caused by carotid artery dissection, common symptoms include ipsilateral headache in 68–92% of cases, focal cerebral deficits in 49–67% of cases, and cranial nerve palsies in 12–14% of cases [123].

Pathophysiology

Often, the syndrome occurs due to cervical-carotid dissection that can be caused by a motor vehicle accident (MVA), penetrating trauma to the upper chest or neck or iatrogenically [122, 129]. Such damage to the motor neuron pathway along its anatomical course will result in the signs and symptoms of Horner syndrome.

Iatrogenic Horner syndrome occurs with multiple types of procedures due to the extensive pathway of the sympathetic system along the spinal cord and carotid artery. Procedures involving manipulation of the neck, such as in chiropractic manipulation or endotracheal tube placement have the risk of causing iatrogenic Horner syndrome. The association with thyroid surgery described above is thought to be due to the contiguous localization of the oculosympathetic ganglion with neurovascular supply to the thyroid gland, complicating the isolation of thyroid structures during removal without causing Horner syndrome [126]. Other possible etiologies include postoperative hematoma compressing the sympathetic pathway, ischemia to the neurons, and stretching during retraction [130]. Minimally invasive video-assisted thyroidectomy is also thought to be associated with the occurrence of Horner syndrome, due to the limited mobility afforded to the endoscopic tools used in the procedure by the region of anatomy [126].

One example of surgical intervention resulting in a pediatric case of Horner syndrome is from a case report of pulmonary hydatid cyst removal in a 10-year-old girl whose ptosis recovered in 3 months and anisocoria recovered in 6 months [131].

Treatment

Treatment of Horner syndrome secondary to cervical-carotid dissection with antiplatelet or anticoagulant medication can reduce the risk of stroke. Often, heparin bridged with warfarin to an INR of 2.0–3.0 for 3–6 months is used until the dissection resolves of its own accord, which occurs in 85–90% of cases [123]. Antiplatelet drugs such as aspirin or clopidogrel are also used frequently, either alone or in combination [132]. Between the two therapies, a recent randomized controlled trial of 250 patients with carotid or vertebral dissection determined that the recurrence of stroke on either therapy at 3 months was lower than found in previous studies, and that there was no significant difference between antiplatelet or anticoagulant medication in regards to the rare outcomes of recurrent ipsilateral stroke or death [132]. Patients who fail medical management of carotid artery dissection may be closely monitored or undergo surgical intervention, such as intravascular stenting [123].

Head Injury

In the United States, head trauma is a frequent cause of emergency room visits. In 2013, the American College of Surgeons' National Trauma Data Bank reported that 36% of adult trauma admissions involved head injury [133]. Typically, the demographic of head trauma patients is composed of young males [134]. Head injuries are most commonly caused by motor vehicle accidents, and non-restrained passengers have a greater severity of injury [2, 50, 135]. Patients with the most severe ocular injury often present with a GCS score less than or equal to eight [2, 135]. Patients who lose consciousness following closed head injury are more likely to have permanent neurologic injury [50].

A variety of neuro-ophthalmic injuries can result from closed head trauma. In a retrospective review of 181, patients with closed head trauma and no preexisting ocular disease, primary ophthalmic complaints included: blurred or decreased vision (46%), diplopia (30%), headaches (13%), trouble reading (6%), ocular irritation (3%), oscillopsia (2%), pupil irregularity (2%), sagging eyelids (2%), and photopsia (2%) [50]. Constricted visual field loss was most frequently observed (41% of reported visual field defects), but any part of the visual pathway may be injured [50].

In the evaluation of head injury and its visual complications, the ophthalmologist should consider skull base fractures, intracranial contusions, arterial or venous injury, direct penetrating trauma to visual pathways, and TBI.

Skull Base Fractures

Epidemiology and Mechanism

A skull base fracture extends through any of the cranial floor bones: the orbital plate of the paired frontal bones, cribriform plate of the ethmoid bone, occipital bone, sphenoid bone, and petrous or squamous portions of the paired temporal bones [133, 136]. Skull base fractures are most often caused by high impact, accidental closed head trauma [137]. Approximately 7–16% of all closed head trauma result in basilar skull fracture [133]. Iatrogenic injury during skull base surgery is a less frequent cause of skull base fracture.

Accidental Trauma

Blunt head trauma causes over 90% of skull base fractures [137]. Motor vehicle accidents are the most frequently reported mechanisms, often involving unrestrained passengers in high-speed collisions [138, 139]. In a review of 81 cases of basilar skull fracture, 59% of patients were in vehicular accidents, 35% were injured by high velocity falls from a height, and 6% were assaulted [140]. These high impact mechanisms of skull base fracture are consistently cited throughout the literature [133]. The majority of patients are young and male [140].

Penetrating trauma, such as injury from a gunshot, is a less common mechanism of skull base fracture [133, 137]. Skull base fractures from assault with projectile weapons have increasing incidence in urban settings [141].

The force and direction of impact predicts the type of skull base fracture pattern and associated complications. Most commonly, a fracture involves the anterior skull base and is associated with direct, frontal impact [133]. A high velocity, lateral force of impact may produce a fracture that extends from the anterior skull base to the middle and posterior skull base, or a fracture in the coronal plane through the central skull base [133, 138, 142]. Isolated fractures of the posterior skull base are commonly from lateral or posterior head injury [133].

Because surrounding bony structures heavily protect the skull base, significant trauma is needed to produce a skull base fracture [141]. Such large-force trauma is likely to present with multiple injuries. Complex facial or orbital fractures are often comorbid with basilar skull fracture [133, 137].

Iatrogenic Trauma

Iatrogenic skull base fracture is most frequently associated with complications of functional endoscopic sinus surgery (FESS) [143, 144]. Less than 1% of FESS are complicated by skull base injury with CSF leak [144]. The skull base damage most often affects the lateral lamella of the cribriform plate or the posterior ethmoid roof [143].

Additional procedures that have been implicated in skull base fracture are septoplasty, otologic surgery including removal of vestibular schwannoma, transsphenoidal pituitary resection, craniofacial resection, and transcranial approaches to access the optic chiasm or cavernous sinus [143, 145, 146].

Anatomy of the Skull Base and Clinical Implications in Skull Base Fracture

The skull base forms the floor of the anterior, middle, and posterior cranial fossae. The contents of each fossa have important clinical implications in skull base fracture (see Table 12.5: skull base openings and their contents, and Figs. 12.18 and 12.19). The clinical presentation can vary greatly based on the location and severity of the fracture [137]. Patients with basilar skull fracture should be evaluated for dural laceration with CSF leak,

Table 12.5 Skull base openings and their contents

Location in skull base	Opening	Contents
Anterior	Cribriform plate	Branches of olfactory n. (CN I)
Middle	Optic canal	Optic n. (CN II), ophthalmic a.
	Superior orbital fissure	Oculomotor n. (CN III), trochlear n. (CN IV), ophthalmic division of trigeminal n. (CN V1), abducens n. (CN VI), superior ophthalmic v.
	Foramen rotundum	Maxillary division of trigeminal n. (CN V2)
	Foramen ovale	Mandibular division of trigeminal n. (CN V3), accessory meningeal a., lesser superficial petrosal n., emissary veins
	Foramen spinosum	Middle meningeal a. (branch of external carotid a.), meningeal branch of CN VII
	Foramen lacerum	A. of the pterygoid canal, n. of pterygoid canal, venous drainage
	Carotid canal	Internal carotid a., sympathetic plexus
Posterior	Internal acoustic meatus	Facial n. (CN VII), vestibulocochlear n. (CN VIII), labyrinthine a. and v.
	Jugular foramen	Internal jugular v., glossopharyngeal n. (CN IX), vagus n. (CN X), accessory n. (CN XI), inferior petrosal sinus, posterior meningeal a.
	Hypoglossal canal	Hypoglossal n. (CN XII), venous plexus of hypoglossal canal
	Foramen magnum	Spinal v., anterior spinal a., posterior spinal a., spinal cord, accessory n. (CN XI), vertebral a.

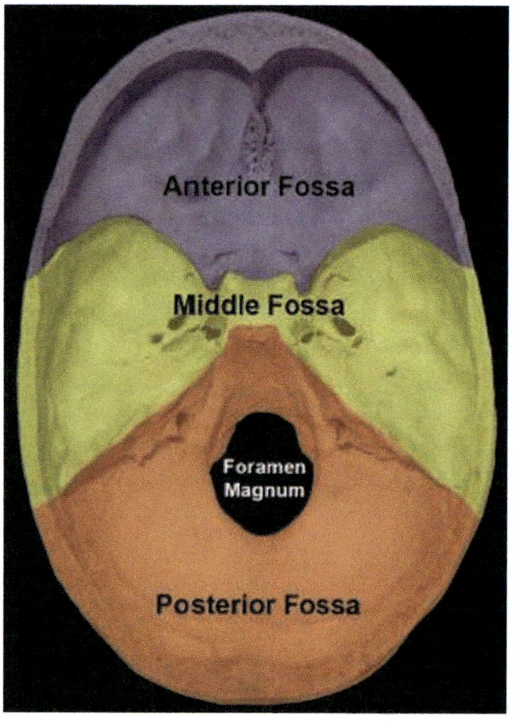

Fig. 12.18 Anterior, middle, and posterior cranial fossae. From Baugnon and Hudgins [133]. Reproduced with permission from Elsevier

infection, contusions, pneumocephalus, brain laceration, encephalocele, meningoencephalocele, intracranial hematomas, cranial nerve palsy, and neurovascular injuries [50, 133, 136, 141, 147].

For a summary of skull base fracture locations and complications, see Table 12.6.

Anterior Skull Base Fracture

The anterior skull base, formed by the orbital portion of the frontal bones and the ethmoid bone, is the most common site of basilar skull fracture [138]. The anterior skull base begins at the posterior wall of the frontal sinus and extends posteriorly to the anterior clinoid processes and planum sphenoidale. Due to its location and structure, the anterior cranial fossa absorbs extrinsic force directed to the mid-facial skeleton or anterior cranial vault. It limits energy transfer and damage of the more posterior cranial contents [138].

The olfactory nerve fibers pass through the thin cribriform plate of the ethmoid bone, and are commonly disrupted with traumatic anterior

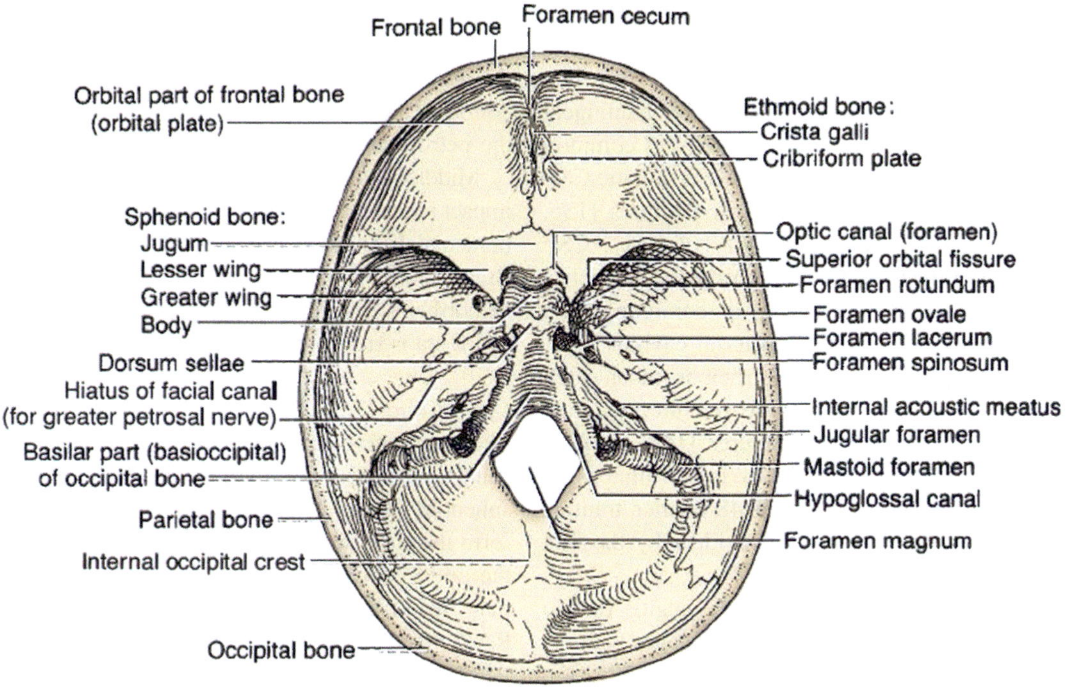

Fig. 12.19 Skull base anatomy. From BRS Gross Anatomy, 7th edition. Reproduced with permission from Wolters Kluwer

skull base fracture or during transethmoidal surgical approaches to the anterior skull base [148]. Patients with anterior skull base fracture can present with anosmia due to olfactory nerve damage, epistaxis from damage to anterior and posterior ethmoidal arteries, or frontal lobe contusion [133, 137].

There is a close spatial relationship of the anterior skull base with the paranasal sinuses and the orbit. Given the high impact trauma needed to cause anterior skull base fracture, the paranasal sinuses and orbit may also be injured [133, 141]. If there is damage to the optic nerve or intraorbital structures, patients may have decreased visual

Table 12.6 Location of skull base fracture and frequently associated complications

Location	Complication
Anterior skull base	Anosmia (CN I injury) Intraorbital injury CSF rhinorrhea/meningoencephalocele
Middle skull base	Vascular injury: ICA occlusion, dissection, pseudoaneurysm, aneurysm, carotid-cavernous fistula CN injuries: II, III, IV, V, VI Horner's syndrome
Posterolateral skull base (temporal bone)	Vascular injury: ICA CN injuries: VII, VIII CSF otorrhea/meningoencephalocele
Posterior skull base	Venous vascular injury or vertebrobasilar injury CN injuries: IX, X, XI, or XII Craniocervical junction and cervical spine injuries

Table adapted from Baugnon and Hudgins [133], with permission from Elsevier acuity, proptosis, enophthalmos, orbital hematoma, diplopia, chemosis, increased intraocular pressure, or other visual findings [137].

High impact trauma can cause meningeal tears, and closed head injury is the most common etiology of CSF leaks [136, 143]. Traumatic CSF leak occurs in 10–45% of skull fractures [136, 139, 140, 149]. In the majority of cases, CSF fistula manifests as CSF rhinorrhea, in which a meningeal tear results in a communication between the intracranial and nasal cavities [133, 137, 140, 149]. CSF rhinorrhea is most often caused by anterior skull base fracture, and less often by temporal bone fractures [149]. 80% of patients with CSF rhinorrhea following basilar skull fracture present within 48 h after trauma, and about 95% of cases are evident by the first 3 months of injury [133].

CSF leak poses a risk for meningitis due to communication of the disrupted meninges with the flora of the nasal or middle ear cavities [133, 136]. Meningitis has been reported in about 10–15% of patients with CSF rhinorrhea [149]. The risk of meningitis increases with time. There is a 1% risk of meningitis in the first 24 h after injury with CSF fistula. The meningitis risk increases to 9% after one week and 18% after 2 weeks [133, 149].

CSF hypotension is a complication of chronic CSF leak. The patient may have optic disc edema, enophthalmos, diplopia, orthostatic headaches, posterior neck pain, nausea, or vomiting. CSF may be identified on MRI by subdural fluid collections, pachymeningeal enhancement, venous engorgement, pituitary hyperemia, and downward displacement of the brain [150]. CSF hypotension has an opening pressure less than 60 mmHg.

Middle Skull Base Fracture

The middle skull base begins anteriorly at the greater wing of the sphenoid bone and ends posteriorly at the clivus. The greater wing of the sphenoid bone forms the anterior floor of the middle skull base, and the anterior petrous bone forms the posterior floor. The middle skull base has many important structures that are susceptible following fracture (see Table 12.5: skull base openings and their contents). Vascular complications are most frequently reported following middle skull base fracture. In particular, the internal carotid artery is susceptible due to its course in the cavernous sinus and carotid canal of the petrous bone.

Middle skull base fractures occur from high impact injury, and there are often serious associated intracranial injuries, such as DAI (see: Traumatic Brain Injury section) or multi-compartmental hemorrhage. The temporal lobe in the middle cranial fossa is susceptible to contusion injuries [148].

Optic Canal

The optic nerves exit the orbit through the optic canals, which pass through the lesser wing of the sphenoid bone. The anterior clinoid processes form the roof of the optic canal. Compression of the optic nerve from middle skull base fractures may result in decreased visual acuity and a RAPD (see: Section "Optic Nerve Trauma").

Superior Orbital Fissure

The superior orbital fissure is the space between the lesser and greater wings of the sphenoid bone. Multiple cranial nerves (III, IV, V1, VI) and the superior ophthalmic vein pass through the superior orbital fissure and may be injured in middle skull base fracture. CN III, IV, and VI palsies lead to various degrees of ophthalmoplegia (see: Section "Oculomotor System").

Other important foramina in the middle skull base are the foramen rotundum, foramen ovale, and the foramen spinosum. The foramen rotundum is posterior and inferior to the base of the superior orbital fissure and transmits the maxillary division of the trigeminal nerve (V2). The foramen ovale is posterior and lateral to the foramen rotundum and transmits the mandibular division of the trigeminal nerve (V3). The foramen spinosum is further posterior and lateral and transmits the middle meningeal artery.

Sella Turcica

The sella turcica of the sphenoid bone is in the central part of the middle skull base. It is located posterior and medial to the two orbits, between the anterior and posterior clinoid processes. The hypophyseal fossa, a depression within the body of the sphenoid bone, holds the pituitary gland.

The optic chiasm is inferior to the sella turcica. Due to its anatomical relationship, fractures of the sella turcica can result in chiasmatic compression, laceration, contusion, hematoma, or ischemic compromise [133, 151]. Traumatic chiasmal syndrome describes the consequences of sagittal midline skull base fractures through the sella turcica. Patients have complete or partial bitemporal hemianopsia that is consistent with optic chiasm injury [152]. Optic chiasm lesions are rare, and have been observed in only 4.4% of patients with visual complications following head trauma [153]. It is best diagnosed by MRI [154]. Additional neurologic features observed in traumatic chiasmal syndrome are diabetes insipidus from interruption of the hypothalamic-pituitary apparatus, panhypopituitarism, intrasellar hematoma, pneumatocele, or cranial nerve defects [151–153]

Internal Carotid Artery

The internal carotid artery (ICA) course has four parts: cervical (ascending through the neck), petrous (crossing the temporal bone), cavernous, and cerebral (see Fig. 12.20). The cervical part ascends the neck in the carotid sheath without any branches, and enters the petrous bone through the carotid canal. The petrous part gives off the caroticotympanic and pterygoid branches. It travels along the petrous bone and then enters the cavernous sinus between the anterior and middle clinoid processes, medial to the abducens nerve. The cavernous part has small branches to the wall of the cavernous sinus, hypophysis, and the semilunar ganglion of the trigeminal nerve. In its last segment, the ICA enters the middle cranial fossa and branches into the ophthalmic artery, anterior choroidal artery, and posterior communicating artery (PcommA). It finally bifurcates into the anterior and middle cerebral arteries, and these terminal branches form part of the Circle of Willis (See: Vascular Trauma).

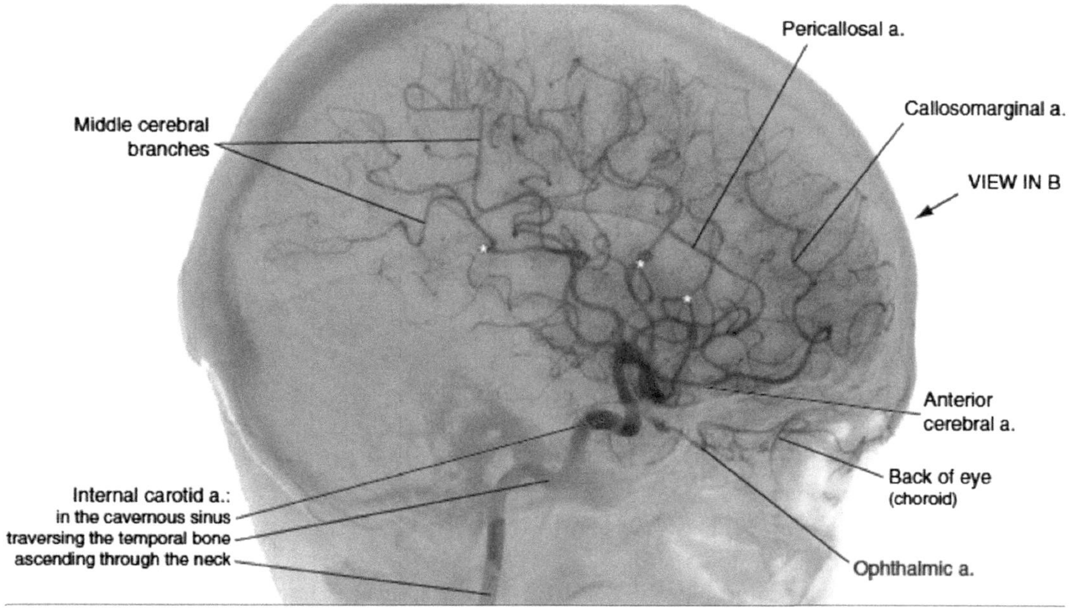

Fig. 12.20 Course of the internal carotid artery, as demonstrated with an arterial phase of a right internal carotid angiogram, lateral view. Nolte [168], 6th Ed. Reproduced with permission from Elsevier

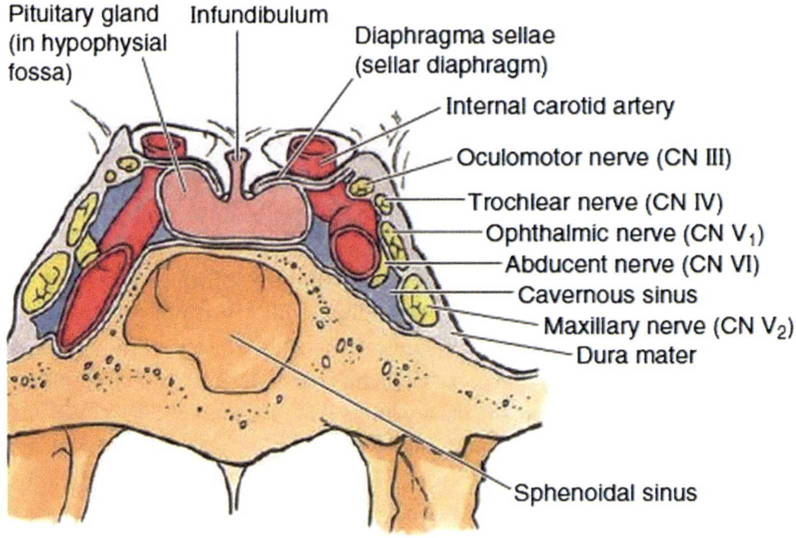

Fig. 12.21 Cavernous sinus anatomy. From Moore Clinically Oriented Anatomy. 6th Ed. Reproduced with permission from Wolters Kluwer

The cavernous and petrous segments of the ICA are most susceptible to basilar skull fracture due to proximity to the skull base. ICA injury carries severe risk of stroke, pseudoaneurysm, and death [137]. The ICA carries postganglionic sympathetic fibers. If the postganglionic sympathetic fibers traveling on the ICA are injured, patients can develop partial Horner Syndrome with miosis and ptosis [133]. Anhidrosis is an unlikely manifestation of Horner syndrome from middle skull base fracture, because sympathetic nerve fibers responsible for sweating travel separately with the external carotid and maxillary arteries [155].

Cavernous Sinus

The cavernous sinus is a paired structure located within the sphenoid bone on either side of the sella turcica. It contains CN III, IV, V1, V2, VI, the cavernous portion of internal carotid artery, and postganglionic sympathetics traveling on the ICA (see Fig. 12.21). Cranial nerve neuropathies may follow trauma involving the cavernous sinus [133]. CN VI is most susceptible due to its medial location in the cavernous sinus. Comparatively, CN III, IV, V1 and V2 are located in the lateral cavernous sinus, where the dural attachments of the cavernous sinus are protective [156].

The cavernous sinus has multiple venous connections, creating an overall low-pressure venous system (see Fig. 12.22) [156]. The anterior and posterior intercavernous sinuses create a communication between the right and left cavernous sinuses. Anteriorly, the superior and inferior ophthalmic veins and the sphenoparietal sinuses drain into the cavernous sinus. Posteriorly, the cavernous sinus drains into the superior and inferior petrosal sinuses, which will ultimately drain into the sigmoid sinus, transverse sinus, and internal jugular vein. Superiorly, the superficial, middle, and inferior cerebral veins approach the cavernous sinus. Inferior to the cavernous sinus, the emissary veins drain into the pterygoid plexus. If there is an ICA injury in the region of the cavernous sinus, there is risk of carotid-cavernous fistula (CCF) formation with backup of blood into the venous system (see carotid-cavernous fistula section later in this chapter) [137, 157].

Petrous bone

The petrous bone is commonly involved in middle skull base fractures [137]. The most frequent clinical presentation of petrous bone fracture is conductive hearing loss due to middle ear and ossicular chain damage [137]. Patients may

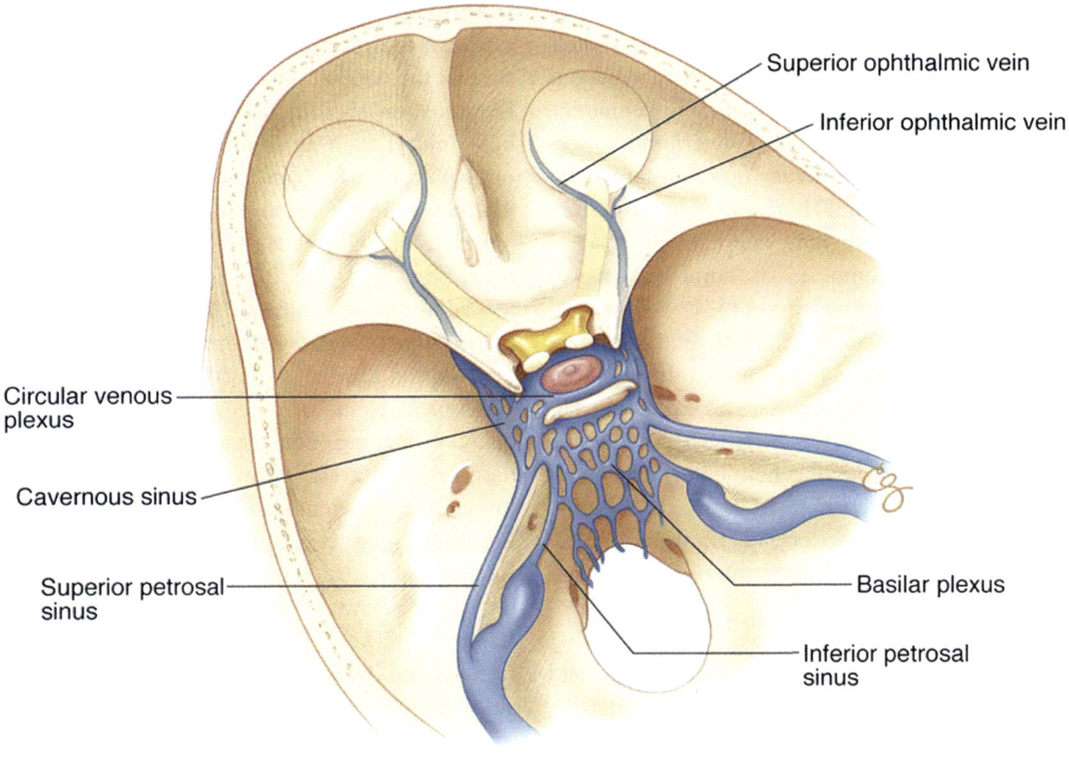

Fig. 12.22 Anatomy of the cavernous sinus drainage system. From BCSC Neuro-ophthalmology. Reproduced with permission from American Academy of Ophthalmology

also have postauricular hematoma (Battle's sign), hemotympanum, or CSF otorrhea. There may be vascular injury to the ICA or to the superior petrosal sinus, which courses along the medial border of the petrous bone in the petrous ridge [148].

There may be associated cranial nerve injury, especially sensorineural deafness, vertigo, or tinnitus from CN VIII injury or facial palsy from CN VII injury. CN VI palsy is less common with middle skull base fracture, but it can occur if the middle skull base fracture extends to the petrous apex and sphenoid sinus [155]. Such an extensive fracture would produce traumatic petrous apex syndrome, involving CN V, VI, VII, and VIII. The CN VI palsy is often caused by benign stretching injury and usually spontaneously resolves in a few months (See: Oculomotor Injury Section) [158].

Posterior Skull Base Fracture

The posterior skull base begins anteriorly at the clivus and it is formed by the occipital bone and the posterior temporal bone. The posterior cranial fossa holds the cerebellar hemispheres, midbrain, pons, and medulla. The cerebellum is separated from the temporal and occipital lobes by the tentorium cerebelli.

The posterior skull base is the least likely location for skull base fracture. The majority of posterior skull base fractures involve the petrous and occipital bones [133, 137]. The severity of traumatic impact and coup-contrecoup injury may cause parieto-occipital contusions and associated visual field defects [50].

Epidural hematoma (EDH) is the most common complication seen with posterior skull base fractures. The venous sinuses, particularly the sigmoid sinus, jugular bulb, and transverse sinus, are susceptible in this region [133]. If a posterior skull base fracture lacerates the posterior venous sinuses, it can cause a posterior fossa venous EDH [137]. There is high risk of rapid hematoma expansion, and acute clinical deterioration secondary to fourth ventricular or brainstem compression (see: Epidural Hematoma section) [133]. Venous sinus injury may alternatively lead to venous sinus thrombosis or dural AV fistula (See: Venous Injury section) [133].

The posterior skull base has several important foramina. The jugular foramen is at the posterior end of the petro-occipital fissure, extending laterally from the posterior occipital condyle. The sigmoid sinus and jugular bulb enter the jugular foramen at its posterior end. CN IX, X, XI enter the foramen at its anterior end. Damage to these cranial nerves is life-threatening. Deficits can include dysphagia, loss of the gag reflex, orthostatic hypotension, vocal cord paresis causing airway obstruction, upper GI dysmotility, and paralysis of sternocleidomastoid and trapezius muscles [133, 159].

The hypoglossal foramen carries CN XII, the meningeal branch of the ascending pharyngeal artery, and hypoglossal venous plexus. The hypoglossal foramen is adjacent to the occipital condyles. Fracture through this region is rare, and could result in ipsilateral tongue deviation and atrophy from CN XII palsy [133, 155].

The foramen magnum transmits the brainstem, medulla, CN XI, vertebral and posterior spinal arteries, and the exit of the spinal cord. The clivus extends to the foramen magnum, and there is a high mortality associated with clivus fracture due to the proximity of the clivus to the brainstem and spinal cord [142, 160]. Bilateral CN VI palsy is a sign of clival fracture because the Dorello canal is located within the clivus [133, 137]. In addition, the basilar artery and other nearby cranial nerves are susceptible to injury. Clivus fracture is very rare, occurring in only 2% of all cranial fractures with an estimated incidence of 0.21–0.56% [133, 160]. Reported mortality following clival fracture varies from 24 to 80% [160].

Diagnosis of Skull Base Fracture

Physical examination may be limited due to the state of the patient following high impact trauma. Examination should look for evidence of skull base injury, such as cranial nerve deficits, periorbital ecchymosis, and hemotympanum [133]. There should be a close examination for CSF otorrhea or rhinorrhea, which is diagnostic of dural break and skull base injury [141]. Damage to adjacent structures, such as the globe, extraocular muscles, and lacrimal drainage system, should also be assessed.

Clinical examination should be paired with detailed imaging. For primary diagnosis, a standard non-contrast head CT can rule out intracranial hematomas or other acutely life-threatening conditions [137]. This can be followed up by more detailed imaging as described below. In cases of posterior skull base fracture, a repeat CT scan should be conducted to rule out late-developing hematomas from venous sinus injury [137].

Imaging for Skull Base Fracture

High-Resolution CT

High-resolution CT (HRCT) with multiplanar reformats in the axial, coronal, and sagittal planes is considered the best means to image skull base fractures and understand the extent of damage [136, 137, 142, 161]. Multiplanar reconstruction has improved skull base fracture detection rates, and has a reported sensitivity as high as 92% and a specificity of 100% [133, 145]. Its level of detail is useful for surgical planning [136, 161]. HRCT predicts CSF leak with an 87–92% reported accuracy [136, 145, 162]. However, HRCT has limitations for CSF leak because it may identify bony defects that are not actively leaking CSF [136, 143].

The fracture is identified on HRCT as a non-corticated, non-interdigitating lucency in the skull base. There may be adjacent pneumocephalus, sinus or mastoid opacification, air-fluid levels, or intraorbital emphysema (see Fig. 12.23) [133].

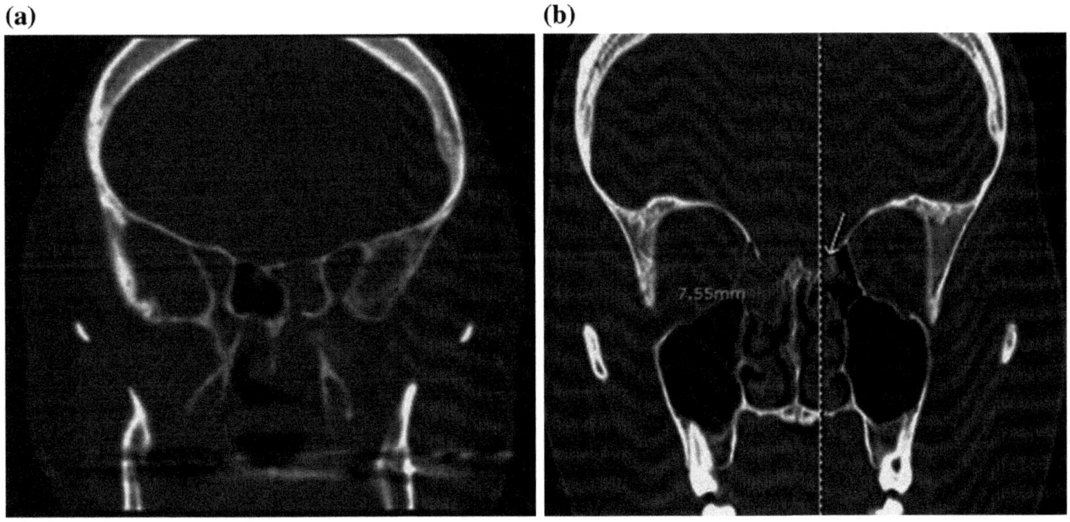

Fig. 12.23 **a** Coronal reconstruction on HRCT of a patient with a basilar skull fracture in the area of the sphenoid. The bony defect and filling of the sinus with fluid is seen. **b** Coronal reconstruction on HRCT of a patient with bilateral basilar skull fractures with bony displacement (*arrow*). From Lin and Lin [136]. Reproduced with permission from Elsevier

CT Angiography

CT Angiography (CTA) is routinely used for all patients with complex skull base fractures that involve the carotid canal or cavernous sinus [133, 157]. Findings that prompt further evaluation with CTA include clinical or radiologic evidence of thromboembolic disease such as stroke, fractures through the carotid canal, air within the cavernous sinus, intracanalicular air, enlarged superior ophthalmic veins, or fractures through the clivus [133]. Alternatives to CTA are carotid angiography, digital subtraction angiography (DSA), and magnetic resonance angiography (MRA). Vascular imaging is critical in a preoperative work-up to rule out carotid pseudoaneurysms and CCFs prior to surgery [136].

CT Venography

CT Venography (CTV) is used for all skull base fractures that involve the transverse sinus, superior sagittal sinus, jugular foramen, or other major venous landmark. If there is sinus involvement, HRCT shows increased density in the venous sinuses, which can represent venous sinus thrombosis or extra-axial hemorrhage [133]. Both CTA and CTV should be performed urgently if HRCT indicates vascular involvement.

MRI

If a patient has clinical features of cranial nerve palsy, MRI is required to assess for neural compression [142]. The soft tissue detail provided by MRI is useful for examining early and late complications of basilar skull fracture, such as infection, concussion, and herniation [142]. MRI is also useful for providing additional details about the skull base fracture because CSF appears hyperintense on T2-weighted imaging [136]. However, MRI has a high false positive rate for localizing fractures and CSF fistulas because CSF is difficult to differentiate from mucosal thickening and fluid within a sinus [136, 149]. Therefore, CT is preferred for early investigations of head injury and MRI is only used as a secondary evaluation of soft tissue detail [137].

Evaluation for CSF Leak

The diagnosis of CSF leak is critical in basilar skull fracture management. CSF leak is evidence of a dural break. Its presence and associated risk for meningitis dictates the treatment plan for basilar skull fracture. Localization of a CSF fistula is needed prior to surgical interventions.

The initial evaluation for CSF leak is clinical. Patients are asked to perform valsalva or positional maneuvers to see if CSF rhinorrhea or otorrhea is produced from the high-pressure maneuvers [137]. If CSF rhinorrhea or otorrhea is suspected, the secretions are collected for laboratory testing with β-2 transferrin or β-trace protein testing. In addition, all patients with suspected CSF leak will undergo HRCT to localize the site [149]. HRCT may be followed by other imaging tests, such as CT cisternography, MR cisternography, intrathecal fluorescein injection, or radionuclide cisternography if the fracture site is not easily localized [133, 137].

β-2 Transferrin Test

The β-2 transferrin test is the gold standard for identifying CSF in fluid [136]. β-2 transferrin is produced by neuraminidase activity in the brain and is abundant in CSF. Detection of beta-2 transferrin in nasal or aural secretions, where it is not normally present, provides an indirect and noninvasive diagnosis of CSF leak [149]. Only 0.5 mL of rhinorrhea or otorrhea fluid is needed for testing [143], and the test has a reported sensitivity of 99% and a specificity of 97% [163]. The test can be used for an early diagnosis or to rule out latent CSF leaks that may appear weeks or months following trauma [137, 143].

On its own, the β-2 transferrin test is limited because it cannot provide information about the location of the CSF fistula [143]. If there is a positive β-2 transferrin test and HRCT identifies a single potential fracture site, this is strong evidence for the site of CSF leak [145]. If HRCT shows two possible sites of osseous defect, CT cisternography should be performed to conclusively identify the site of CSF leak [145]. If the β-2 transferrin test is negative, the test should be repeated. A series of two negative tests is enough to rule out CSF leak [133].

β-trace Protein Test

The β-trace protein (BTP) test is an alternative to the β-2 transferrin test [136]. BTP is produced in the leptomeninges and the epithelial cells of the choroid plexus. It is the second most abundant protein in CSF, at a concentration 35-fold more than in plasma. BTP is present in very small concentrations in nasal secretions, so detection of BTP can indirectly diagnose CSF rhinorrhea. Compared to the β-transferrin test, BTP detection requires less time and cost. However, the test cannot be used for patients with bacterial meningitis or reduced GFR, which affects BTP levels [149].

CT Cisternography

CT cisternography (CTC) can confirm that a basilar skull fracture identified on HRCT correlates with an active CSF leak [149]. It is useful for identifying the location if HRCT shows multiple fracture sites that could possibly be linked to CSF leak [133, 143]. CTC is also recommended if there is a high probability of CSF fistula (i.e., positive β-2 transferrin test) but HRCT did not identify a bony defect [137, 162].

A CT is performed following administration of intrathecal iodinated contrast [143]. CTC can only be undertaken in a patient who has an active CSF leak or a leak that can be elicited with maneuvers such as Valsalva or bending down [133, 149]. The CT represents one point in time, so intermittent CSF leaks may not be identified. The sensitivity of the test varies from 48 to 98% based on flow rate of the CSF leak [162]. Reliability of the test is also affected by location of CSF leak. CTC has best visibility for CSF fistula in the frontal or sphenoid sinus because the sinuses act as reservoirs of the iodinated contrast [143].

Magnetic Resonance Cisternography

Magnetic Resonance Cisternography (MRC) is an alternative to CTC for localizing active CSF fistulas [149]. It cannot identify intermittent leaks, and has a reported accuracy of 89 and 87%

sensitivity across both active and inactive leaks [143, 145]. MRC is typically reserved for patients with complex trauma, multiple fracture sites, or high suspicion of encephalocele or meningoencephalocele [145].

Intrathecal Fluorescein Injection

CSF fistula can be diagnosed with intrathecal injection of sodium fluorescein solution followed by a minimally invasive endoscopic examination with special filters or UV sources to identify areas of fluorescein leak [137, 143]. Intrathecal fluorescein injection is not FDA approved for use in the United States [136]. The test has use for finding CSF leaks that have small CSF output, but it is limited by several factors. The test's reliability varies based on size of defect, timing of intrathecal injection, rate of leak, and rate of CSF turnover [149]. If there is a high rate of turnover and leak, then fluorescein may be diluted by the time of endoscopic exam. Skull base exposure is limited for patients that have not had previous sinus or skull base surgery [143]. Reported complications from sodium fluorescein solution include mild tinnitus, headache, nausea, vomiting, pulmonary edema, confusion, seizure, coma, and death [149]. These side effects are minimized with lower concentrations of sodium fluorescein [143, 149].

Radionuclide Cisternography

With radionuclide cisternography, pledgets are placed intranasally and then the patient receives an intrathecal injection of a radiotracer [143]. After several hours, pledgets are removed and analyzed for radioactivity. Because the pledgets are held in place for several hours, the test is useful for low-volume or intermittent leaks that are not well identified with CT or MR cisternography. However, the test can only identify the presence of CSF leak and cannot make determinations about the location. Sensitivity varies from 62 to 76% and there is a false positive rate up to 33% [143, 145, 162].

Management of Skull Base Fracture

Management of basilar skull fracture is individualized to the patient based on the patient's clinical presentation and severity of basilar skull fracture [143]. In cases of polytrauma, the management of other injuries may need to be prioritized over the skull base fracture [141].

A closed basilar skull fracture with no associated vascular or nerve damage does not require surgical repair. Basilar skull fractures with dural break, indicated by CSF leak, have two primary management options: conservative and surgical management. The presence and duration of CSF leak, size and quality of fracture, and evidence of additional intracranial injuries play a key role in the decision for nonsurgical or surgical management.

Conservative Management

The goal of conservative management is to decrease intracranial pressure and rate of CSF leakage. The patient is often maintained in the ICU for observation during this time [137]. Conservative measures include bed rest, head elevation, and carbonic anhydrase inhibitors [133, 164]. Sinus precautions are in place to prevent increased pressure in the sinuses, which could contribute to CSF leak. Sinus precautions involve avoidance of nose blowing, drinking straws, and incentive spirometers [136]. Patients are given stool softeners to prevent Valsalva maneuvers [133].

For a stable patient with CSF leak, conservative management is encouraged because traumatic CSF leaks are associated with a high rate of spontaneous closure, ranging from 50 to 90% and often observed within one week of traumatic injury [133, 136, 139, 140, 149]. In a retrospective review of 735 patients with skull base fracture, 28 out of 34 patients with CSF leak resolved following 2–10 days of conservative management [164]. In a report describing 92 patients with skull base fracture, conservative management led to spontaneous resolution of 26 out of 29 cases of CSF otorrhea or otorrhinorrhea [146]. Given these promising statistics, the majority of patients can avoid unneeded surgery and its associated risks. After resolution of CSF leak, the patient should continue to be monitored for recurrent CSF leak or a late meningoencephalocele [136].

CSF diversion
CSF diversion is initiated if the CSF leak does not resolve following 7 or more days of conservative management [165]. Lumbar drain puncture or external ventricular drain may be used [164]. Lumbar drain is less invasive and preferred for CSF diversion, but external ventricular drain is useful if patients require continuous intracranial pressure monitoring [149]. CSF diversion has variable success for terminating CSF leak. Success is closely related to the severity of the injury and size of skull base defect [164].

Antibiotic Prophylaxis
The need for antibiotic prophylaxis for a patient with skull base fracture and CSF leak is currently debated [136]. In a 2011 Cochrane review regarding the efficacy of antibiotic prophylaxis for meningitis prevention, the compiled data from five randomized controlled trials did not provide clear evidence to support antibiotic prophylaxis [166]. There was no significant difference between antibiotic prophylaxis groups and controlled placebo groups regarding the incidence of meningitis, meningitis-related morality, or the all-cause mortality. The review indicated that previously published RCTs were limited in size and researcher bias, and request that more research is needed before a stronger evaluation regarding antibiotic prophylaxis can be made [166].

Surgical Management

Surgery Following Conservative Management
If a CSF leak persists following 1 week of conservative management, surgical management is favored. At this point, there is a low likelihood of spontaneous resolution of the CSF leak, and the risk of meningitis increases to 9% [133, 136, 149, 165].

Early Surgical Management
There are several circumstances in which surgery for skull base fracture should be undertaken early in the patient's treatment course.
The size of a fracture dictates its prognosis. Large skull fractures with bone displacement greater than 1 cm require surgical repair [133, 136, 167]. Severe compound, comminuted, depressed fractures or fractures with large extensions are unlikely to spontaneously heal and should be surgically closed [133, 136, 165]. The location of the fracture and CSF fistula is also an important factor. Fractures of the cribriform plate or near the midline are more likely to develop infection and require repair [136, 165, 167]. CSF leak caused by temporal bone trauma or iatrogenic causes are less likely to stop spontaneously, and physicians should have a lower threshold for recommending surgical closure [146]. If a CSF leak is recurrent or delayed, there is also low likelihood of spontaneous closure and these are good candidates for surgical dural closure [149, 165].

An entire assessment of the patient can reveal reasons for surgical management. Encephalocele or meningoencephalocele secondary to basilar skull fracture should be urgently treated [133, 136, 137]. The herniation prevents spontaneous closure of the dural defect, and is associated with a high risk of recurring meningitis from exposure to sinus bacteria [165].

Life-threatening intracranial pathology may arise secondary to basilar skull fracture or the inciting high impact trauma. Surgical emergencies include tension pneumocephalus, compressive intracranial hematoma, other significant vascular injury, or cranial nerve injury [133, 136, 137, 165]. When immediate open intracranial repair is required for another cause, basal skull fracture and dural repair may be conducted at the time if the patient is clinically stable with good neural status and there is no concern for intracranial edema [133, 136, 149].

The timing of early surgical management is individualized based on the clinical state of the patient. If surgery is needed for life-threatening intracranial injury, it should be performed as soon as the patient is clinically stable for surgery [165]. For patients that require fracture repair and dural closure for severe fracture types, the risks of surgery are reduced if the procedure is postponed until resolution of acute post-traumatic cerebral edema [167]. When the cerebral parenchyma is edematous, it is more vulnerable to injury and operations that are performed too early could be fatal [165].

Surgical Approach

There are a variety of surgical approaches to repair of basal skull fractures and CSF fistula. Endoscopic techniques have become the standard of care, but craniotomy may still be used depending on the location and severity of skull base fracture [143, 149]. CSF fistula is closed at the same time as surgical repair of skull base fracture [165]. In the operating room, the identified site of dural break is exposed, the recipient bed is prepared, and graft material is placed to tightly seal the CSF leak [136, 137, 143]. Any associated intracranial or maxillofacial injuries should also be repaired at this time [137, 139]. For extensive trauma with a large amount of soft tissue and bony damage, bone grafts or free flap reconstruction may be employed [136, 141].

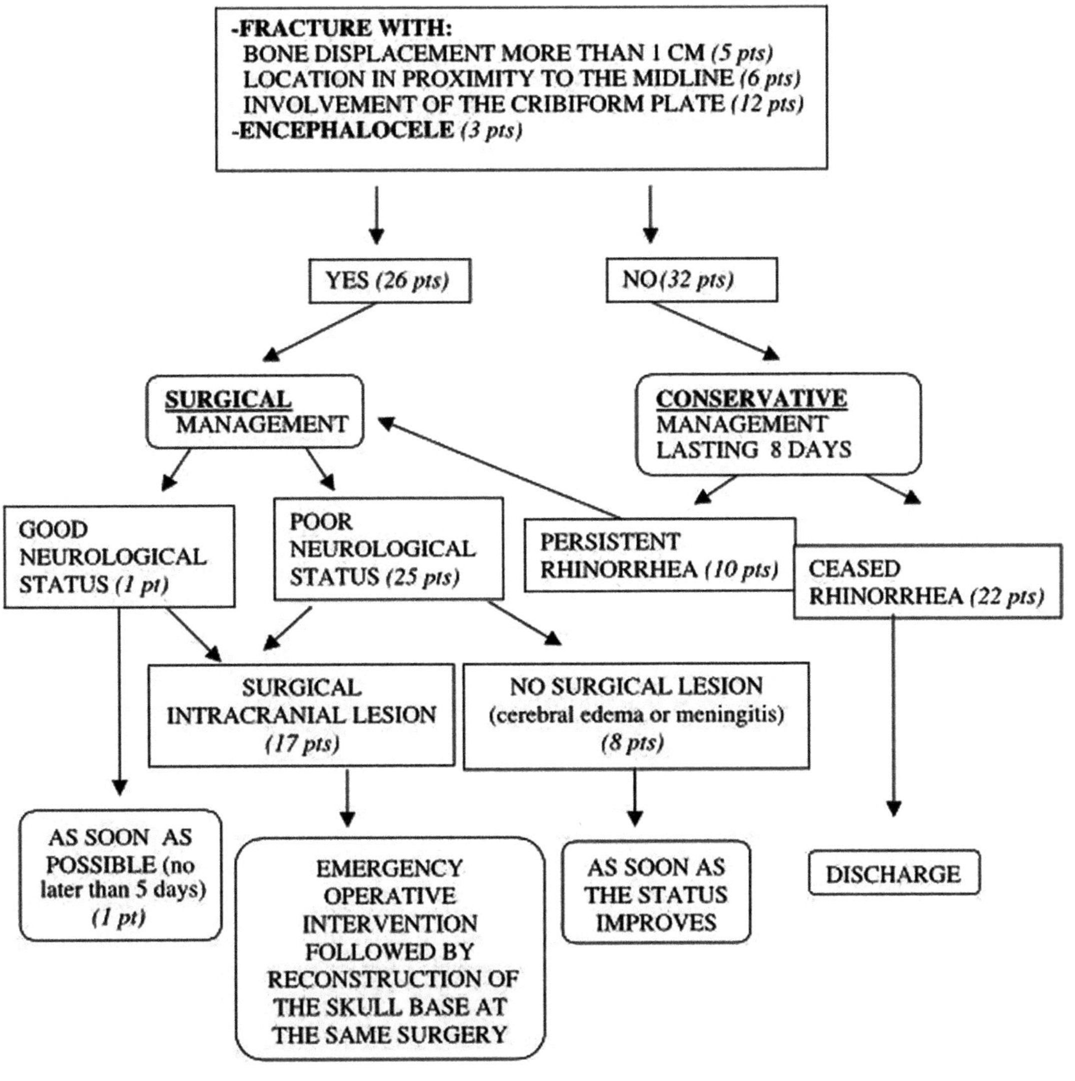

Fig. 12.24 Management of post-traumatic CSF fistula. From Rocchi (2005). Severe craniofacial fractures with frontobasal involvement and cerebrospinal fluid fistula: indications for surgical repair. Surgical neurology. Reproduced with permission from Elsevier

Complications
Complications following repair of CSF fistula include recurrent CSF leak, sinusitis, vision changes, intracranial hypertension, cavernous sinus thrombosis, seizure, meningitis, subdural hematoma (SDH), pneumocephalus, intracranial abscesses, and death [136, 149, 165]. A movement toward endoscopic repair of CSF fistulas has decreased the risk of major complications from 1 to 2.5% to less than 1% [149].
Outcomes
The refinement of endoscopic and extracranial techniques has led to improved success rates for CSF fistula repair and neurosurgical repair of skull base fractures. The success rate for CSF repair via craniotomy is estimated at 70–80%. Success rates for endoscopic repair are reported to be 90% or greater and avoid the risks of craniotomy [143, 149]. A CSF fistula treatment algorithm can be seen in Fig. 12.24.

Penetrating Trauma to the Visual Pathways

Intracranial penetrating trauma may be caused by low velocity mechanisms such as stab wounds or high-velocity mechanisms such as gunshot wounds. Low velocity penetrating injury only damages structures in its course. Comparatively, high-velocity penetrating trauma causes direct injury along its trajectory, as well as diffuse damage from a fast release of forces due to a rapidly increased intracranial pressure [141]. As a result, gunshot wound injuries typically involve radial fracture lines extending from the site of penetrating injury, comminuted, and displaced fracture fragments [141].

If the course of penetrating injury disrupts the visual pathways, it may result in corresponding visual field defects. The visual pathway involves the route of the optic nerve to the optic chiasm, optic tracts, lateral geniculate body, and optic radiations. It ends at the visual cortex in the occipital lobe. The anatomy of the visual pathways and predicted visual field defects based on the site of lesion are summarized in Fig. 12.25 and Table 12.7.

Vascular Trauma

The brain is a region of high metabolic activity. Without its own oxygen or glucose stores, the brain is dependent on cerebral perfusion. Irreversible damage can occur to the brain with only a few minutes of ischemia [168]. Ischemic damage is a common cause of visual dysfunction.

Arterial Supply to the Brain

Internal Carotid Arteries
The internal carotid arteries provide 80% of the blood supply to the brain (see Table 12.8) [168].

The ICA terminates at the skull base by bifurcating into the anterior cerebral artery (ACA) and middle cerebral artery (MCA). The ACA travels superior to the optic nerve and enters the longitudinal fissure. Its branches arch posteriorly, following corpus callosum to supply the medial frontal and parietal lobes (see Fig. 12.26).

The MCA courses into the lateral sulcus with branches to the insular cortex, and then it courses to supply the lateral surface of the cerebral hemisphere with branches to the temporal lobe, parietal lobe, and superficial portions of the frontal lobe and occipital lobe (see Fig. 12.26). Small MCA branches, the lenticulostriate arteries, penetrate the cerebrum to supply deep structures.

Vertebral-Basilar Artery System
The remaining 20% of blood supply to the brain and spinal cord is from the vertebral-basilar artery system, which supplies the posterior aspect of the intracranial contents, as described in the Table 12.9.
The right vertebral artery is a branch from the innominate artery and the left vertebral artery is a branch from the subclavian artery. The vertebral arteries ascend through foramina on the lateral cervical spinal process, and enter the skull through the foramen magnum. The two vertebral arteries give rise to the posterior spinal artery, anterior spinal artery, and posterior inferior cerebellar artery. The vertebral arteries join near

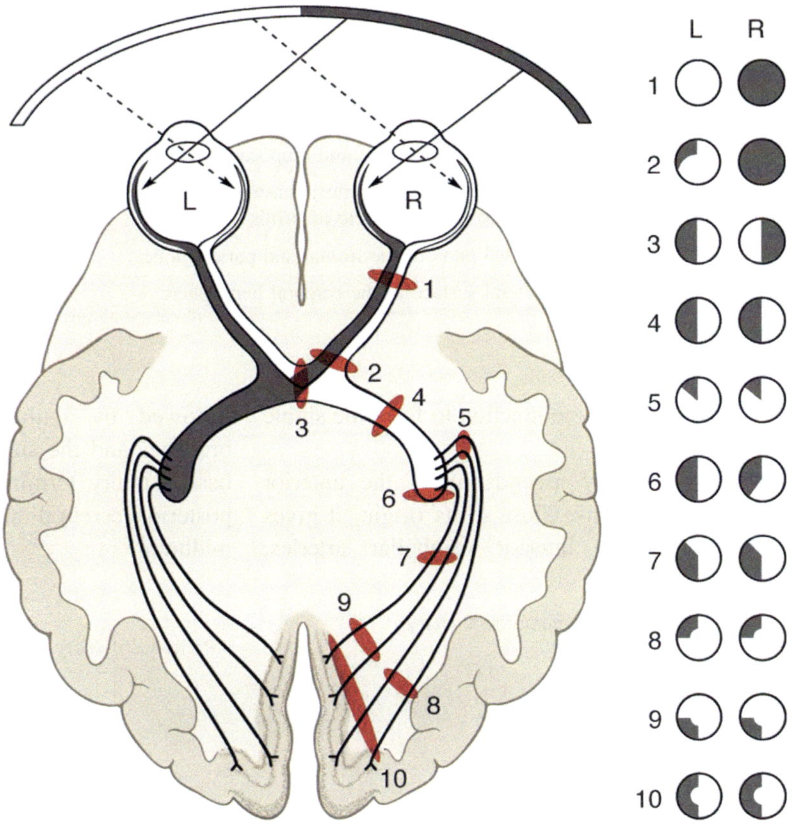

Fig. 12.25 Visual pathways and visual field defects associated with lesions at various locations. From BCSC Neuro-Ophthalmology. Reproduced with permission from American Academy of Ophthalmology

Table 12.7 Result of lesions to visual pathways, as depicted in Fig. 12.25

Label in figure	Site of lesion	Visual field defect
1	Optic nerve	Ipsilateral loss of vision
2	Optic nerve at its junction with the optic chiasm	Junctional scotoma: ipsilateral loss of vision and contralateral superior temporal hemianopia
3	Optic chiasm, medial aspect	Bitemporal hemianopia
4	Optic tract	Contralateral homonymous hemianopia
5	Optic radiation, temporal lobe (Meyer's loop)	Contralateral homonymous superior quadrantanopia
6	Lateral geniculate nucleus	Contralateral incongruous homonymous hemianopia (sectoranopia)
7	Optic radiation, parietal lobe	Contralateral homonymous inferior quadrantanopia
8	Occipital lobe, inferior	Contralateral homonymous superior quadrantanopia, macular sparing
9	Occipital lobe, superior	Contralateral homonymous inferior quadrantanopia, macular sparing
10	Majority of occipital lobe, sparing the posterior tip	Contralateral hemianopia, macular sparing

Table 12.8 Areas supplied by branches of ICA

ICA branch	Area supplied
Ophthalmic a.	Eye, orbital contents, ocular adnexa
Anterior choroidal a.	Optic tract, choroid plexus of inferior horn of lateral ventricle, portions of internal capsule, thalamus, amygdala, and hippocampus
Posterior communicating a.	Thalamus, hypothalamus, anastomosis with posterior cerebral artery (vertebral artery system) to form Circle of Willis
Anterior cerebral a.	Medial parts of the frontal and parietal lobes
Middle cerebral a.	Lateral surface of the cerebral hemisphere

Adapted from Nolte [168]

the medullary-pontine junction to form the single basilar artery.

The basilar artery ascends along the anterior surface of the pons. Close to its origin, it gives off the anterior inferior cerebellar arteries, followed by multiple small pontine arterial branches and the superior cerebellar artery. The basilar artery terminates by branching into the posterior cerebral arteries at the level of the midbrain.

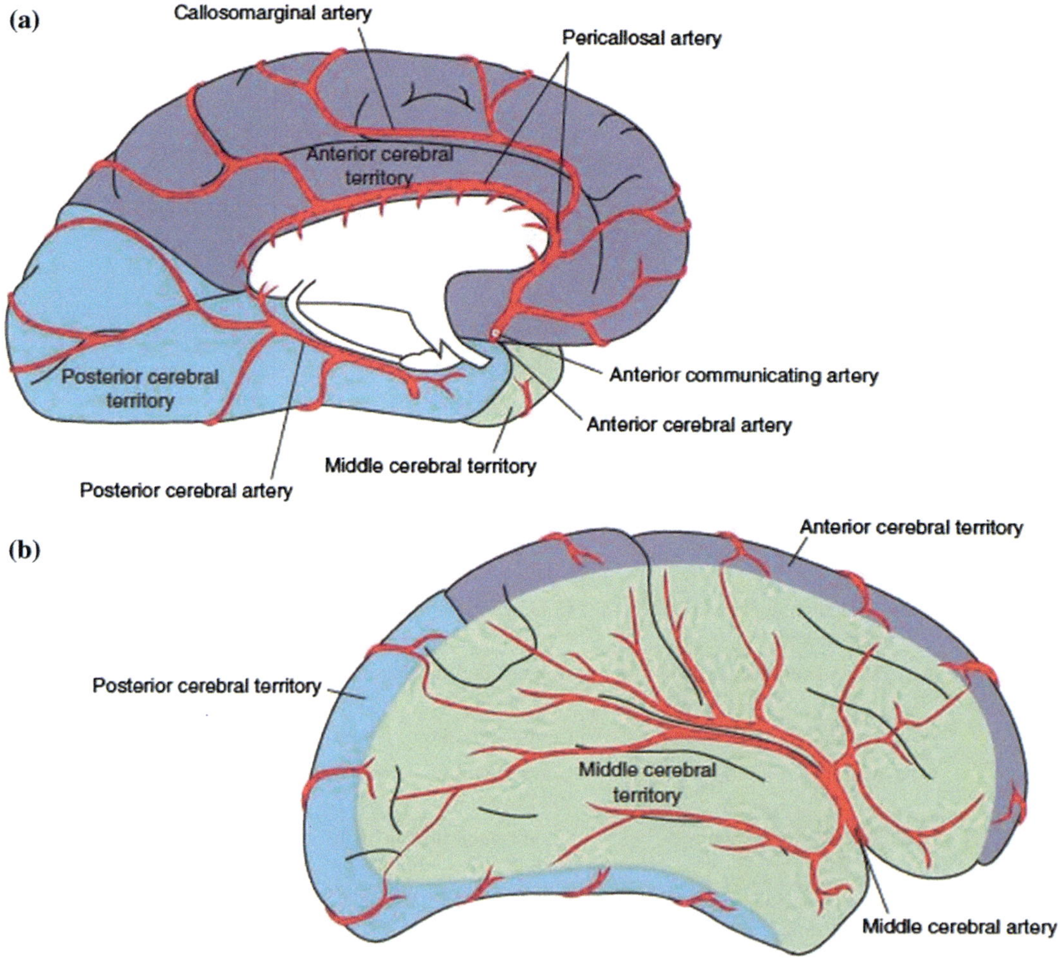

Fig. 12.26 From Nolte [168]. 6th Ed. Figure 6-4 "Arteries on the medial and lateral surfaces of the brain, with their areas of supply indicated". Reproduced with permission from Elsevier

Table 12.9 Areas supplied by the vertebral-basilar arterial system

Vertebral a. branches	Area supplied
Posterior spinal a.	Posterior third of spinal cord
Anterior spinal a.	Anterior two-thirds of spinal cord
Posterior inferior cerebellar a.	Inferior surface of cerebellar hemisphere, lateral medulla, choroid plexus of fourth ventricle
Basilar a. branches	**Area supplied**
Anterior inferior cerebellar a.	Anterior portions of inferior surface of the cerebellum, parts of caudal pons
Pontine aa.	Pons, midbrain
Superior cerebellar a.	Superior surface of the cerebellum, caudal midbrain, rostral pons
Posterior cerebral a.	Medial and inferior surfaces of temporal and occipital lobes (including primary visual cortex), rostral midbrain, posterior diencephalon, choroid plexus of the third ventricle, body of lateral ventricle

Adapted from Nolte [168]

Circle of Willis

The Circle of Willis forms an anastomosis between the ICA and vertebral-basilar systems, therefore providing a safety net in the case of vascular occlusion. The posterior cerebral artery (PCA) from the vertebral-basilar system connects to the PcommA from the ICA (see Fig. 12.27).

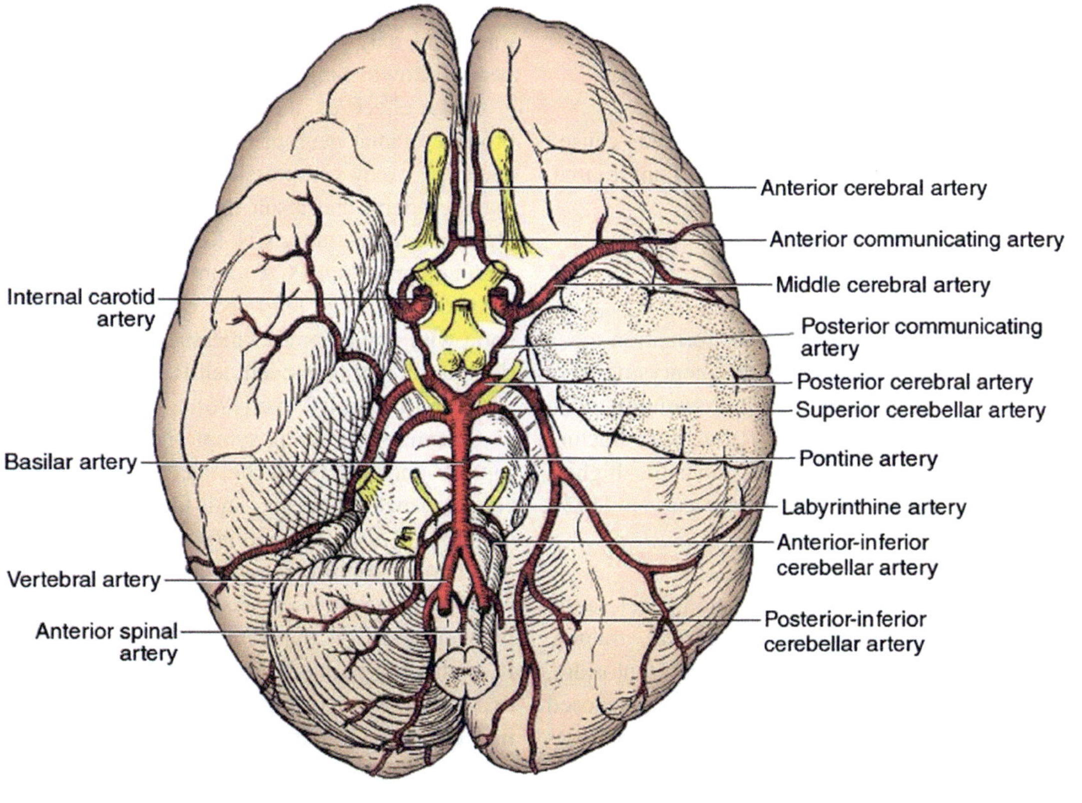

Fig. 12.27 Circle of Willis. From BRS Gross Anatomy 7th ed. Reproduced with permission from Wolters Kluwer

Traumatic Arterial Injury: Traumatic Aneurysms

Traumatic intracranial aneurysms are rare, representing less than 1% of all intracranial aneurysms [169]. They are more prevalent in children than adults, and it is estimated that 30% of traumatic aneurysms occur in patients less than 20 years old [15, 170]. There is a severe risk of delayed intracranial hemorrhage (ICH), and ruptured traumatic aneurysms have a mortality rate of about 50% [171, 172].

Traumatic aneurysms are "false" aneurysms. There is a complete disruption of the arterial wall, and a false lumen is formed by a surrounding hematoma [169]. Such aneurysms often have a poorly defined shape and irregular neck.

Traumatic aneurysms most frequently form at the skull base or on distal, small cerebral branches [169]. The majority (90%) of traumatic aneurysms occur in the anterior fossa. Those in the posterior fossa likely involve the posterior inferior cerebellar artery and are associated with an occipital bone fracture [15].

Mechanism

Traumatic aneurysms are most commonly caused by penetrating trauma, followed by blunt trauma, and iatrogenic trauma [15].

Penetrating Trauma

Penetrating intracranial injury can directly damage vessels walls and induce formation of a traumatic aneurysm. Traumatic aneurysms have been associated with gunshot wounds, stab wounds, and bone fragments from skull fracture [15, 169, 172]. Stab wounds have the highest probability of causing traumatic aneurysm [173].

Blunt Trauma

Shearing forces from acceleration-deceleration injuries can cause indirect arterial trauma. A vessel may directly strike the falx, tentorium, or skull base as a result of high-velocity closed head trauma [15, 174]. Motor vehicle accidents and falls from heights are cited as the most common mechanisms to cause traumatic aneurysm [170, 175].

Iatrogenic Trauma

There is a risk of traumatic aneurysm from intracranial surgery, endoscopic skull base surgery, and endovascular procedures [15]. Less commonly, traumatic aneurysm has been reported following endarterectomy, surgical radical neck dissection, chiropractic neck manipulation, angiography, repeated subdural taps, and endoscopic ventriculostomy [15, 172].

Clinical Presentation

Traumatic aneurysm may be asymptomatic, or it can present with symptoms of a mass effect or aneurysm rupture. The timeline of traumatic aneurysm clinical presentation varies based on the location and size of aneurysm. Symptoms may become evident only a few minutes after injury, especially if early rupture occurs. Alternatively, symptoms can also develop slowly over time, and may not be identified until months to years following injury [169].

Mass effect of the traumatic aneurysm can produce cranial neuropathies. Intracavernous ICA aneurysms may compress the optic nerve or ophthalmic artery, and result in ipsilateral vision loss [15]. In a case study, CN III palsy was the presenting sign of left PCA traumatic aneurysm. The symptoms included left upper eyelid ptosis, anisocoria with pupil diameter measuring 3 mm on the right and 5 mm on the left, left RAPD, and limited adduction of the left eye [175].

Common presenting symptoms of aneurysmal rupture include headache, decreased level of consciousness, seizure, and focal neurological deficits [172]. Depending on its location, aneurysmal rupture may result in subarachnoid hemorrhage. Severe epistaxis is a sign of rupture of aneurysms on the petrous or intracavernous ICA and can be fatal. The epistaxis results from expansion of hemorrhage medially and inferiorly into the sphenoid sinus [15].

Iatrogenically caused traumatic aneurysm may present with intraoperative hemorrhage. Postoperative clinical symptoms suggestive of ICH include headache, signs of neurological decline such as coma, epistaxis, or cranial nerve palsy [171].

Diagnosis

Due to nonspecific clinical presentation in the setting of head trauma with possible other intracranial injuries, the diagnosis of traumatic aneurysm requires a high degree of suspicion. In the case of acute neurological deterioration following head injury, traumatic aneurysm should be investigated with radiographic studies [169].

CT Scan

A CT scan is used as the initial diagnostic study because it can be quickly performed in an emergency (Fig. 12.28). It can demonstrate acute ICH in the case of ruptured aneurysm [172]. However, associated hemorrhagic brain lesions related to blunt head trauma or metallic artifacts from penetrating trauma may interfere with visualization [169]. CT scan should be followed with angiography if CT identifies ICH, skull fracture, or if there is continued clinical suspicion for an aneurysm [174]. Follow-up imaging with angiography is especially important in cases of penetrating trauma for which development of traumatic aneurysm is more likely.

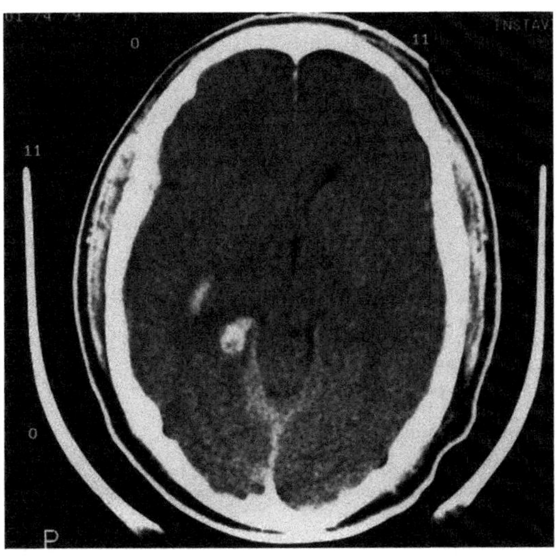

Fig. 12.28 Non-contrast head CT demonstrating subarachnoid and intraparenchymal hemorrhage. From Horowitz et al. [176]. Reproduced with permission by Elsevier

CT Angiography (CTA)

CTA has become the preferred method for the initial evaluation of intracranial vascular injury because it is better to use in emergencies and with acute, unstable patients. The reported sensitivity and specificity of CTA approaches 100% [169]. CTA studies are limited if there are metallic artifacts.

Digital Subtraction Angiography (DSA)

DSA is the gold standard for diagnosing aneurysm, although CTA is preferred in emergencies [170]. DSA is used to confirm and document the location of aneurysms initially identified with CTA. On DSA, traumatic aneurysms are identified due to delayed filling and emptying of the aneurysmal sac [169]. An arteriogram image can be seen in Fig. 12.29.

The timeline of imaging is important. Traumatic aneurysms may take some time to develop. If an early angiographic study is negative, it should be repeated 2–4 weeks after the injury to rule out delayed formation of an aneurysm [169]. There have been several documented reports of patients with normal angiographic studies immediately after trauma who then experienced delayed hemorrhage weeks following trauma and repeat angiographic studies identified delayed traumatic aneurysms [172].

Management

Early management of traumatic aneurysm is advised due to the risk of aneurysmal rupture and high associated mortality rate [169]. Traumatic aneurysm is managed with neurosurgical or endovascular methods designed to remove the aneurysm from the general circulation. Endovascular approaches include detachable balloons or embolization with detachable coils [172]. Surgical approaches include aneurysm clipping or excision of the aneurysm with anastomosis or bypass of the affected artery [15, 176]. The appropriate treatment option is based on the location of aneurysm and its structure.

(a) (b)

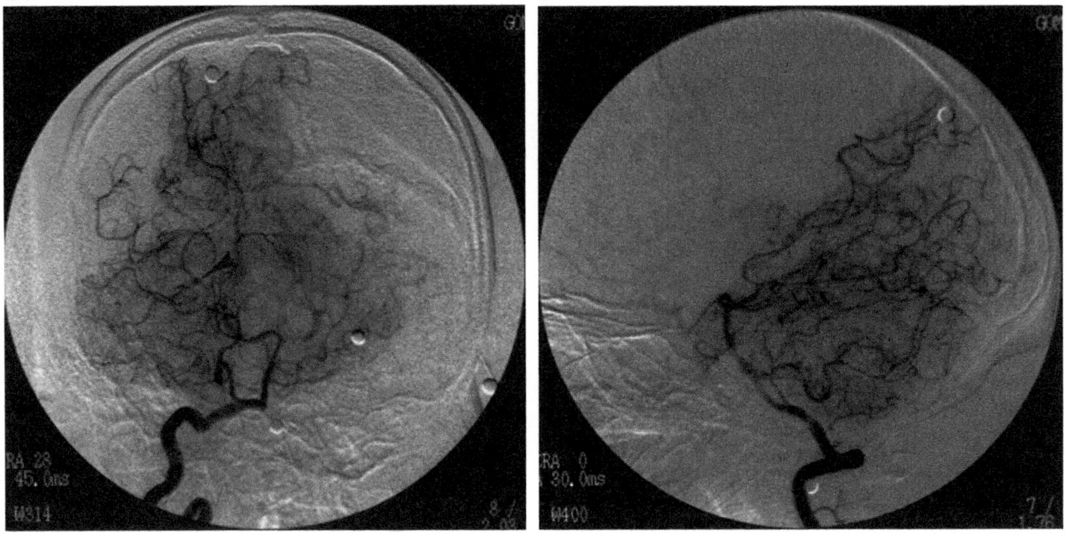

Fig. 12.29 AP (**a**) and lateral (**b**) right vertebral artery arteriogram demonstrating a PCA aneurysm (*arrowhead*). From Horowitz et al. [176]. Reproduced with permission from Elsevier

Carotid-Cavernous Fistula and Cavernous Sinus Syndrome A CCF is an abnormal connection between the carotid artery or its branches and the venous networks of the cavernous sinus. CCF arising secondary to trauma is rare. They have been reported in about 0.2% of craniomaxillofacial trauma cases [177, 178]. Although the overall incidence of CCF following trauma is low, CCF is the most common post-traumatic intracranial vascular anomaly [156].

The CCF is an opening for high arterial pressure to enter the typically low-pressure venous system of the cavernous sinus (see: Skull Base Fracture section for description of cavernous sinus anatomy). With the high-pressure system, there is potential for reversal of blood flow within the superior ophthalmic vein. Subsequent venous congestion within the orbit is termed cavernous sinus syndrome.

CCFs may be high-flow (direct) or low-flow (dural) fistulas. High-flow connections are between the internal carotid artery and cavernous sinus, whereas low-flow connections involve small arterial branches of the ICA [179]. The high-flow, direct fistulas are most commonly seen after severe head trauma.

Mechanism

Shearing forces in high-velocity blunt trauma or direct penetrating trauma can cause tears or lacerations in the muscular wall of the ICA, and lead to formation of a CCF. A variety of mechanisms have been attributed to CCFs, including bony injury from adjacent skull base or maxillofacial fractures, penetrating trauma from gunshot wounds or intracranial stab wounds, and acceleration–deceleration injuries [148, 156, 173, 177, 178, 180, 181].

Iatrogenic causes of CCF have also been documented following endoscopic and neurosurgical procedures in close proximity to the intracranial vasculature [156].

Several comorbid conditions have been associated with a higher risk of developing CCF. These include atherosclerotic disease, pregnancy, and musculoskeletal and collagen vascular anomalies such as Ehlers–Danlos syndrome, osteogenesis imperfecta, and fibromuscular dysplasia [156]. Additionally, arteriovenous malformations and preexisting ICA aneurysms are risk factors for CCF [156].

Clinical Presentation

The symptoms of CCF are secondary to blood shunting from the high-pressure arterial system to the low-pressure venous system, with resultant venous congestion. The timeline of symptoms varies. A high-pressure CCF can present acutely within hours of injury, or it can have a delayed presentation if the initial trauma to the

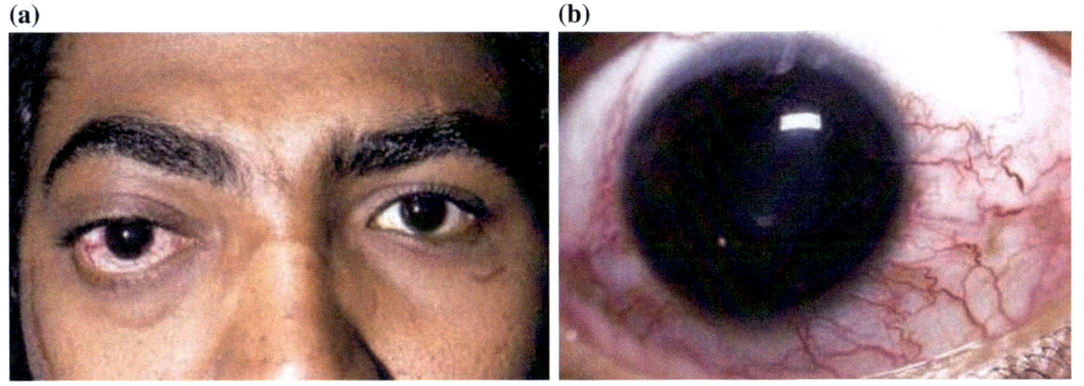

Fig. 12.30 Proptosis (**a**) and arterialization of vessels (**b**) in CCF. *Reproduced with permission from* Chaudhry et al. [183]. Open access article. "This 25-year-old man presented with chief complaints of right eye proptosis, decreased vision and elevated intraocular pressure (**a**). Closer examination revealed dilated episcleral vessels. Based on history and imaging studies, diagnosis of CCF was made (**b**)"

arterial wall was minor [156, 178]. There have been case reports of CCF presenting months after traumatic injury [177, 180].

Venous congestion is often first evident in the orbits, which are affected by reversed blood flow in the superior and inferior ophthalmic veins [156]. In a review of CCF, 88% of patients with CCF reported visual disturbances including diplopia, progressive vision loss, and orbital pain [182]. The most common presenting symptoms include proptosis, orbital bruits, and chemosis [142, 148, 182]. Chemosis results from dilated episcleral and bulbar conjunctival vessels, which may be described as "corkscrew" in appearance (see Fig. 12.30) [183]. Extraocular muscle palsies result from involvement of the cavernous sinus. The lateral rectus muscle is often impaired first due to the medial location of CN VI in the cavernous sinus [156]. Patients may have increased IOP, anterior segment ischemia, choroidal effusions with risk of acute angle-closure glaucoma, distended retinal blood vessels, papilledema, optic nerve atrophy, and peripheral visual field defects [156, 180].

Common extraocular symptoms of venous congestion include headache, nausea, and vomiting [177]. Patients often report hearing buzzing, pulsating, or swishing sounds [180].

If CCF is not treated, patients develop vision loss [177]. There are multiple associated causes of vision loss, including retinal hypoxia and optic nerve atrophy. CCF can also lead to fatal complications such as subarachnoid hemorrhage or severe epistaxis [156].

Diagnosis

CTA and MRA

CTA and MRA are noninvasive studies used for the initial evaluation of a patient with suspected CCF. These studies may demonstrate proptosis, extraocular muscle enlargement, superior ophthalmic vein dilation, or dilation of cortical or leptomeningeal vessels. Absence of these findings does not rule out CCF [142].

Digital Subtraction Cerebral Angiography

Four-vessel digital subtraction cerebral angiography is the gold standard test for conclusive diagnosis of CCF (see Fig. 12.31) [156]. Angiographic studies determine the exact location and configuration of the CCF, and help to guide surgical management.

Other studies

Doppler studies can demonstrate arterialized blood flow in the ophthalmic veins [178]. CT without contrast may be useful for describing the anatomy surrounding the cavernous sinus. It can identify bony fractures that may have caused the CCF, and can demonstrate dilation of the superior ophthalmic vein [156].

Management

Timely management of CCF is required to prevent vision loss and hemorrhagic consequences. The goal of treatment is to close the fistula while preserving the cerebral vascular supply. This is

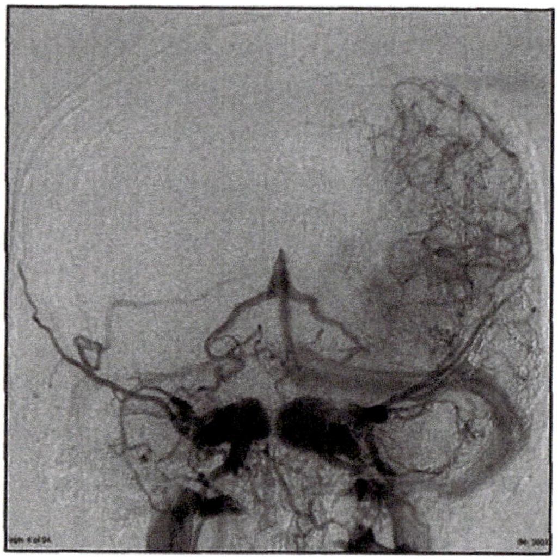

Fig. 12.31 Digital Subtraction Angiography. From Gallucci [180]. Diagnostic angiogram, frontal view. The right side of the figure shows the enlarged left carotid-cavernous fistua. The left side of the figure shows normal filling of the right cavernous sinus. Reproduced with permission from Wolters Kluwer

achieved with endovascular balloon or coil embolization [142, 177, 184].

Early endovascular management has a high success rate for reversing visual and oculomotor disturbances (see Fig. 12.32) [180, 184]. More than 80% of CCF patients will have a complete resolution of symptoms if treated early [178]. Complications of endovascular embolization are reported in 2–5% of cases, and include cerebral infarction, decreased visual acuity, diabetes insipidus, retroperitoneal hematoma, femoral vein thrombosis, and ophthalmoplegia [178].

Venous Drainage of the Brain

The venous system of the brain involves a system of superficial and deep cerebral veins that drain into the dural venous sinuses. The superficial veins are on the surface of the cerebral hemispheres. The superior superficial veins drain into the superior and inferior sagittal sinuses. The superior sagittal sinus is also responsible for absorbing CSF through the arachnoid villi and granulations. The inferior superficial veins drain into the transverse and cavernous sinuses. The deep veins converge to form the vein of Galen, and enter into the straight sinus. The dural venous sinuses ultimately drain into the internal jugular veins (see Fig. 12.33).

Traumatic Venous Injury: Traumatic Cerebral Venous Sinus Thrombosis (CVST)

Cerebral venous sinus thrombosis (CVST) is rare in the general population, causing only 0.5–1% of strokes [185]. TBI increases the risk for CVST. In a retrospective study of 240 patients with TBI, 16.7% of patients with TBI had evidence of a CVST [186].

Mechanism

Formation of a CVST is influenced by both extravascular and intravascular factors.

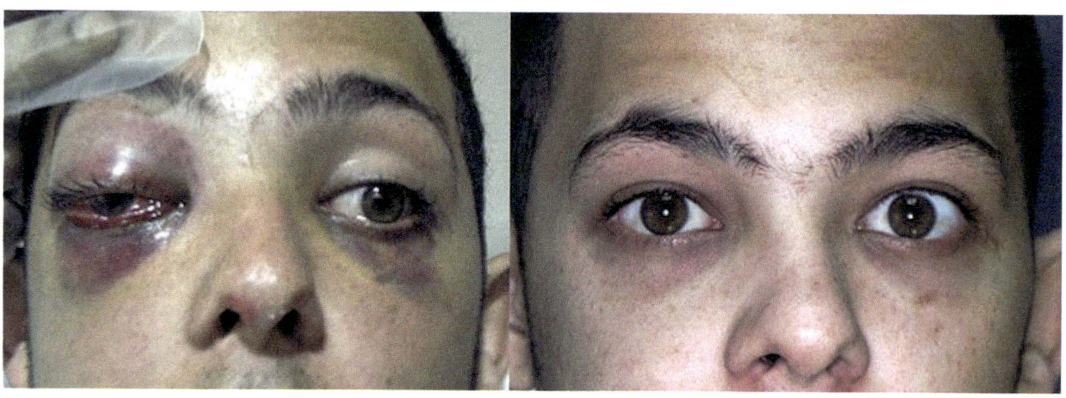

Fig. 12.32 CCF before (*left*) and 4 weeks after (*right*) endovascular coiling of the fistula. Right-sided proptosis and chemosis gradually subsided. Mild enophthalmos resulted from displacement of medial orbital wall. From Schutz et al. [178]. Reproduced with permission from John Wiley and Sons

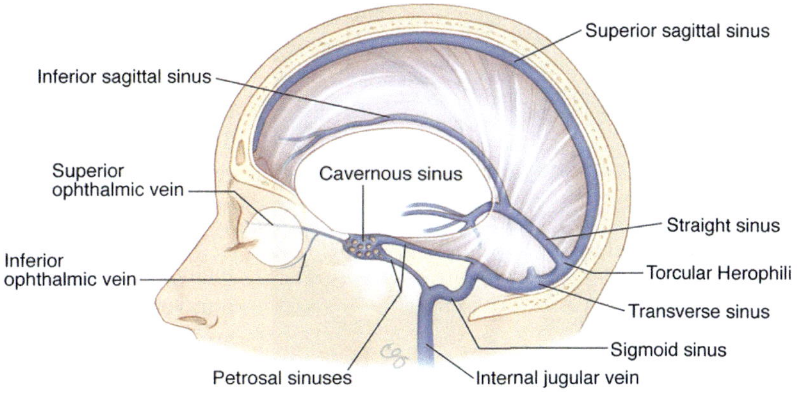

Fig. 12.33 Cerebral venous sinuses. From BCSC Neuro-Ophthalmology Figs. 1–15. Reproduced with permission from American Academy of Ophthalmology

Endothelial venous damage may be caused by direct, extravascular compression on venous sinuses by a skull fracture or hematoma [186]. Intravascularly, head injury patients may be in a hypercoagulable state if increased intracranial pressure was managed with dehydration therapy such as Mannitol [185].

Clinical Presentation

CVST is difficult to diagnose because symptoms are nonspecific and mild in early stages [186]. The rate of symptomatic progression is typically slow, and occurs over days to weeks. The slow evolution is related to the gradual growth of a venous thrombus and the multiple collaterals of the venous system [187]. Multiple cranial nerves can be affected by CVST (Table 12.10).

Increased intracranial pressure secondary to decreased CSF drainage through the superior sagittal sinus can contribute to the clinical picture. Patients have progressive headache and vomiting [185]. They may have papilledema with associated visual signs of transient visual obscuration and visual field constriction beginning in the inferonasal quadrants [188].

Table 12.10 CN involvement in CVST [187, 189]

Location of CVST	Cranial nerves commonly involved
Transverse or sigmoid sinus	III–VIII
Petrosal sinus	V
Jugular vein	IX–XI

If the thrombus extends to the cortical veins, venous infarction is likely and there is potential for hemorrhagic transformation. Infarction, localized edema, or hemorrhage can result in focal deficits, seizures, or impaired consciousness [188]. A thrombus in the deep venous system can cause loss of consciousness [187].

Diagnosis

Unenhanced CT is used in the initial evaluation of CVST. Reported signs of CVST include the dense vein sign, empty delta sign, and cord sign. There may also be localized cerebral swelling, edema, and venous infarction with or without hemorrhage [187]. Unenhanced CT findings have a low sensitivity and specificity for CVST, and confirmatory testing with MRI and MRV or CTV is necessary if there is clinical suspicion for CVST [187].

With CVST, MRI will reveal an absence of flow voids in the affected venous sinus [187]. There are several features on venography to indicate CVST [185]. Stenosis of the venous sinuses will appear as a local filling defect, sudden venous thinning, or visualization of the distal venous end (Fig. 12.34). Venous thinning is present when the diameter of a vein is less than half the normal diameter of the distal end in the same venous sinus. In severe cases, there may be complete nonvisualization of the venous sinuses.

Management

CVST is managed with systemic anticoagulation [190]. After thrombus resolution, patients may be maintained on oral aspirin [185]. MRV or CRV

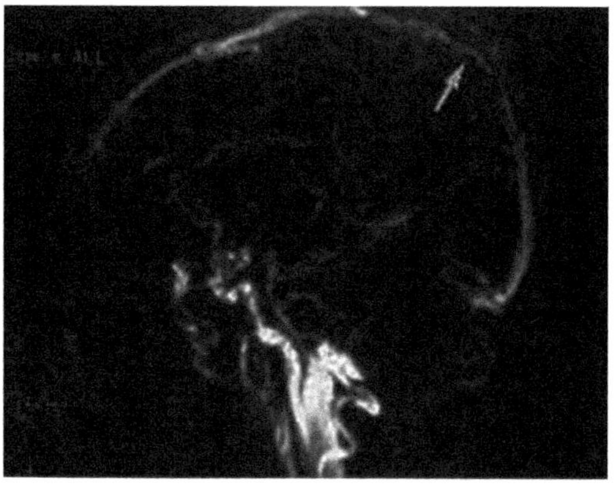

Fig. 12.34 Sagittal slice from the phase contrast MRV study reveals signal drop out within a partially occluded posterior superior sagittal sinus (*arrow*). There is also some reduction of flow within the anterior straight sinus. From Connor and Jarosz [187]. Reproduced with permission from Elsevier

should be repeated to visualize recanalization of the venous sinus. There is often full recovery following anticoagulation [189].

Traumatic Intracranial Hemorrhage

ICH is defined as bleeding within the intracranial vault. ICH subtypes are further defined by the anatomic site of the bleeding: subarachnoid, intraparenchymal, epidural or SDHs [191]. They may all result from head trauma, and are associated with multiple CNS complications.

Subarachnoid Hemorrhage

Subarachnoid hemorrhage is bleeding within the subarachnoid space. Traumatic subarachnoid hemorrhage (TSAH) is commonly caused by TBI. The reported incidence of TSAH following moderate or severe head injury is 28–61% [192–200] The average age of patients with TSAH is in the mid-1940s, which is about 10 years older than the typical average of head trauma patients [194, 201].

Clinical Presentation

TSAH acutely presents with severe headache, vomiting, altered mental status, and possible loss of consciousness. The symptoms are related to the sudden increase in ICP from hemorrhage [15, 202]. Compared to other patients with head trauma, patients with TSAH tend to have lower Glasgow Coma Scale scores at the time of hospital admission [194]. Head trauma patients with TSAH also have a worse prognosis for complete recovery and greater mortality rates compared to head trauma patients without TSAH [194, 201].

With time, further outcomes of TSAH may include ICH growth causing cerebral herniation, intraventricular hemorrhage resulting in scarring and hydrocephalus, raised intracranial pressure, cerebral vasospasm, cerebral edema, autonomic dysfunction, seizures, and focal neurologic defects [191, 203]. Papilledema is not often associated with blurred vision or visual field changes unless ICP is elevated for a long duration of time [204].

Terson Syndrome

Terson syndrome (TS) is a secondary complication of SAH. The initial description of TS described vitreous hemorrhage following SAH. Over time, the definition has evolved to describe the coexistence of any type of intracranial bleed and any type of intraocular hemorrhage [205, 206]. The reported incidence of TS ranges from 12.1–50%, which vary due to different inclusion criteria from varied interpretations of TS [204–207].

TS most often presents within 24 h of head trauma, but has also been reported occurring days to weeks following head injury [204, 206]. The clinical presentation of TS involves symptoms of IOH. Patients may complain of floaters or overall decreased visual acuity depending on the extent of intraocular hemorrhage. Ocular involvement is often bilateral, but may be asymmetrical [204]. TS indicates a poor prognosis for SAH patients. The mortality rate for SAH patients with TS is higher when compared to SAH patients without TS [202]. Diagnosis of TS is best made by fundoscopic examination (Fig. 12.35), although this may be difficult in acutely ill or unstable trauma patients. CT scan or MRI may show a crescent-shaped hyperintensity on the retina [206]. Ocular ultrasound can be valuable when the view of the retina is poor due to vitreous hemorrhage, and may indicate associated retinal detachment in TS [208].

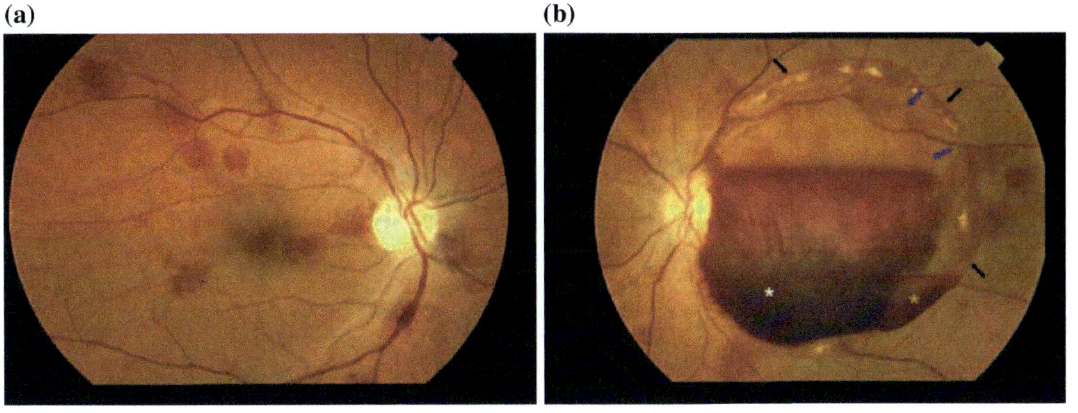

Fig. 12.35 Terson Syndrome. **a** Right fundus with scattered superficial and deep retinal hemorrhages in the posterior pole. **b** Left fundus with macular sub-internal limiting membrane (ILM) hemorrhage (*white asterisk*) and subhyaloid hemorrhage (*orange asterisk*). *Arrows* designate a "double ring sign" characteristic of simultaneous sub-ILM and subhyaloid hemorrhage [210]. The inner ring is caused by detachment of the ILM from the sub-ILM hemorrhage (*blue arrows*) and the outer ring is formed by the detached posterior hyaloid from the subhyaloid hemorrhage (*black arrows*). From Srinivasan and Kyle [210]. Reproduced with permission from Nature Publishing Group

About half of TS patients experience spontaneous regression of the intraocular hemorrhage within weeks to months following injury, and there is a good prognosis for complete visual recovery [202, 205, 207]. Patients should be followed for secondary complications of TS, such as elevated intraocular pressure, epiretinal membrane formation, perifoveal traction, and retinal detachment [204, 208]. If vitreous hemorrhage does not begin clearing spontaneously by 3–12 months after injury, a pars plana vitrectomy (PPV) should be performed to remove the hemorrhage [204, 209]. If PPV is performed early for non-clearing vitreous hemorrhage, there is good prognosis for visual recovery [208, 209].

Diagnosis

CT scan is the best imaging modality to identify acute intracranial bleeds. The advancement of CT scan technology greatly improved detection of TSAH [197, 211]. The sensitivity of fifth generation CT scan for diagnosing SAH is reported as 68–100% and the specificity is 93.9–99.4% [197, 211].

Lumbar puncture is the gold standard for diagnosing SAH. Macroscopic blood in the CSF, termed xanthochromia, identifies the presence of SAH even if hemorrhage is not yet evident on CT scan [202, 211]. LP should be performed if CT scan is negative but there is a high clinical suspicion for SAH.

Intraparenchymal Hemorrhage

Intraparenchymal hemorrhage (IPH) describes hemorrhage into the brain parenchyma. The hemorrhage can possibly extend into the ventricles and the subarachnoid space.

Clinical Presentation

The earliest symptom of IPH is often headache, resulting from rapidly increased ICP [212]. Patients may also experience stiff neck, vomiting, stiff neck, or seizures. Patients with a severely reduced level of consciousness have a worse prognosis [15].

Headache is followed by focal deficits, which often evolve over a period of minutes to half an hour [212]. Table 12.11 describes the ophthalmic outcomes of IPH based on location of lesion.

Diagnosis

An early head CT will show hyperdense accumulation of intraparenchymal blood [191]. MRI is useful for following evolution of hemorrhage.

Epidural Hematoma

In epidural hematoma (EDH), there is bleeding externally in the dural membrane. EDH is reported in 1% of all head trauma cases and 10%

Table 12.11 Ophthalmic outcomes of intraparenchymal hemorrhage

Frontal lobe	– If affecting precentral gyrus or deep white matter: conjugate deviation of eyes to side of lesion – If resulting midline shift: contralateral CN III compression with contralateral pupillary dilation
Parietal lobe	– Contralateral complete or incomplete homonymous hemianopia – Visual neglect of contralateral hemifield – Asymmetric oculomotor response to horizontally moving targets – Abnormal optokinetic tape/drum response with movement toward side of lesion
Temporal lobe	– Contralateral complete or incomplete homonymous hemianopia – Prone to swelling and brainstem compression → ipsilateral dilated pupil from CN III compression
Occipital lobe	– Contralateral complete or incomplete homonymous hemianopia; for incomplete, the field defect is congruous – If significant tissue destruction, abnormal optokinetic tape/drum response with movement toward side of lesion
Lateral basal ganglia, putamen, and internal capsule	– Contralateral homonymous hemianopia – Conjugate deviation of eyes to side of lesion – If R-sided lesion: left hemifield visual neglect
Caudate	– Conjugate deviation of eyes to side of lesion – Conjugate gaze paresis to side opposite lesion – Ipsilateral central Horner's syndrome
Thalamus	– Paralysis of upward gaze – Tonic downward and medial deviation – Acute esotropia – Dysconjugate gaze with limited abduction of one or both eyes – Conjugate gaze deviation away from side of lesion – Skew deviation – Pupils: small, anisocoric, poorly reactive to light – Visual neglect
Midbrain	– Oculomotor disturbances (primarily vertical gaze) – Abnormal pupillary size and reactivity
Pons	Disturbances generally seen if large, midline hemorrhage: – Pupils: pinpoint and poorly reactive, less often dilated and fixed – Oculomotor disturbances (horizontal and vertical gaze) – Bilateral horizontal gaze paresis with vertical, bobbing eye movements – Ocular myoclonus
Medulla	– Horizontal nystagmus – Ipsilateral Horner syndrome
Cerebellum	– Oculomotor disturbances: ipsilateral abducens nerve paresis, skew deviation, INO, nystagmus, ocular dysmetria, macrosaccadic oscillations – Pupils: small, poorly reactive – Horner's syndrome

Table based on Walsh and Hoyt Clinical Neuro-Ophthalmology Ch. 40, pgs 2143–2151

of severe head trauma cases, with a 20% mortality rate [213, 214]. It is often associated with mild to moderate head trauma, with Glasgow Coma Scale (GCS) between 13 and 15 [214].

Mechanism

The common mechanisms of traumatic EDH include high-velocity falls, motor vehicle accidents, and assaults [214]. EDH develops from

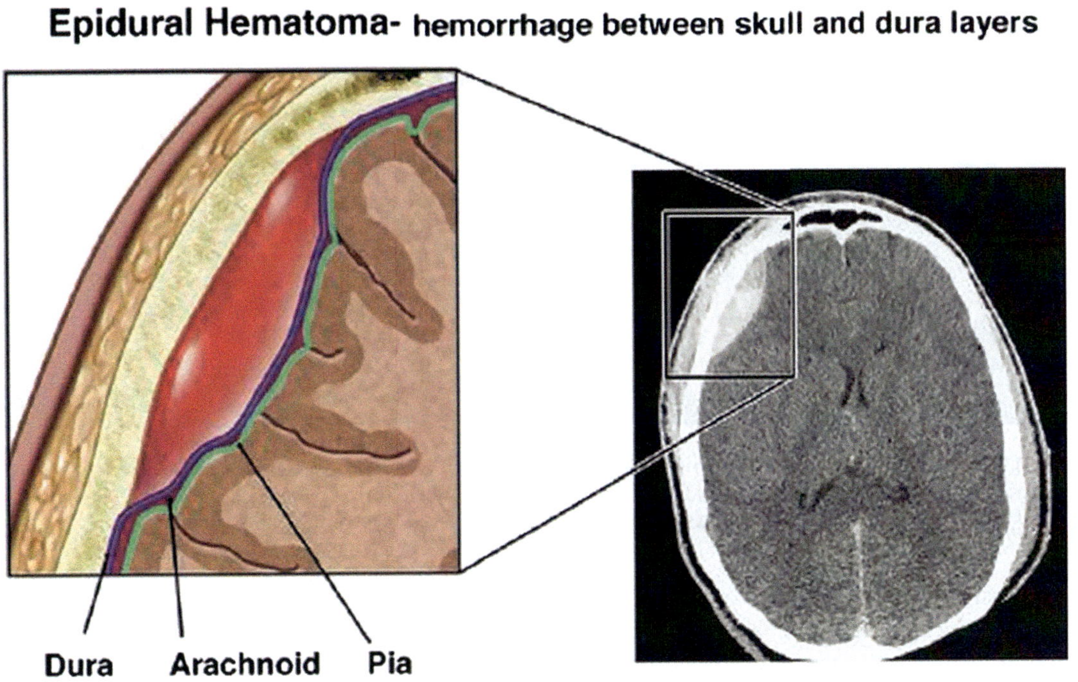

Fig. 12.36 Epidural hematoma anatomical and CT scan correlates. From Freeman and Aguilar [191]. Reproduced with permission from Elsevier

rupture of vessels that run in the periosteal layer of the dura, and bleeding separates the dura from the calvarium (see Fig. 12.36).

Temporoparietal trauma commonly injures the middle meningeal artery, frontal trauma injures the anterior ethmoidal artery, and posterior fossa trauma often injures the transverse or sigmoid sinuses. Posterior fossa EDH is comparatively rare, reported in 0.1–0.3% of all cranial traumatic conditions, and often caused by posterior skull base fracture (see: Skull Base Trauma section) [213–215]. EDH progresses at a slower rate in cases of posterior fossa injury because the hematoma is venous in origin.

In traumatic EDH, rupture of vessels is caused by skull fracture from the precipitating head injury [133, 191]. The frequent site of fracture leading to EDH is the pterion, an area of weakness where the frontal bone, greater wing of the sphenoid bone, squamous temporal bone, and parietal bone join [148]. Pterion fracture may damage the nearby anterior branches of the middle meningeal artery.

Clinical Presentation

The classic presentation of an EDH describes a "lucid interval" during which the patient appears awake and alert, followed by a loss of consciousness and rapid neurological decline secondary to mass effect [213]. One study identified this clinical picture in 47% of patients [214].

Additional signs and symptoms of EDH include scalp hematoma suggestive of underlying cranial fracture, headache, vomiting, transient or complete loss of consciousness, amnesia, and epistaxis [134]. Three is a risk of cerebral herniation, which may present with pupil-involving third nerve palsy in the case of uncal herniation, as the EDH increases in size [191]. Posterior cranial fossa EDH has a more indolent clinical presentation, and may present with occipital scalp hematoma, diplopia from CN VI compression, cerebellar signs, and nuchal rigidity [215].

Diagnosis (CT)

An unenhanced head CT is the best modality to quickly diagnose EDH. CT scan is useful for

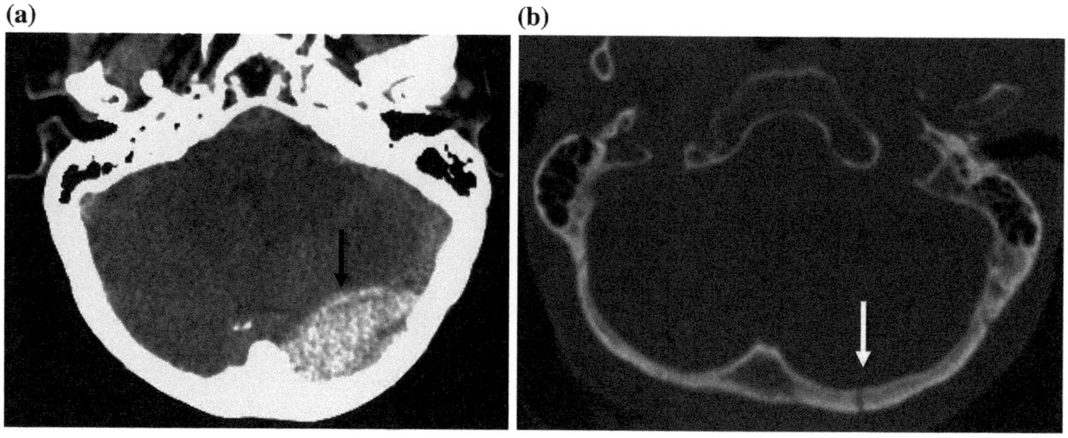

Fig. 12.37 **a** Axial soft tissue window through the posterior fossa demonstrating a large epidural hematoma (*black arrow*), causing mass effect on the fourth ventricle. **b** Bone window CT demonstrates underlying occipital bone fracture (*arrow*). From Baugnon and Hudgins [133]. Reproduced with permission from Elsevier

demonstrating hematoma size and quality, associated intracranial lesions, and evidence of a midline shift, which suggests urgent need for neurosurgical intervention [216, 217]. CT will demonstrate a biconvex hyperdensity that can cross the midline (see Figs. 12.37 and 12.38). As

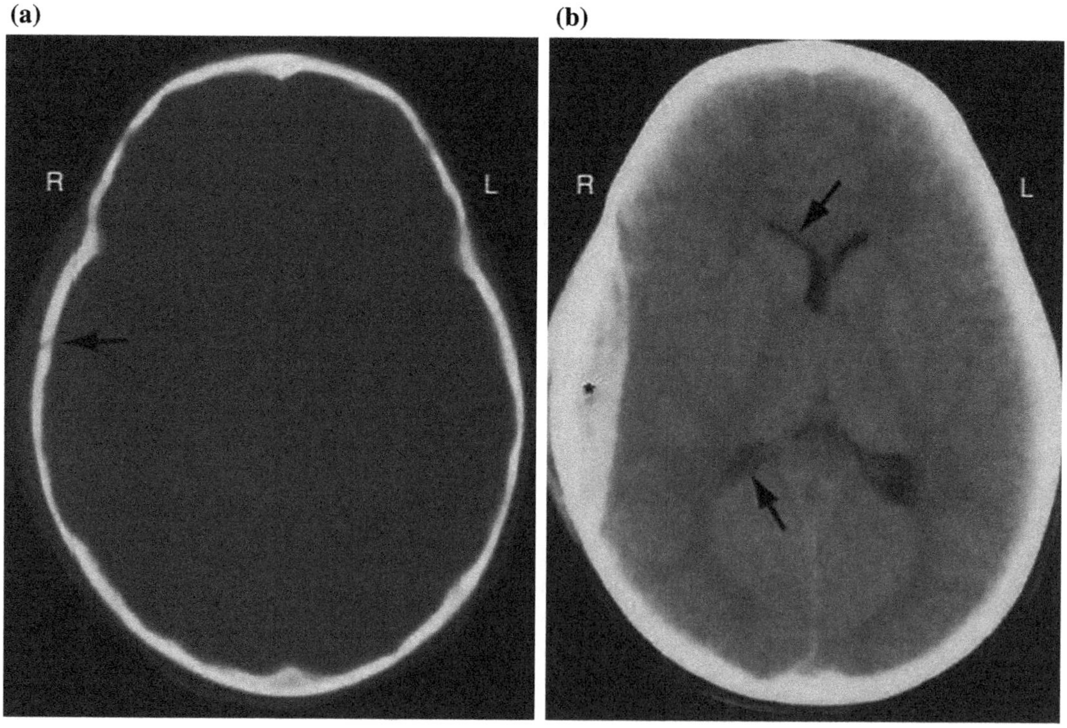

Fig. 12.38 Epidural hematoma in a 3-year-old girl following head injury in MVA. **a** CT set to show bony details reveals a fracture of the right temporal bone (*arrow*). **b** CT set to reveal soft tissue details reveals a lens-shaped hyperdensity (*) and compression of the right lateral ventricle (*arrows*). From Nolte [168]. 6th Ed. Reproduced with permission from Elsevier

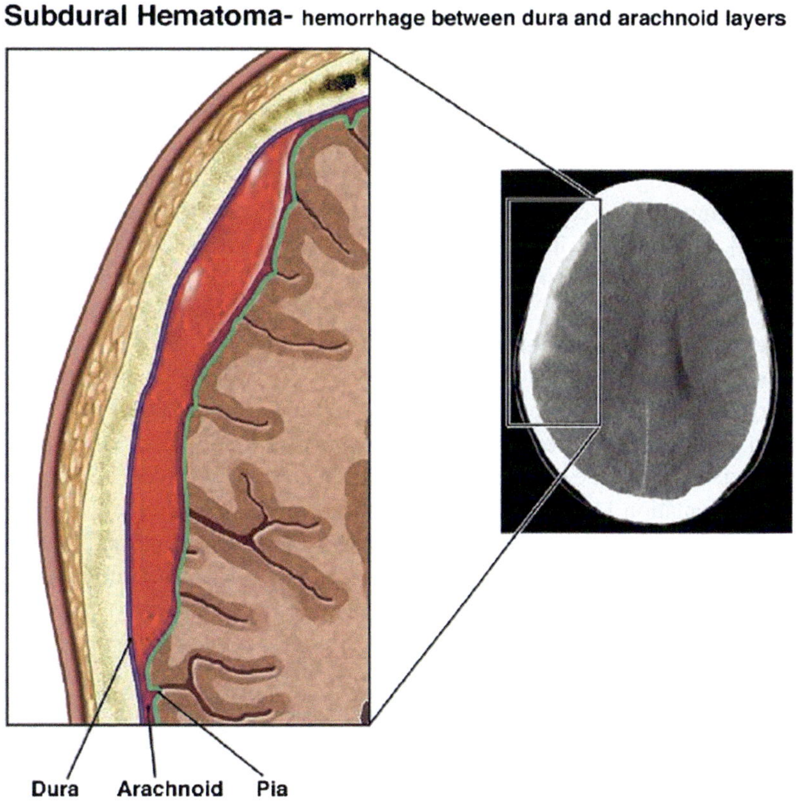

Fig. 12.39 Subdural hematoma anatomical and CT scan correlates. From Freeman and Aguilar [191]. Reproduced with permission from Elsevier

the blood continues to rapidly accumulate, relatively hypodense areas will be seen within the hematoma indicating non-coagulated fresh blood [213].

MRI can also be used to view an EDH, although it is not ideal in emergency situations due to the possibility of ferromagnetic metallic foreign bodies and the length of time it takes to obtain the images. It is best for assessing adjacent parenchymal injury, and can identify dural venous sinus thrombosis that could be associated with posterior fossa EDH [213].

Subdural Hematoma

In SDH, there is bleeding under the dural membrane, often caused by tears of the cerebral bridging veins as they enter the dural sinus (see Fig. 12.39) [168, 191].

SDH occurs in about 30–49% of severe head injuries [218, 219]. Severe head injury is defined as Glasgow Coma scale less than 9 on admission. Traumatic SDH has one of the highest associated mortality rates of all types of head trauma, reported between 40 and 90% [220]. Compared to EDH, SDH has a higher association of intraparenchymal brain damage and worse prognosis [218].

Mechanism

The most common mechanisms of traumatic SDH include blunt assault, gunshot wounds, high-velocity falls, and motor vehicle accidents [216, 219]. Forces from rapid acceleration–deceleration injuries, in which the venous sinuses move with the skull but the brain lags behind, can cause tears in the bridging veins [168].

Clinical Presentation

Patients with SDH may present with headache, seizures, and other signs of raised intracranial pressure [191]. If the patient has unreactive pupils, this may signify transtentorial herniation

[220]. Pupillary involvement with SDH is associated with a higher mortality rate [219].

Diagnosis (CT)

Like EDH, an unenhanced head CT is the primary imaging modality for diagnosis of SDH, appearing as a crescent-shaped hyperdensity [191]. Unlike EDH, it does not usually cross the midline.

General Management of Intracranial Hemorrhage

Urgent neurosurgical management may be needed based on the extension of ICH, severity of associated traumatic head lesions, and GCS score on presentation [191]. SDH greater than 10 mm wide or causing midline shifts greater than 5 mm should be urgently evacuated [221]. Smaller SDHs require surgical evacuation if a comatose patient had a decrease in GCS score by 2 points or more from the time of injury, anisocoria or fixed pupils, or ICP greater than 20 mmHg [222]. Urgent craniotomy is recommended for EDH greater than 30 mm regardless of GCS score, or for comatose patients with anisocoria or fixed pupils [221].

Surgical intervention prior to clinical deterioration has better outcomes with decreased mortality rate and increased likelihood of good functional outcome [167, 222–228] Clinical deterioration describes the life-threatening compressive effects of ICH on brain structures, including cerebral herniation, and it is signified by a decline in GCS to a comatose state.

For patients with SDH or EDH, rapid transport to a hospital with neurosurgery has been associated with decreased mortality and better long-term outcome [226, 228]. In a prospective study of 171 SDH and EDH patients, craniotomy within 2 hours of coma onset resulted in significantly decreased mortality (80–47% for SDH and 65–17% for EDH) and improved long-term outcome, as compared to craniotomy delayed over 2 hours after coma onset [223]. A study by Sakas et al. reviewed 40 patients who were surgically managed for IPH, EDH, or SDH due to clinical signs of cerebral herniation with bilateral, non-reactive, mydriatic pupils >4 mm. The patients with neurosurgical intervention delayed more than 3 hours after clinical signs of cerebral herniation had a higher morbidity and mortality (less than 3 h delay: 30% mortality, 3–6 hours delay: 63% mortality, greater than 6 hours delay: 100% mortality) [167].

Medical management is appropriate for small ICH with no focal neurological deficits [221, 222]. Medical management involves close observation in the ICU, ICP pressure monitoring, and serial CT scans [191, 229]. Efforts should be made to maintain the volume status and mean arterial pressure of a patient with ICH to ensure adequate cerebral perfusion pressure [192]. For SAH, calcium channel blockers such as nimodipine improve outcomes by reducing bleeding and vasospasm [198, 201]. A ventriculo-peritoneal shunt may be required for persistently elevated ICP causing headache, papilledema and visual loss [230].

Traumatic Brain Injury

TBI is a major cause of mortality and long-term loss of quality of life. According to surveillance data from the CDC's National Center for Injury Prevention and Control, approximately 1.7 million people in the United States suffer traumatic brain injuries each year [231]. Within this group, there are 52,000 deaths, 275,000 hospitalizations, and 1,365,000 Emergency Department visits. The rate of TBI is higher in younger age groups and males, although the need for hospitalization is more frequent in patients aged greater than 75 years old [231]. Most TBI is caused by falls (35.2%), followed by unknown causes (21%), motor vehicle and traffic accidents (17.3%), being struck by or against objects (16.5%), and assault (10%) [231].

The definition of TBI is not standardized, although it typically describes external mechanical injury to the brain resulting in primary and secondary outcomes. Mechanical injury may involve blunt or penetrating trauma. In war veterans, the main mechanism is blast-induced TBI from prolonged, close contact with explosive weapons [232].

Primary TBI describes the immediate impact of trauma with possible damage to the skull and brain parenchyma. Primary TBI includes basilar skull fractures, ICH, penetrating injury, contusions and DAI. For a discussion of basilar skull fractures, ICH, and penetrating head trauma, refer to earlier in the chapter.

Secondary TBI describes the long-term neuropsychiatric and functional impairment that follows TBI. Frequently reported sequelae include headache, dizziness, irritability, impaired concentration, memory deficits, fatigue, depression, anxiety, judgment problems, noise sensitivity, and visual disturbances [233]. Ophthalmic complications associated with secondary TBI include photophobia, oculomotor deficits, and visual field loss. Secondary TBI has been reported months to years following the inciting traumatic event [233, 234]. It results from the combined effect of systemic hypotension, intracranial hypertension, hypoxia, seizure, infection, and inflammatory responses following primary TBI [203].

Primary Injury

Contusions

Contusions are very common in TBI. In a prospective study by Choi et al. of 135 survivors of severe TBI, 89% of TBI patients had cerebral contusions [193]. Contusions are often associated with coup-contrecoup injury and form at sites of brain parenchyma that may hit against the cranial fossa, falx cerebri, or tentorium cerebelli during high-velocity closed head trauma [235, 236]. In the study by Choi et al., the most frequent regions for contusion were frontal (59%) and temporal (46%) [193].

Visual field deficits have been reported following contusions. Contusions within the temporal lobes produce incongruous homonymous hemianopia, namely superior quadrantanopia. Contusions in the posterior parietal and occipital regions produce congruous, or symmetric, homonymous hemianopia [1]. See Fig. 12.25 for a summary of visual field deficits in various locations along the visual pathway. The majority of visual field loss is stable at follow-up.

Contusions can be seen as hyperintense lesions on CT scan (see Fig. 12.40) [35]. Surrounding regions of hypointensity indicate vasogenic edema [236].

Diffuse Axonal Injury

DAI is a severe form of TBI. It is found in 50% of trauma patients and identified as the major cause of unconsciousness and persistent vegetative state following head trauma [237–239].

DAI describes widespread axonal damage from shearing forces during rapid rotational

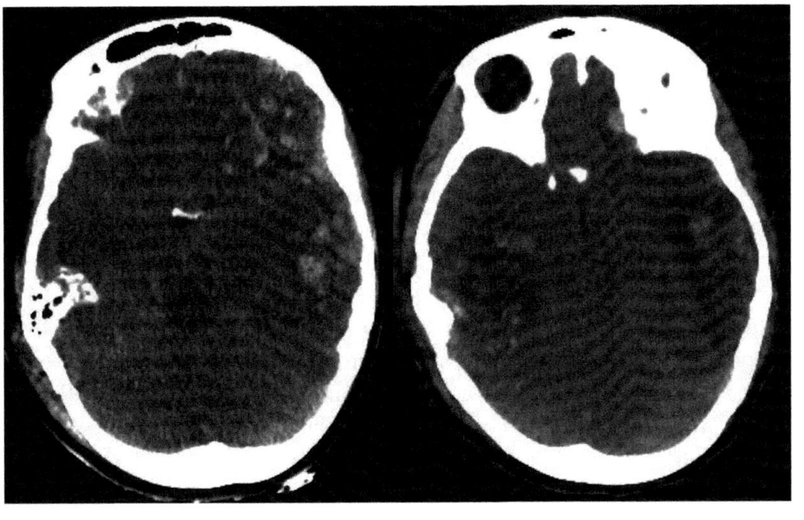

Fig. 12.40 Axial CT showing multiple acute parenchymal contusions, seen as hyperdense foci within the orbital frontal regions and temporal lobes. From Currie et al. [236]. Permission received from British Medical Journal

movement, especially fast acceleration or deceleration, which stretch and deform brain parenchyma and vasculature [240, 241]. DAI most greatly affects interfaces of different tissue density [242]. Most frequently, damage may be localized to the corpus callosum, grey–white matter junctions, deep white matter, periventricular regions, hippocampal regions, and the brainstem [236, 238].

An early diagnosis of DAI in the acute setting of trauma has long-term implications for reducing patient morbidity. If neuropsychological rehabilitation is initiated during the initial recovery period, the duration and presence of post-traumatic neuropsychiatric symptoms are reduced [233, 243]. MRI is the best imaging modality for DAI. Sensitivity with T1-weighted MRI is 58% and T2-weighted MRI is 95% [244]. Comparatively, CT has a low sensitivity (15%) for DAI [244, 245]. MRI can identify small intracranial blood collections and axonal injury in patients with normal-appearing CT scans [241, 246].

Following TBI, foci of low signal intensity on T1 and high signal intensity on T2 are evident in white matter tracts, especially near white-grey junctions [236, 244, 247]. The foci relate to areas of nonhemorrhagic parenchymal lesions and axonal shearing injuries, and they may persist into the chronic stage of TBI (see Fig. 12.41) [248, 249]. FLAIR sequences provide enhanced visualization of nonhemorrhagic lesions, which appear hyperintense [236].

In early DAI, hyperintensity on diffusion-weighted imaging (DWI) is attributed to regions of cytotoxic edema, and these hyperintense lesions are seen to decrease over time [247].

Compared to T2-weighted imaging, high field strength T2*-weighted gradient-echo (GRE) imaging can better identify microhemorrhage in both acute and chronic stages of TBI [236]. Microbleeds are seen as hypointense lesions [6]. If available, susceptible-weighted imaging (SWI) has improved sensitivity for detecting microhemorrhage, and it has been shown to detect four times as many hemorrhagic lesions as T2*-weighted GRE [250].

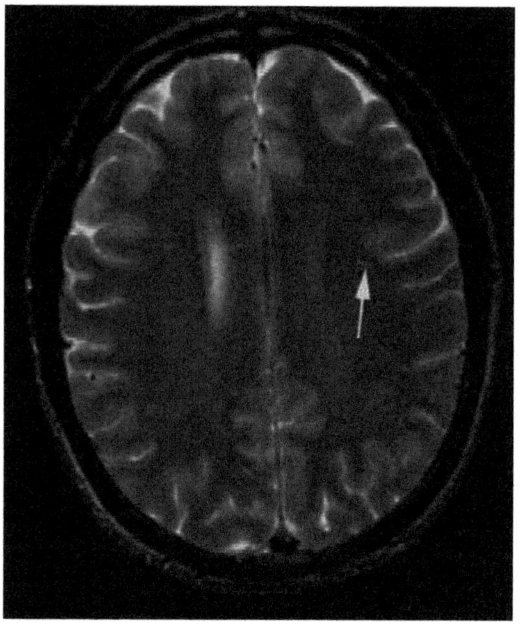

Fig. 12.41 "Fast spin-echo T2-weighted image of an otherwise healthy young man 3 months after head trauma, demonstrating presumed gliosis in the periventricular white matter (*arrow*)". From Johnston et al. [249]. Reproduced with permission from Wolters-Kluwer

Secondary TBI: Ocular Manifestations

These patients often benefit from referral to a low vision specialist with experience handling the visual sequelae of TBI, as discussed below.

Photophobia

Photosensitivity is a frequent long-term visual outcome of TBI, identified in about 50% of TBI patients [232, 251, 252]. Photosensitivity decreases over a long period of time, and for the majority of patients, it does not begin to resolve until one year following TBI [253]. In the majority of patients with TBI, photosensitivity will never completely improve back to their baseline. Factors contributing to a worse prognosis for recovery of photosensitivity include dry eye, migraines, and loss of consciousness at the time of trauma [253].

The interaction of three neural circuits has been linked to photophobia (Fig. 12.42) [254]. Ganglion cells send light-related signals to the

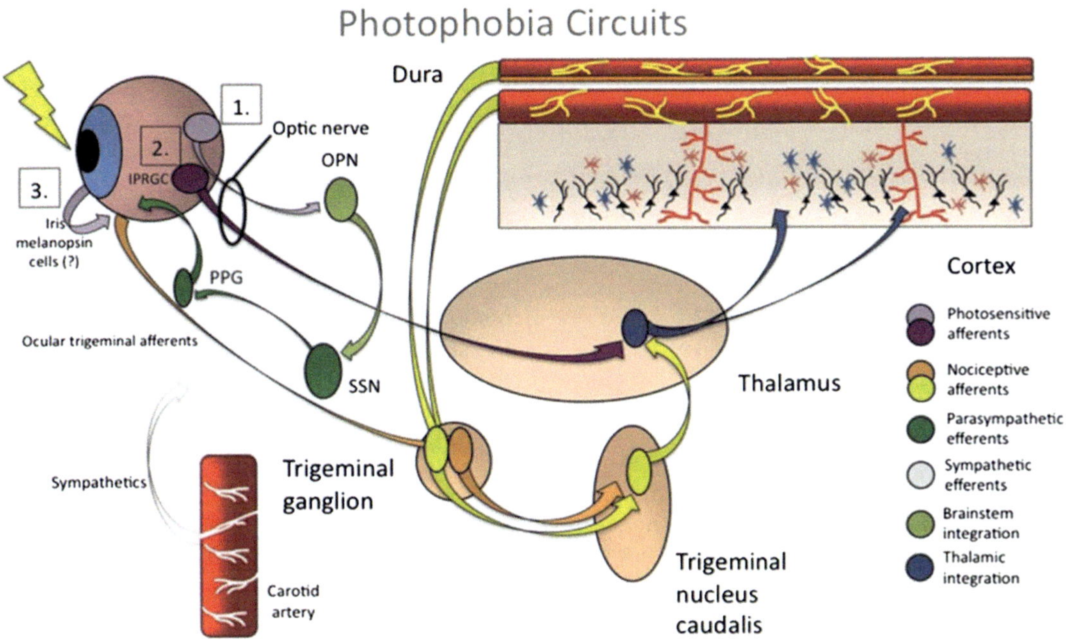

Fig. 12.42 Proposed pathway for chronic photophobia. From Katz and Digre [254]. Reproduced with permission from Wolters Kluwer

olivary pretectal nucleus (OPN), which activates the superior salivatory nucleus (SSN) and the pterygopalatine ganglion (PPG). The pathway causes ocular vasodilation and activation of ocular trigeminal afferents heavily expressed on blood vessels. The trigeminal afferents then project to the trigeminal nucleus caudalis, thalamus, and cortex. Melanopsin-containing, intrinsically photosensitive ganglion-like cells have been identified in rodent iris, and have been shown to facilitate light activation of the trigeminal blink reflex even after optic nerve transection. Intrinsically photosensitive ganglion cells send signals directly to the thalamic pain centers, which have an output to sensory and association cortex.

Various filters may be used to alleviate symptoms. One filter that has shown promise in addressing chronic photosensitivity associated with migraine is FL-41, a rose-tinted lens [254]. FL-41 seems to work best for patients with sensitivity to fluorescent lighting because it filters mostly the 480 nm wavelength [254]. This is the maximum sensitivity of the intrinsically photosensitive RGC, also known as a melanopsin ganglion cell, thought to be responsible in the signal pathway for photophobia. This wavelength is between the blue (420 nm) and green (530 nm) maximum sensitivity wavelengths.

Chronic use of dark sunglasses indoors is not recommended because it maintains a dark-adapted state, further exacerbating photophobia when the sunglasses are not in use [253, 255]. Additionally, grey lenses transmit the 480 nm wavelength to a greater extent than FL-41 lenses (Fig. 12.43). Dark sunglasses do not need to be restricted from use in outdoor sunlight environments [254].

Oculomotor Deficits

TBI is associated with ocular misalignment, especially at near [256]. Findings may include large exophoria, decreased fusion ranges, receded near point of convergence, defective smooth pursuit and saccadic eye movements, decreased amplitude of accommodation, and monocular

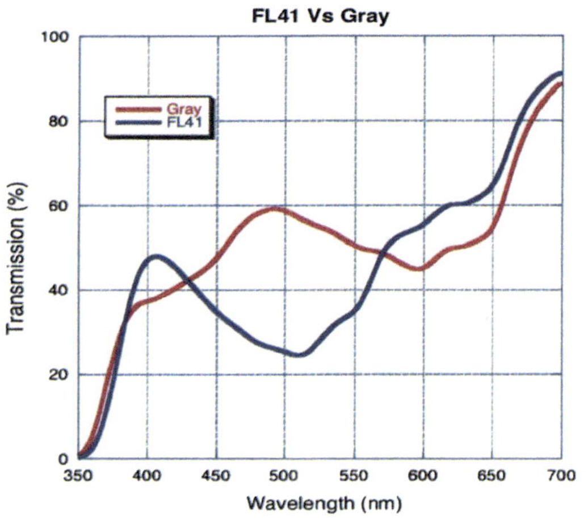

Fig. 12.43 Spectral transmission of the FL-41 tint across the visible spectrum compared to the spectral transmission of a neutral gray tint. The neutral gray tint is similar to that one might observe in an ordinary pair of over-the-counter sunglasses. Its transmission is fairly flat, or neutral, across most of the visible spectrum. Comparatively, FL-41 attenuates wavelengths in the *blue-green* spectrum, very close to the peak sensitivity of melanopsin (480 nm). It may be this property of FL-41 that patients with photophobia find therapeutic. *Source* Katz and Digre [254]. Reproduced with permission from Elsevier

accommodative facility [50, 232, 253, 257, 258]. As a result of these deficits, TBI patients have reading difficulties, including reduced reading speeds [232, 258]. Convergence insufficiency bothersome to the patient can usually be addressed with base in prism glasses used for reading. In addition, patients may use a ruler or other straight edge to help with maintaining their reading position. Internuclear ophthalmoplegia has also been observed following TBI [257]. Traumatic ocular motor cranial nerve deficits are discussed in another section in this chapter.

Visual Field Defects

The visual pathway is frequently affected in TBI and the location of the head trauma and contusions will directly impact the resultant visual field defect. Approximately 30–35% of TBI patients have reported visual field defects [50, 51, 258, 259]. In an autopsy study of 45 severe TBI patients, axonal injury involved the optic chiasm, optic tracts, or optic radiations in 87% of cases [237].

In a retrospective study of 188 closed head trauma patients, the most common types of visual field loss, identified with Goldmann perimetry visual field testing and tangent screen testing, were functional (tunnel) fields, arcuate defects, and homonymous hemianopia [50]. Other visual field defects that have been described secondary to TBI include quadrantanopia, bitemporal hemianopia, central scotoma, and complete homonymous hemianopia [1, 51, 259]. Following significant head trauma with impaired visual fields, patients should be counseled on capacity to drive, depending on the driving laws in their region of residence.

Oculomotor System

Overview of Anatomy

The Orbit

Detailed anatomy of the orbit is discussed in the Eyelid and Orbital Trauma chapter. The seven bones that form the bony orbit include frontal, zygomatic, maxillary, ethmoid, sphenoid, lacrimal, and palatine. The orbital roof separates the orbit from the frontal sinus and intracranial cavity. It is comprised of the orbital plate of the frontal bone and the lesser wing of the sphenoid. The lesser wing of the sphenoid also makes up part of the medial wall with the lacrimal bone, the orbital plate of the ethmoid, and the frontal process of the maxilla. The maxilla along with the palatine bone and orbital plate of the zygomatic bone make up the floor of the orbit. Finally, the zygomatic bone and the greater wing of the sphenoid make up the lateral wall. Important neurovascular structures pass through the orbital apex via the optic canal (within the lesser wing of the sphenoid), and the superior and inferior orbital fissures (delineated by the greater wing of the sphenoid) (Fig. 12.44).

The Extraocular Muscles

Seven muscles make up the extraocular musculature, consisting of four rectus muscles, two oblique muscles, and one palpebral muscle. The

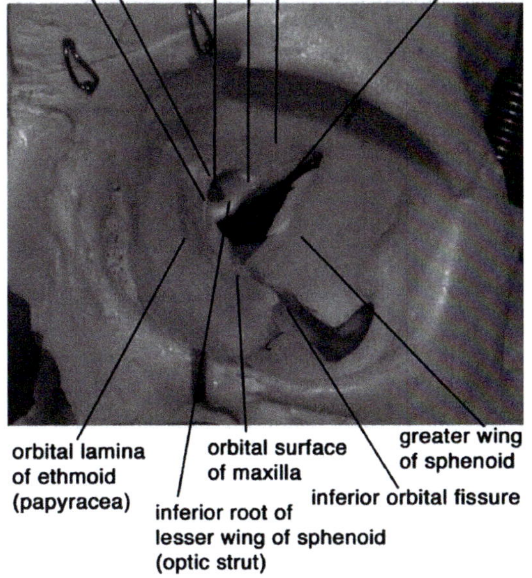

Fig. 12.44 Anterior view of the anatomy of the bones and landmarks of the left orbit. The optic canal and the superior and inferior orbital fissures allow for the passage of neurovascular structures into the orbit. From Linnau et al. [260]. Accessed January 31, 2016. Reproduced with permission from Science Direct

four rectus muscles include superior, inferior, medial, and lateral. The rectus muscles as well as the levator palpebrae superioris (levator muscle) originate from the annulus of Zinn, a tendinous ring at the orbital apex. The superior oblique originates from the periosteum of the body of the sphenoid bone, above and medial to the optic foramen, travels through the trochlea in the anterior superomedial orbit, and inserts on the sclera superiorly, beneath the insertion of the superior rectus. The inferior oblique originates from the anterior medial inferior orbital rim periosteum of the orbital plate of the maxillary bone, and inserts on the posterior inferior temporal surface of the sclera, at the level of the macula. The levator palpebrae superioris originates from the lesser wing of the sphenoid bone, superior to the annulus of Zinn. The body of the muscle courses over the superior rectus anteriorly until a point close to the Whitnall ligament, where it has attachments to the Müller's muscle posteriorly and travels anteriorly to become the levator aponeurosis, which inserts onto the anterior surface of the tarsus and pretarsal orbicularis.

The Ocular Motor Cranial Nerves, in Brief

There are three ocular motor cranial nerves that control eye movements: the third, or oculomotor nerve, the fourth, or trochlear nerve, and the sixth, or abducens nerve. These nerves arise from their nuclei located in the midbrain and pons, then course through the subarachnoid cistern and the cavernous sinus before entering the orbit via the superior orbital fissure to reach their designated targets, namely, the extraocular muscles. Details of their route from their origin in brainstem nuclei to their targets of innervation are described below.

The Orbital Apex

The posterior one third of the conical orbit, approximately 13–17 mm, is referred to as the orbital apex [260]. The annulus of Zinn, formed by the tendons of the extraocular muscles, surrounds the optic nerve and is a prominent landmark of the orbital apex (Fig. 12.45). Via the superior orbital fissure, structures that pass out-

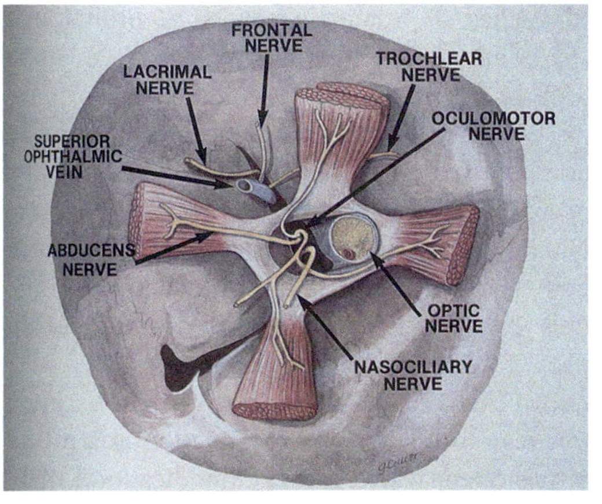

Fig. 12.45 Anterior view of the right orbital apex, including the Annulus of Zinn, the extraocular muscles, and their nerves. Except for the lacrimal, frontal, and trochlear nerves and the superior ophthalmic vein, the majority of the neurovascular structures that supply the orbit pass through the Annulus of Zinn. From Yeh and Foroozan [4]. Reproduced with permission from Ovid

side the annulus of Zinn include the lacrimal and frontal nerves of the ophthalmic branch of the trigeminal nerve, the trochlear nerve, and the superior ophthalmic vein. The superior orbital fissure also transmits the superior and inferior divisions of the oculomotor nerve, the nasociliary nerve, and the abducens nerve, which pass inside the annulus of Zinn. The optic nerve and ophthalmic artery enter the orbit via the optic canal and traverse inside the annulus of Zinn.

The concentration of important nerves, muscles, and vasculature in close proximity to one another in the orbital apex make traumatic injury to this region particularly devastating. Orbital apex damage often occurs in severe, forceful injuries to the face, skull base, or other skull bones by extension [260]. The findings of ophthalmoplegia, dysesthesia, or pain in the territory of the ophthalmic division of the trigeminal nerve, and optic neuropathy are suggestive of orbital apex syndrome occurring in the region of the annulus of Zinn. Cases without optic nerve involvement are termed superior orbital fissure syndrome [240]. In some cases of orbital apex syndrome, the only finding may be a RAPD, signifying damage to the optic nerve [260].

Unfortunately, iatrogenic orbital apex syndrome is a fairly common complication in procedures involving the nasal sinuses or deep orbit. In studies of traumatic causes of orbital apex syndrome, iatrogenic injury comprised up to 35% of cases and was the most common cause [4]. While most cases of trauma were blunt and non-penetrating, orbital apex syndrome can occur in rare cases with penetrating trauma without bony fractures, especially if a foreign body is retained in the orbit [4]. Neuroimaging is thus crucial for evaluation of potential orbital apex syndrome, and high-resolution MRI is the test of choice for evaluation of the soft tissues in this region, unless a ferromagnetic foreign body is suspected, which is a contraindication to MRI [4]. High-resolution CT with thin cuts (1 mm) of the orbital apex allows special attention to detect bony abnormalities of the sphenoid, temporal, and the orbital plate of the frontal bone to avoid complications of skull base disruptions that could develop over time [260]. Management consists of relieving the etiology of the syndrome, if possible. For a detailed discussion of optic canal and orbital apex fractures, please see the skull base trauma section of this chapter.

Cranial Nerve III: The Oculomotor Nerve

Anatomy

The oculomotor nerve (third nerve) arises from its nucleus in the periaqueductal portion of the midbrain at the level of the superior colliculus (Fig. 12.46). The nerve fascicle then projects anteriorly through the midbrain, spreading slightly laterally through the red nucleus and cerebral peduncle (Fig. 12.46). The nerve then emerges from the interpeduncular fossa on the ventral side of the midbrain and enters the subarachnoid cistern. In the cistern, the nerve passes between the PCA and superior cerebellar artery (SCA), traverses inferior to the PcommA and inferior and medial to the uncus before entering the cavernous sinus (Fig. 12.46). The third nerve subsequently runs superiorly and laterally, deep to the dura propria layer, just superior to the trochlear nerve, before exiting the cavernous sinus at the orbital apex (Fig. 12.46). The third nerve bifurcates into the superior and inferior division before entering the orbit via the superior orbital fissure, passing through the annulus of Zinn. The superior division of the third nerve divides to innervate the levator muscle and superior rectus; the inferior division innervates the medial rectus, lateral rectus, inferior rectus, and inferior oblique.

Parasympathetic pupillary fibers travel from the Edinger Westphal nucleus in the midbrain and follow the path of the third nerve, traveling slightly medially and peripherally. The peripheral orientation of the fibers makes them susceptible to compressive injury. The parasympathetic fibers then follow the inferior division, synapse in the ciliary ganglion inferior lateral to the optic nerve, and briefly piggyback on to the nerve to the inferior oblique before reaching the posterior ciliary nerves, which ultimately innervate the iris sphincter muscle (pupillary constrictor).

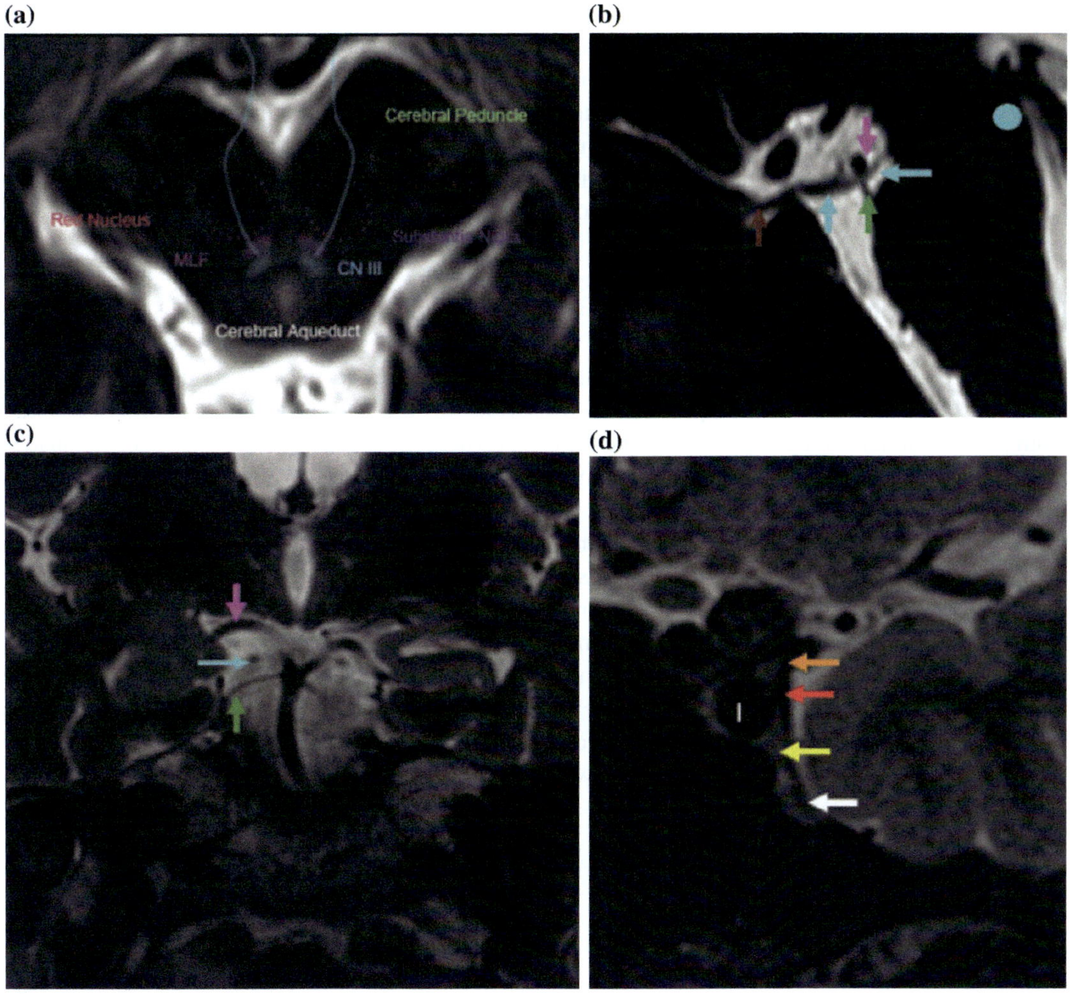

Fig. 12.46 Anatomy of CN III. **a** The oculomotor nuclei are demonstrated by the *solid light blue ovals* seen here at the level of the *red* nucleus, denoted by the *red dotted outline*. The medial longitudinal fasciculus (MLF) is shown by the *solid light purple* ovals. The substantia nigra (*purple dotted outline*) and cerebral aqueduct (*white dotted outline*) are also demonstrated. **b c** and **d** The course of the oculomotor nerve from the nuclei (*blue dot* in **b**) is outlined with the following *arrows* highlighting its segments: *light blue arrow* cisternal segment, *brown arrow* dural cave segment, *orange arrow* cavernous segment of CN III. The structures in close proximity to CN III along its course are indicated as follows: *green arrow* superior cerebellar artery, *pink arrow* posterior cerebral artery, *red arrow* cavernous segment of CN IV, *yellow arrow* ophthalmic division of the trigeminal nerve, and *white arrow* maxillary division of the trigeminal nerve. The cavernous portion of the internal carotid artery (denoted by the letter "I" in image **d**) can be seen medial to the neurovascular structures running along the lateral wall of the sinus. From Tantiwongkosi B, Hesselink J. Imaging of Ocular Motor Pathway. Neuroimaging Clinics of North America [serial online]. August 1, 2015;25 (Orbit and Neuro-ophthalmic Imaging):425–438. Reproduced with permission from Clinical Key

Traumatic Third Nerve Palsy

Clinical Presentation

Complete third nerve palsy consists of ptosis, a fixed dilated (mydriatic) pupil, and limitation of adduction, infraduction and supraduction. In primary position, there is usually exotropia and hypotropia of the affected eye due to unopposed activity of the lateral rectus and superior oblique muscles, innervated by the sixth and fourth nerves, respectively.

Trauma to the third cranial nerve is the second most common mechanism of dysfunction, occurring by compression, stretch and contusion, or transection [240]. Traumatic closed head injury affecting the third nerve tends to be more severe than in cases where the fourth or sixth cranial nerve are affected, typically due to motor vehicle accidents [261].

Mechanisms of Injury

At the origin of the third nerve, injuries to the nucleus occur when the dorsal midbrain suffers traumatic impact against the tentorial incisura, or from severe trauma that results in DAI. The third nerve, having the shortest course of the three ocular motor cranial nerves, is vulnerable in the cisternal space where it passes in close proximity to the SCA and PcommA. Cisternal aneurysms account for up to 14% of CN III palsies overall, where aneurysms of the PcommA are the most common (Figs. 12.47 and 12.48). Impingement on the nerve by these aneurysms affects the peripheral parasympathetic fibers that run along CN III. Pupil involvement (mydriasis) with CN III palsy (Fig. 12.47) suggests a compressive rather than microvascular etiology, which spares the pupil in approximately 68–80% of cases [240]. Ruptured aneurysms can cause direct hemorrhagic damage to the nerve or lead to uncal herniation, while unruptured aneurysms are thought to cause compressive mechanical distortion, edema and fibrosis of the nerve itself [240].

The third nerve is vulnerable to damage by stretch and contusion where it attaches to the dura posterior to the cavernous sinus and adjacent to the posterior clinoid processes [15]. Asynchronous movement of the brainstem, supratentorial structures, and the skull base can cause rootlet avulsion or stretching, especially with downward displacement of the brainstem [262], or contusion at the site where it crosses the posterior petroclinoid ligament [263]. Traumatic avulsion of the third nerve can be from severe trauma with basilar skull fracture with other neurological dysfunction, or from minor trauma without affecting other cranial nerves [263]. Transtentorial herniation of the uncus may cause

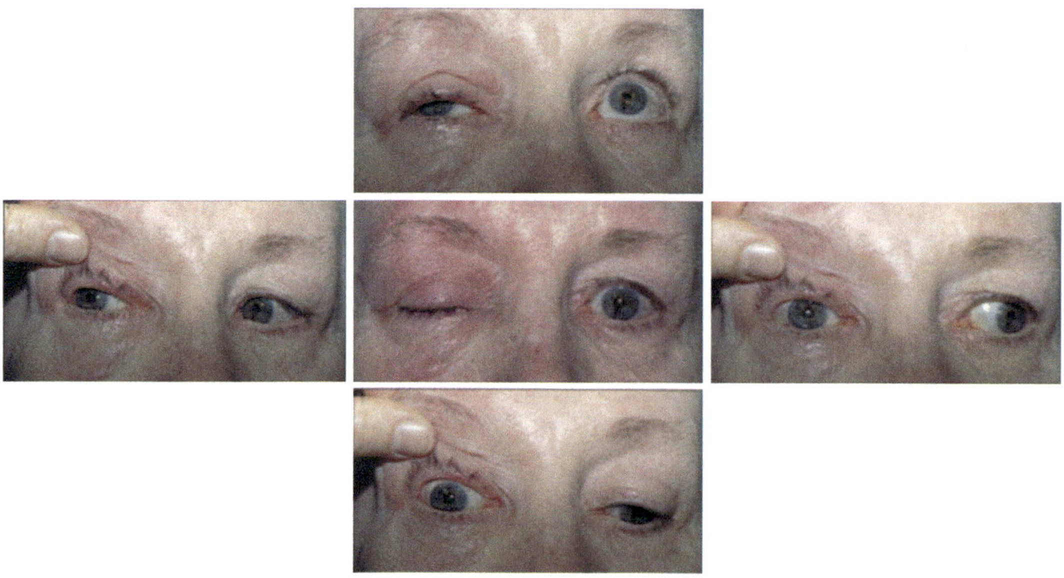

Fig. 12.47 Right third nerve palsy seen on examination of eye movements. The complete right-sided ptosis obscures the gaze initially and requires manual retraction to examine attempted movements of the eye. From Perlmutter D, Moster M. Paresis of Isolated and Multiple Cranial Nerves and Painful Ophthalmoplegia. Book Chapter. 9.16, 927–936.e1 Ophthalmology [e-book]. Philadelphia, Pennsylvania: Saunders; 2013. Available from: Discovery eBooks, Ipswich, MA. Reproduced with permission from Clinical Key

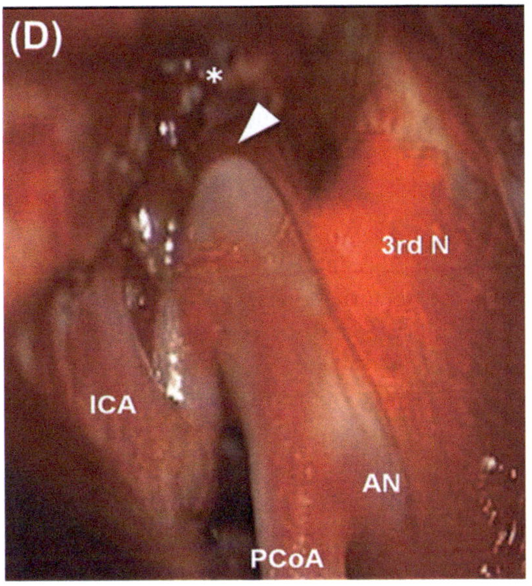

Fig. 12.48 Aneurysm of the Posterior Communicating Artery Directly Stretching CN III. Demonstrates a posterior communicating artery aneurysm (AN) with its neck (*arrowhead*) visible after removal of the clinoid process (at the *asterisk*). The aneurysmal dilation stretched the oculomotor nerve (3rd N). *ICA* internal carotid artery. *PCoA* posterior communicating artery. From Nagatani K, Otani N, Seno S, Takeuchi S, Wada K, Mori K. Diagnostic pitfalls associated with a large true posterior communicating artery aneurysm: a case report. British Journal Of Neurosurgery [serial online]. October 2013;27 (5):687–689. Available from: MEDLINE with Full Text, Ipswich, MA. Accessed April 26, 2016. Reproduced with permission from Taylor Francis Online

compression of the third nerve and this is discussed in more detail below.

In the cavernous sinus, CN III dysfunction can be due to traumatic CCF. Both direct and indirect subtypes often present with ophthalmoplegia involving the third, fourth and sixth nerves, usually with other findings such as dilated, tortuous conjunctival vessels, chemosis, and proptosis. Isolated ocular motor dysfunction has been shown to be the presenting finding in approximately one third of indirect CCF cases [240]. Further discussion of CCF is found in the Head Injury section of this chapter.

Diagnosis

Traumatic third nerve palsy is a clinical diagnosis with findings described above. Various etiologies may be confirmed with neuroimaging. Subarachnoid hemorrhage associated with suspected ruptured aneurysm is detected on non-contrast head CT. Imaging with CTA or MRA may detect vascular injuries such as aneurysms or findings consistent with CCF. Conventional angiogram in these cases can be diagnostic and therapeutic (see: Traumatic Aneurysm and Carotid-Cavernous Fistula sections). Fracture of the skull base may be detected with CT of the head and face with thin sections in the area or suspicion. If there is no contraindication to MRI, T1 weighted fat suppressed post contrast images may evaluate lesions of the ocular motor cranial nerves within the orbital apex and cavernous sinus. Additional T2 weighted fast imaging employing steady state acquisition (FIESTA) or constructive interference in steady state (CISS) sequences allow detailed imaging of the cranial nerves within the cisternal space. Intraparenchymal contusion is characterized using non-contrast CT to evaluate hemorrhage, as well as T1, T2 weighted and gradient-echo (GRE) imaging.

Management

The offending etiology should be promptly treated to relieve compressive injury of the third nerve, if possible. Diplopia from traumatic third nerve palsy should be managed conservatively with monocular occlusion, prism lenses, or possibly with botulinum toxin injected into the lateral rectus (which is usually unnecessary). Often the complete ptosis occludes the visual axis initially, allowing for relief of diplopia until the ptosis recovers. Partial recovery often occurs after about five months [263]. Overall, the recovery from trauma is "slow and prolonged" and after 6–12 months surgical interventions may be considered.

Third Nerve Involvement in Uncal Herniation

Epidemiology

In a large study of 1400 patients with third nerve palsy, 186 (13%) were attributed to uncal herniation. Of the 186, etiology for herniation was due to SDH in 95, EDH in 44, and IPH in 33

Table 12.12 Pupillary findings in patients with third nerve palsy due to herniation

Total cases	Fixed pupil	Fixed and minimally reactive	Limited reaction or unequal	Spared	Smaller	Oval
184	42%	59%	32%	9%	4%	4%

Pupil findings versus cause and location of third nerve palsy. From Keane [266]. Available from: MEDLINE with Full Text, Ipswich, MA. Reproduced with permission from Cambridge Journals

[257]. SDHs have been found to occur in up to 29% of patients with traumatic brain injuries overall and have also been reported to be responsible for up to 41% of fixed dilated pupils presenting acutely [264, 265]. In a 2010 study by Keane et al., third nerve palsy with uncal herniation was due to trauma in 69% of cases. SDH was the cause for transtentorial herniation in 67% of cases [266].

The most common causes of traumatic third nerve palsy from secondary herniation include falls (40 of 60 cases, or 66.7%), assault (20 of 30 cases, or 66.7%), and automobile accidents (23 of 134 cases, or 17.2%) [266]. SDHs are most commonly caused by falls in elderly patients over age 75 [264]. This likely occurs because progressive cortical atrophy associated with aging increases cortical bridging vein susceptibility to shearing forces in acceleration.

Clinical Presentation

In cases of transtentorial herniation, patients are often obtunded precluding examination of extraocular motility. The affected pupil becomes dilated and poorly reactive to light. Table 12.12 demonstrates the pupillary findings in 186 patients with herniation. Pupillary reaction to light is affected in almost all cases (91%) [266]. Other findings with increased severity of herniation and further compression of the brainstem include abnormal posturing and decreased Glasgow Coma Scale score.

Mechanism of Third Nerve Injury in Uncal Herniation

Figure 12.49 shows the normal anatomic relationship of the uncus and third nerve in close proximity. Uncal herniation causes mass effect on the third nerve, often secondary to a traumatic hematoma. The expanding hematoma shifts the uncus and adjacent temporal lobe inferomedially over the tentorial incisura (Fig. 12.50). Third nerve injury occurs by two mechanisms: direct compression in the tentorial notch or with stretching and contusion from shifting intracranial contents over the skull base or near the petroclinoid ligament [124, 262, 264].

Diagnosis

Mydriasis in a comatose patient with significant head trauma is worrisome for uncal herniation. While CT may suggest herniation, MRI is the preferred imaging modality for a detailed view of the mass effect and midline shift. The suprasellar cistern will be obscured in mild herniation. Moderate to severe cases will efface the quadrigeminal cistern and cause enlargement of the contralateral cerebellopontine cistern compressing the brainstem (Figs. 12.50 and 12.51) [264].

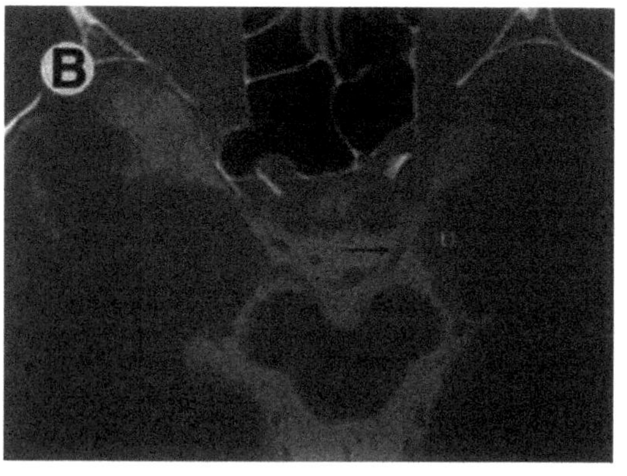

Fig. 12.49 Axial CT demonstrating relationship of CN III (*arrow*) in the cisternal space to the uncus (u). From Eisenkraft B, Ortiz A. Imaging evaluation of cranial nerves 3, 4, and 6. Seminars in Ultrasound, CT, and MRI [serial online]. January 1, 2001;22:488–501. Permission received from Science Direct

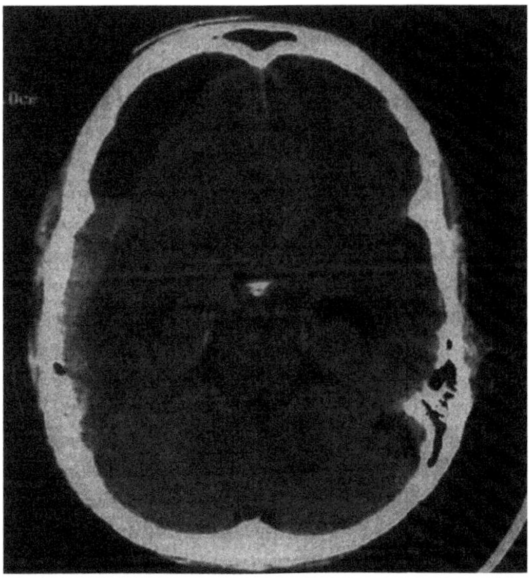

Fig. 12.50 Uncal herniation on unenhanced axial CT due to subdural hematoma. The subdural bleed is seen on the right anterior aspect of the skull causing significant mass effect. From Eisenkraft B, Ortiz A. Imaging evaluation of cranial nerves 3, 4, and 6. Seminars In Ultrasound, CT, And MRI [serial online]. January 1, 2001;22:488–501. Reproduced with permission from Science Direct

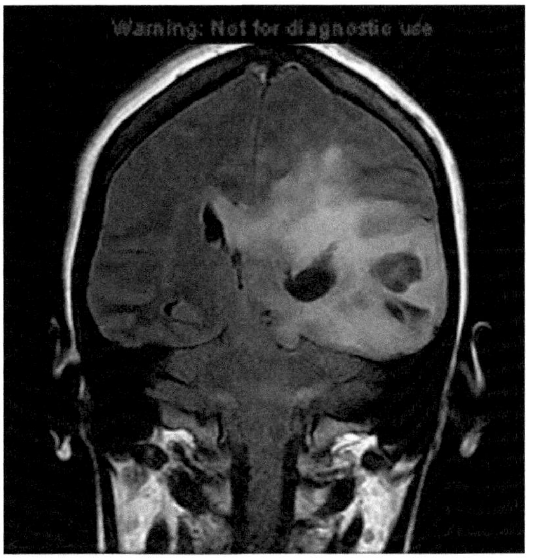

Fig. 12.51 Left temporal hemorrhage causing central and uncal herniation, with resultant brainstem compression. From Young [267]. Reproduced with permission from Clinical Key

Management

Treatment of uncal herniation relies on identification of the underlying cause and if possible, space-occupying lesions should be promptly resected [265]. Craniectomy may be performed in some cases of traumatic subarachnoid hemorrhage [267]. Temporizing measures include decreasing intracranial pressure to prevent further herniation and compression of the brainstem.

Iatrogenic Trauma of CN III

Figure 12.54 demonstrates a cadaveric dissection showing the close proximity of the third nerve to several key brain structures, including the basilar artery. Iatrogenic transection or injury of CN III is reported in surgical procedures that involve structures along the route of the nerve, such as the tentorium, third ventricle, sellar/suprasellar region, and the temporal lobe. In the 2010 study by Keane et al., 10% of traumatic third nerve palsy was iatrogenic [266]. These surgical cases consisted of 87 aneurysm cases, 30 of which were of the basilar artery, and 44 tumor cases, of which 21 were meningiomas and 12 were pituitary adenomas [266]. Postoperative hemorrhage is reported to occur in 0.56% of intracranial procedures and can be another source of pupil-involving third nerve palsy [265].

Surgical excision of tumors along the course of the third nerve The transsphenoidal sinus approach to the sellar/suprasellar region risks pneumatization of surrounding structures, including cranial nerves III through VI in the cavernous sinus [268]. Treatment of pituitary adenomas by endonasal endoscopic approach results in fewer complications than craniotomy from other approaches. Surgical maneuvers frequently spare the third nerves despite being laterally displaced by the tumor [269]. In more adherent lesions, such as epidermoid cyst or meningiomas, subtotal resection may be necessary because of potential damage to the cranial nerves or vascular structures [270].

Temporal lobe tumor resection can be complicated by third nerve paresis, particularly if the lesion invades the interpeduncular fossa [271]. In intracranial procedures with high risk of

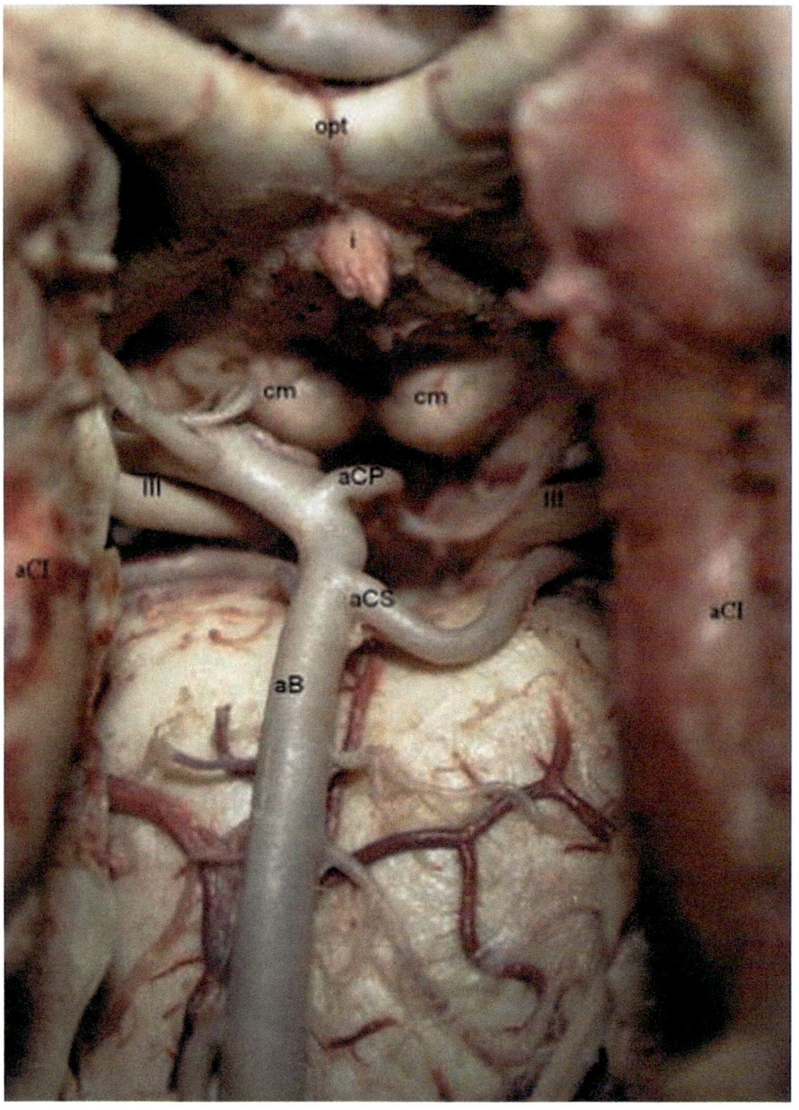

Fig. 12.52 Inferior view of dorsal frontal lobe and pons in a cadaver. *opt* optic chiasm; *i* infundibulum, *cm* mammillary body; *aCP* posterior cerebral artery; *III* oculomotor nerve; *aCS* superior cerebellar artery; *aCI* internal carotid artery; *aB* basilar artery From Buelens E, Wilms G, van Loon J, van Calenbergh F. The oculomotor nerve: anatomic relationship with the floor of the third ventricle. Child's Nervous System: Chns: Official Journal Of The International Society For Pediatric Neurosurgery [serial online]. June 2011;27(6):943–948. Reproduced with permission from Springer

damaging the third nerve, intraoperative nerve monitoring has improved long-term outcomes [272].

Cranial Nerve IV: The trochlear nerve

Anatomy

The trochlear nerve arises from its nucleus in the midbrain at the level of the inferior colliculus, near the junction of the midbrain and pons (Fig. 12.53). In the midbrain, the nerve fibers pass posteriorly from the nuclei and course below the cerebral aqueduct before curving and decussating over the roof of the aqueduct within the superior medullary velum (Fig. 12.54). The nerve then exits on the dorsal aspect of the midbrain below the inferior colliculus on the contralateral side of its nucleus of origin, a unique feature of the trochlear nerve compared to other cranial nerves that exit the brainstem ventrally. In the cisternal space, the trochlear nerves course around the cerebral peduncles and lateral midbrain within the quadrigeminal and ambient cisterns (Fig. 12.54). From there, the trochlear nerve passes into the cavernous sinus where it runs along the lateral wall close to the third nerve

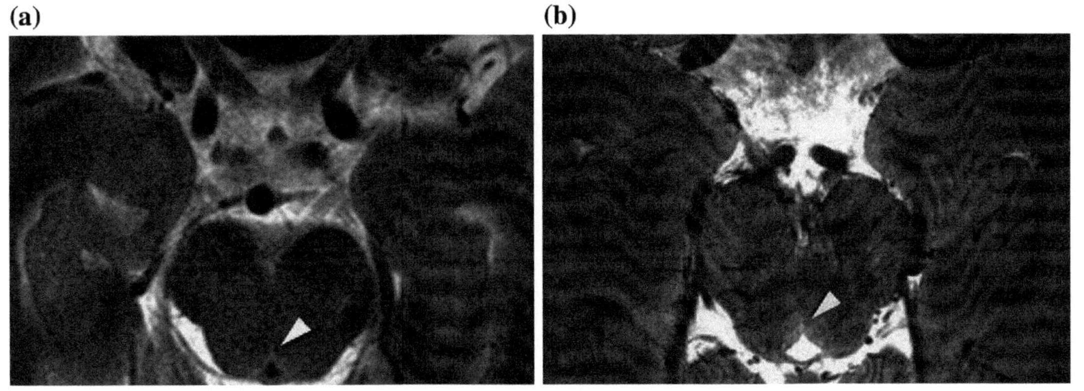

Fig. 12.53 Axial T2 TSE (**a**) and T2 (**b**) imaging of trochlear nerve nucleus (*white arrowhead*) at the level of the inferior colliculi. From Ferreira et al. [262], with permission

superiorly and the ophthalmic division of the trigeminal nerve inferiorly (Fig. 12.54). The trochlear nerve then enters the orbit via the superior orbital fissure, passing superiorly and outside the annulus of Zinn, and proceeding to pass over the optic nerve before innervating the superior oblique muscle. The superior oblique muscle intorts the eye and causes infraduction in adduction.

Traumatic Fourth Nerve Palsy

Epidemiology

Head trauma is the most common cause of acquired trochlear nerve palsy [240]. Kung et al. in 2015 reported 169 of 578 trochlear nerve palsy cases reviewed (29%) were due to head trauma [273].

Clinical Presentation

Damage to the trochlear nerve causes excyclotorsion and limited downgaze in the adducted position, resulting in vertical binocular diplopia from hypertropia of the affected eye.

Pathophysiology

Damage to the nucleus of the trochlear nerve can occur with local ischemia in the setting of trauma when shearing forces destroy the vulnerable paramedian branches of the basilar bifurcation [240]. Unlike the third nerve, trochlear nerve palsy due to aneurysmal dilation is rare, and instead is more commonly due to traumatic vertebral artery dissection [240]. The trochlear nerve has the longest intracranial course, and its unique dorsal exit from the brainstem makes it additionally vulnerable to avulsion and compression by the tentorial edge [274]. The short dorsal fascicles may be injured in isolation from other brainstem structures, making it difficult to distinguish between brainstem and extra-axial nerve disease [15].

Diagnosis

Clinical examination for suspected trochlear nerve palsy involves measuring the vertical deviation with cross-cover testing using prism lenses in all gazes including head tilt. Evaluation involves the Parks three-step test, Maddox rod and double Maddox rod testing, and the upright-supine test for distinguishing a true palsy from skew deviation.

Parks Three-Step Test

The Parks three-step test (Figs. 12.55 and 12.56) determines if the hypertropia is due to trochlear nerve palsy. The first step is to evaluate the eyes in the primary position and determine whether the hypertropia is on the right or left side. The next step is to examine the vertical deviation in right and left gaze to determine which direction increases the hyperdeviation. Finally, the last step is to determine whether a right or left head

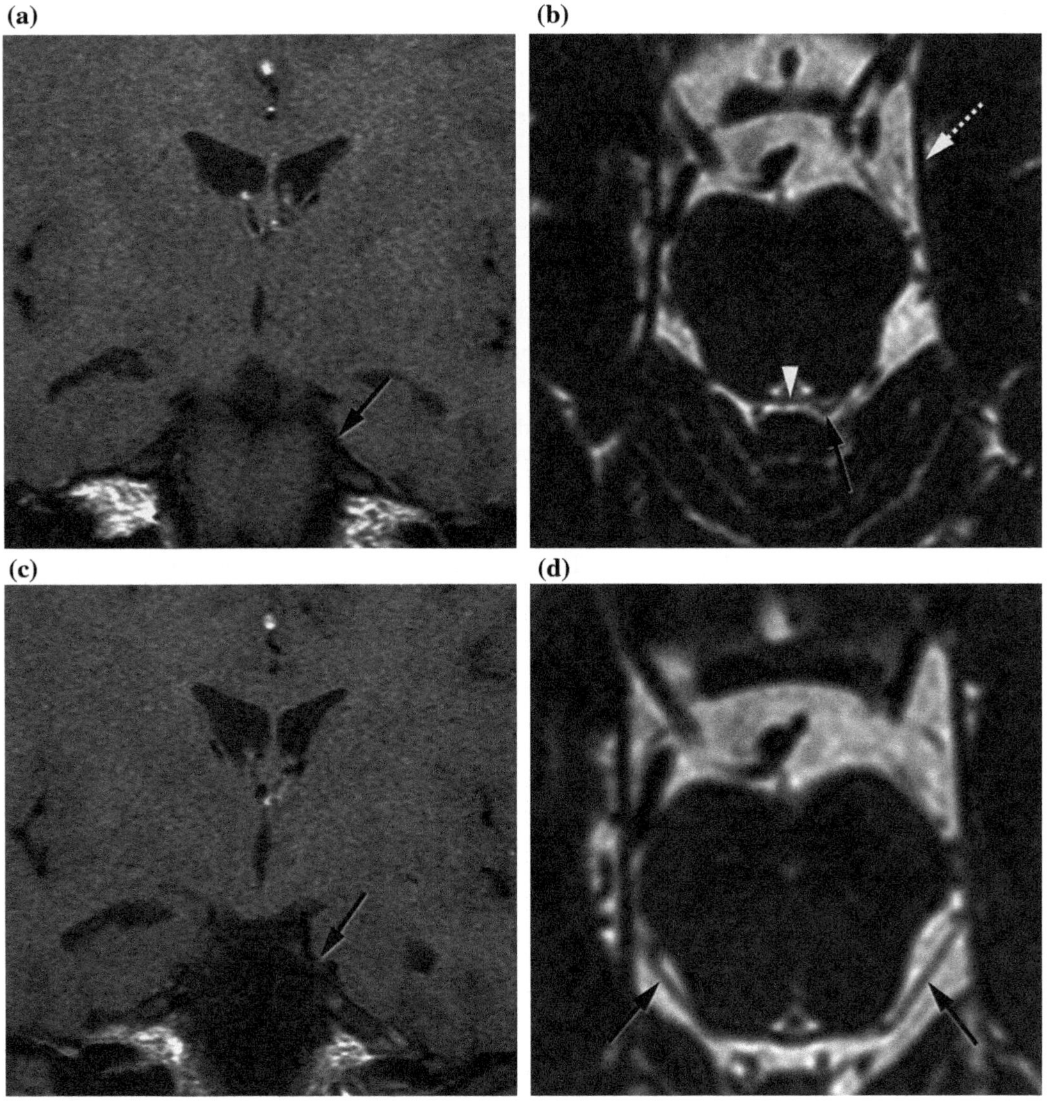

Fig. 12.54 Cisternal portion of Trochlear nerve. **a** and **c** coronal T1 images demonstrating the trochlear nerve (*black arrow*) in the cistern **b** and **d** double oblique axial reconstruction of 3D T2 turbo spin-echo images demonstrating the trochlear nerve (*black arrow*), the superior medullary velum (*white arrowhead*), and the tentorium (*white dashed arrow*). From Ferreira et al. [262]. Reproduced with permission from Science Direct

tilt increases the vertical deviation. An explanation for each of these steps follows:

1. Assess the eyes in primary gaze and eliminate four extraocular muscles based on which eye is elevated or depressed. Paresis of the superior oblique and inferior rectus may cause hypertropia of one eye. Paresis of the superior rectus and inferior oblique may cause depression (or hypotropia) of one eye.
2. Examine the eyes in lateral gaze to exclude another set of four extraocular muscles. The direction of the lateral gaze activates the rectus muscles of the ipsilateral side and the oblique muscles of the contralateral side. Vertical movement in right gaze is accomplished by the right superior rectus and right inferior rectus in the right eye and in the left eye, by the left superior oblique and left inferior oblique muscles. This eliminates the

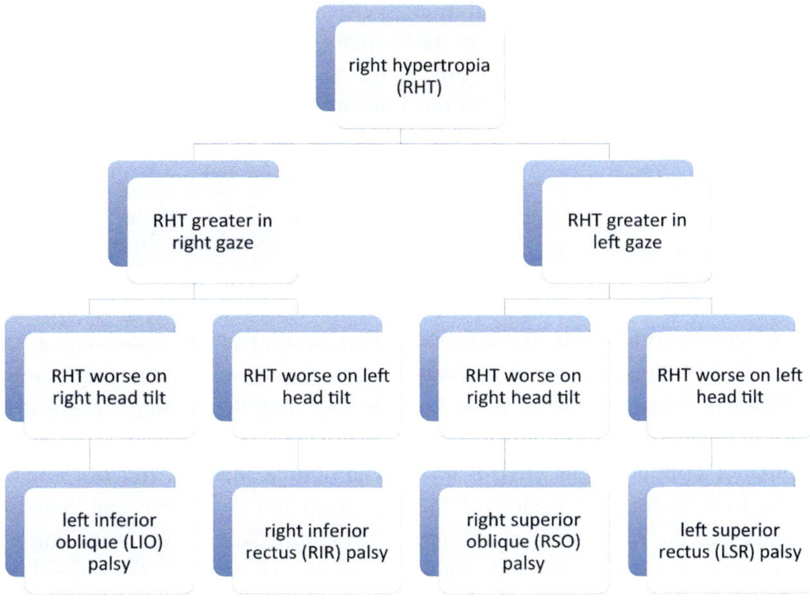

Fig. 12.55 Parks three-step test localization of paretic vertical muscle when there is a right hypertropia (RHT) in primary gaze

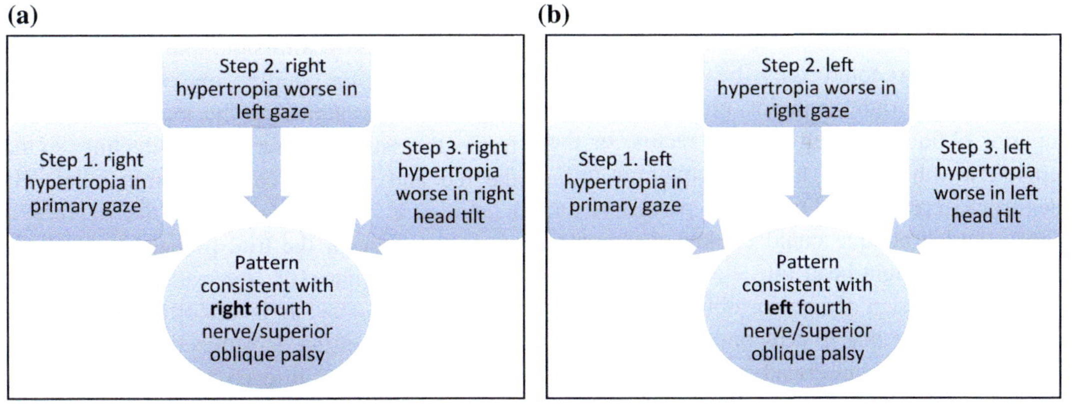

Fig. 12.56 Detecting fourth nerve palsy using the Parks three-step test. **a** Pattern in right fourth nerve palsy and **b** pattern in left fourth nerve palsy

other four extraocular muscles and should leave only two possibly paretic muscles after considering those eliminated in step one.

3. The third and final step will leave one extraocular muscle as the culprit for paresis by eliminating another set of four muscles. Head tilt to one side requires incyclotorsion of the ipsilateral eye, performed by the superior rectus and superior oblique, and excyclotorsion of the contralateral eye, performed by the inferior rectus and inferior oblique.

These steps are explained by the following example:

1. In primary gaze, the right eye is hypertropic.

This suggests the paretic muscle could be one of four: right inferior rectus, right superior oblique, left superior rectus, or left inferior oblique. The following muscles cannot be responsible for the finding: right superior rectus, right inferior oblique, left inferior rectus, and left superior oblique.

2. In left lateral gaze, the vertical deviation is greater.

This suggests the paretic muscle could be one of the following: left superior rectus, left inferior rectus, right superior oblique, or right inferior oblique. The following four muscles cannot be responsible for the vertical deviation: left inferior oblique, left superior oblique, right inferior rectus, and right superior rectus. Exclusion of the left inferior rectus and the right inferior oblique from step one results in only two possible muscles that could be responsible: the left superior rectus and the right superior oblique.

3. In right head tilt, the vertical deviation is greater.

This finding could only be possible with paresis of the right superior rectus, the right superior oblique, the left inferior rectus, or the left inferior oblique. Of the two remaining muscles from steps one and two, only paresis of the right superior oblique could explain the greater hypertropia in right head tilt.

In the discussion of superior oblique palsy, it is important to note that if steps one and two of the Parks three-step test are found to be greater on the same side, then neither the right nor the left superior oblique muscle could be responsible in isolation.

Head trauma will often result in bilateral fourth nerve palsy. Cross-cover testing may reveal hypertropia on one side that switches to hypertropia of the contralateral eye in horizontal gaze or head tilt. The double Maddox rod and the upright-supine test will help distinguish bilateral fourth nerve palsy from skew deviation in this situation.

Maddox Rod Testing

The Maddox rod is a hand held parallel plano-convex cylinder lens with a red filter that converts a point light source to a streak, either vertically or horizontally depending on the orientation. The Maddox rod is used to determine the angle of horizontal or vertical deviation to localize and help quantify severity of muscle paresis. By convention, the red Maddox rod is held over the right eye. Orienting the lines in the vertical plane, a point light source will be seen as a red horizontal line. In the presence of trochlear nerve palsy with excyclotorsion, the line will be oriented diagonally (angled inferonasally) rather than parallel to the floor, and it will be located below or above the point light source seen with the left eye, depending if there is a right or left hypertropia, respectively.

The double Maddox rod test is used to measure cyclotorsion of the eye and can complement the Parks three-step test. With the lines oriented vertically in the 90° plane, a red Maddox rod is placed over the right eye and a clear Maddox rod is placed over the left eye in a trial frame (see Fig. 12.57). If there is a hyperdeviation, the patient will see a red and a white horizontal line, separated vertically from one another. In the presence of excyclotorsion, the red and white lines will not be parallel; one will be oriented diagonally. By adjusting the knobs on the trial frame, the patient is able to rotate the lines so that the red and white streaks appear parallel. The examiner is then able to read the degrees of excyclotorsion off the trial frame. If excyclotorsion is more than 10°, the patient has bilateral fourth nerve palsy. It is important to note that Maddox rod testing is subjective and requires intact visual acuity in each eye, thus limiting its use.

Upright-Supine Test

The upright-supine test can differentiate skew deviation due to disruption of the vestibulo-ocular reflex from true trochlear nerve palsy by measuring vertical prism deviation with alternate cover testing in both the upright and supine positions. Vertical strabismus that decreases by 50% or more from the upright to the supine position suggests a skew deviation instead of trochlear nerve dysfunction with a sensitivity of 80% and specificity of 100% [275]. All patients in the study with trochlear nerve dysfunction had a negative upright-supine test, with change less

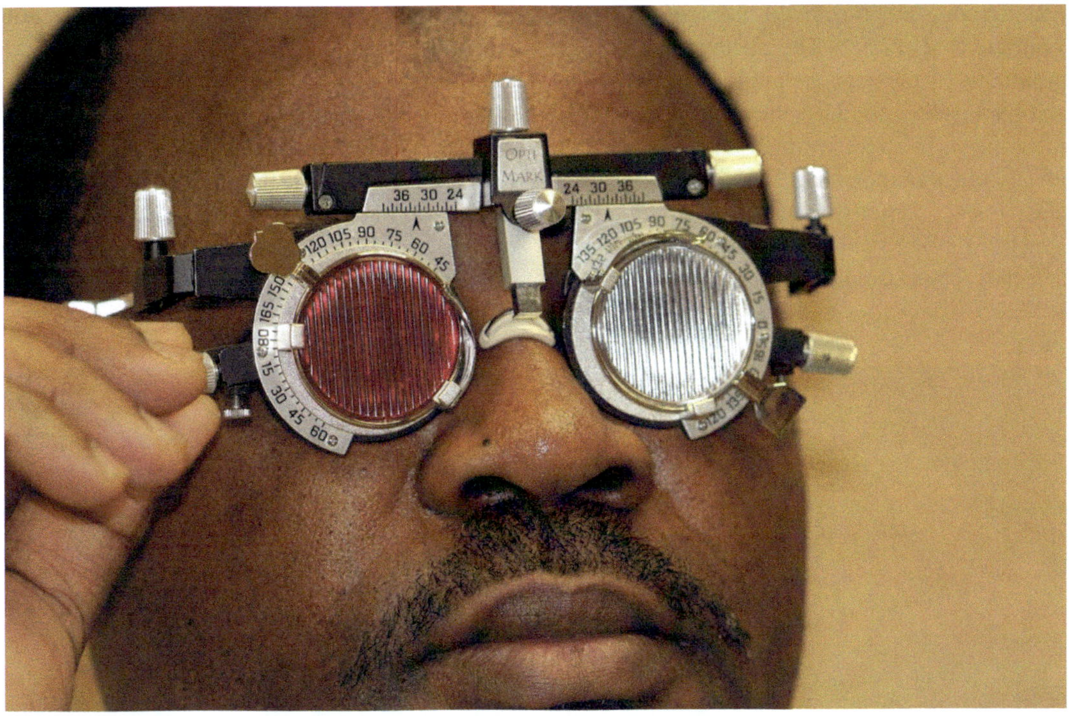

Fig. 12.57 Double Maddox Rod Test. Note the red Maddox rod over the *right* eye and clear Maddox rod over the *left* eye. The patient is turning the knob on the trial frame to correct for excyclotorsion

than 50% from upright to supine position [275]. This test is ideally performed with a fixation target present in the distance in the sitting position and then with a fixed target on the ceiling in the supine position.

Localization of Injury

Owing to the dorsally located trochlear nuclei with short fascicular segments, it can be difficult to localize the injury to the nerve or its fascicles in the brainstem. When the fascicles are injured, the dysfunction is often isolated with similar presentation to subarachnoid nerve segment injury [15]. The rare situation of localization to the dorsal midbrain arises when trochlear nerve palsy is seen in combination with a RAPD without visual loss, via interruption of the pupillary light reflex pathway in this region.

Treatment

As with other acute ocular motor cranial nerve palsies, monocular occlusion is used in the acute setting for relief of diplopia. Recovery occurs over the course of about 6 months. If the vertical deviation causing diplopia is less than 15 prism diopters, Fresnel prisms (flexible plastic prisms adhered to the lens in a pair of spectacle glasses) may be used. Fresnel prism correction higher than 15 prism diopters is not practical due to degradation of visual acuity from the thicker prism. Once the vertical deviation measurements are stable after a period of a few months, the prism correction may be ground into spectacle lenses, which is less likely to affect visual acuity.

Unfortunately, in some patients, symptomatic relief is not achieved after prism correction. This is often due to persistent bothersome excyclotorsion, which may be treated with strabismus surgery of the superior oblique muscle.

Cranial Nerve VI: The abducens nerve

Anatomy

The abducens nucleus is in the dorsomedial caudal pons, close to the pontomedullary junction and underneath the floor of the fourth ventricle (Fig. 12.58). The nucleus lies in close proximity to the medial longitudinal fasciculus and paramedian pontine reticular formation. The facial nerve fascicles wrap around it to form the facial colliculus dorsally. The sixth nerve fascicles travel ventrally near several important structures in the pons. The nerve root then exits at the pontomedullary junction near the pyramids. The nerve then courses in the subarachnoid space ventrally and rostrally, parallel to the clivus, before entering Dorello's fibro-osseous canal. The sixth nerve has the longest subarachnoid course of all the ocular motor cranial nerves, making it particularly susceptible to damage from subarachnoid processes causing raised intracranial pressure, especially in the region of Dorello's canal. The nerve

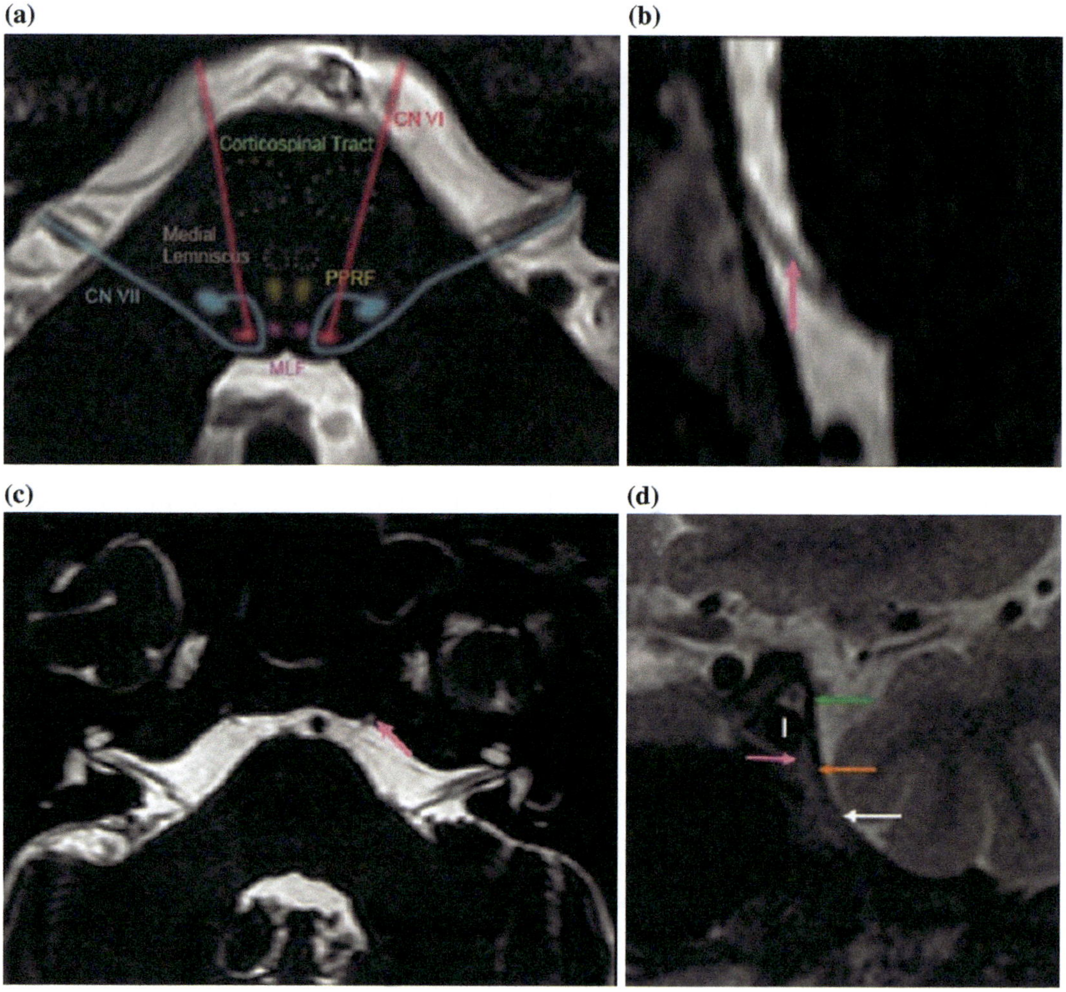

Fig. 12.58 Anatomy of CN VI. **a** *Solid pink dots* and *pink lines* abducens nuclei and fascicles; *solid purple dots* MLF; *solid yellow ovals* paramedian pontine reticular formation (PPRF); *green dashed circles* corticospinal tracts; *yellow dashed circles* medial lemniscus; *solid blue ovals* and *lines* facial nuclei and fascicles. **b** *pink arrow* cisternal segment of abducens nerve **c** *pink arrow* dural cave segment of abducens nerve passing through the Dorello canal. **d** Cavernous sinus: *green arrow* oculomotor nerve; letter "I": internal carotid artery; *pink arrow* cavernous segment of abducens nerve; *orange arrow* ophthalmic division of trigeminal nerve; *white arrow* maxillary division of trigeminal nerve. From Tantiwongkosi B, Hesselink J. Imaging of Ocular Motor Pathway. Neuroimaging Clinics Of North America [serial online]. August 1, 2015;25(Orbit and Neuro-ophthalmic Imaging):425–438. Reproduced with permission from Clinical Key

subsequently passes over the petrous apex, under the petrosphenoid (Gruber's) ligament, and then enters the cavernous sinus. In the cavernous sinus, the abducens nerve proceeds anteriorly within the medial cavernous sinus, in close contact with the internal carotid artery (ICA) and the sympathetic plexus. For this reason, sixth nerve palsy presenting with ipsilateral Horner's syndrome localizes to the cavernous sinus. The nerve then enters the orbit via the superior orbital fissure, within the annulus of Zinn, and proceeds to innervate the lateral rectus muscle.

Traumatic Sixth Nerve Palsy

Epidemiology

In one series of 165 patients presenting with abducens palsy, only 3.1% were due to trauma, though the incidence of unilateral abducens palsy from head trauma had been previously reported as high as 2.7% [276]. In severe cases of head trauma, sixth nerve palsy may be as high as 27%, most commonly due to skull base fractures crossing the petrous ridge [135]. Traumatic middle cranial fossa and transverse sphenoid body fractures are also commonly associated with abducens nerve palsy [158]. Ten percent of traumatic sixth nerve palsy occurs bilaterally, usually associated with more severe findings of cranial and cervical injuries [276]. Iatrogenic etiologies of abducens nerve dysfunction are similar to those for third and fourth nerve palsies, with the addition of procedures involving the cavernous sinus and those that decrease intracranial pressure.

Clinical Presentation

Isolated sixth nerve palsy presents with horizontal binocular diplopia, with ipsilateral impaired abduction and esotropia. Patients will be most symptomatic in ipsilateral lateral gaze and when looking in the distance because there is normally convergence at near. In basilar skull fractures that cross the petrous ridge, cranial nerves VII and VIII are often involved, leading to peripheral facial paresis and hearing loss in addition to sixth nerve palsy.

Pathophysiology

Due to its precarious route, trauma most frequently damages the abducens nerve in cases of raised intracranial pressure or herniation, especially in the vicinity of Dorello's canal, where the nerve is fixed. The immobility of the sixth nerve in Dorello's canal leaves it vulnerable to stretching and even compression by the basilar artery or clivus when the brain moves caudally. Additionally, its passage beneath Gruber's ligament at the base of the posterior clinoid process serves as another susceptible area for contusion and avulsion during head trauma [135].

In the cavernous sinus, the sixth nerve's close relation to the internal carotid artery leaves it at risk of being involved with any extradural carotid aneurysms. Typically, cavernous carotid aneurysms will present with cavernous sinus syndrome rather than isolated unilateral sixth nerve palsy, with the specific findings described in the Head Injury section.

Diagnosis

Patients with sixth nerve palsy may present with partial or complete limitation of abduction. In primary position, there will often be a large esotropia initially. Occasionally, the lateral rectus weakness will be subtle and diagnosis is made based on the observation of slightly slower saccades in abduction of the affected eye. Cross-cover testing reveals ipsilateral esotropia worse on gaze toward the affected side. The etiology of sixth nerve palsy can be detected with neuroimaging with CT for assessment of skull base fractures or MRI for assessment of the brain parenchyma. If there is suspicion for raised intracranial pressure as a cause for bilateral sixth nerve palsy, a dilated fundoscopic examination may reveal papilledema. In this case, urgent intervention is necessary to lower the CSF pressure and prevent permanent cranial nerve palsy or visual loss from persistent papilledema.

Management

Similar to third and fourth nerve palsy, the affected eye in sixth nerve palsy should be managed initially by monocular occlusion and prisms. If the diplopia has not recovered after 6 months, strabismus surgery may be considered for relief.

Summary

After review of this chapter, clinicians will have a thorough understanding of the vast possibilities of injury to the optic nerve, visual pathways, and oculomotor system in assessing trauma patients. Recognition of neuro-ophthalmic clinical signs, knowledge of orbital, cranial nerve and central nervous system anatomy, and detecting radiographic evidence of fractures, hemorrhage, vascular injury, or herniation syndromes will lead to prompt diagnosis and treatment of life threatening sequlae of trauma.

References

1. Elisevich KV, Ford RM, Anderson DP, Stratford JG, Richardson PM. Visual abnormalities with multiple trauma. Surg Neurol. 1984;22:565–75.
2. Kulkarni AR, et al. Ocular manifestations of head injury: a clinical study. Eye Lond Engl. 2005;19:1257–63.
3. Kapur E, et al. Magnetic resonance review of the anatomical structure of the orbital apex and cranio-orbital junction. Med J. 2012;18:191.
4. Yeh S, Foroozan R. Orbital apex syndrome. Curr Opin Ophthalmol. 2004;15:490–8.
5. Dutton JJ. Radiology of the orbit and visual pathways. Saunders Elsevier; 2010.
6. Scheid R, Preul C, Gruber O, Wiggins C, von Cramon DY. Diffuse axonal injury associated with chronic traumatic brain injury: evidence from T2*-weighted gradient-echo imaging at 3 T. AJNR Am J Neuroradiol. 2003;24:1049–56.
7. Wang BH, et al. Traumatic optic neuropathy: a review of 61 patients. Plast Reconstr Surg. 2001;107:1655–64.
8. Steinsapir KD, Goldberg RA. Traumatic optic neuropathy: an evolving understanding. Am J Ophthalmol. 2011; 151, 928–33.e2.
9. Sarkies N. Traumatic optic neuropathy. Eye Lond Engl. 2004;18:1122–5.
10. Steinsapir KD, Goldberg RA. Traumatic optic neuropathy: a critical update. Medscape.
11. Kumaran AM, Sundar G, Chye LT. Traumatic optic neuropathy: a review. Craniomaxillofacial Trauma Reconstr. 2015;8:31–41.
12. McClenaghan FC, Ezra DG, Holmes SB. Mechanisms and management of vision loss following orbital and facial trauma. Curr Opin Ophthalmol. 2011;22:426–31.
13. Hayreh SS, Zimmerman MB. Central retinal artery occlusion: visual outcome. Am J Ophthalmol. 2005;140:376–91.
14. Anderson RL, Panje WR, Gross CE. Optic nerve blindness following blunt forehead trauma. Ophthalmology. 1982;89:445–55.
15. Miller NR, Newman NJ, Biousse V, Kerrison JB. Walsh and Hoyt's clinical neuro-ophthalmology. Lippincott Williams & Wilkins; 2005.
16. Gross CE, DeKock JR, Panje WR, Hershkowitz N, Newman J. Evidence for orbital deformation that may contribute to monocular blindness following minor frontal head trauma. J Neurosurg. 1981;55:963–6.
17. Maegele M. Reversal of isolated unilateral optic nerve edema with concomitant visual impairment following blunt trauma: a case report. J Med Case Rep. 2008;2:50.
18. Crompton MR. Visual lesions in closed head injury. Brain J Neurol. 1970;93:785–92.
19. Warner N, Eggenberger E. Traumatic optic neuropathy: a review of the current literature. Curr Opin Ophthalmol. 2010;21:459–62.
20. Yu-Wai-Man P, Griffiths PG. Steroids for traumatic optic neuropathy. Cochrane Database Syst. Rev. 2013; 6, CD006032.
21. Osborne NN, et al. Optic nerve and neuroprotection strategies. Eye Lond Engl. 2004;18:1075–84.
22. Loane DJ, Faden AI. Neuroprotection for traumatic brain injury: translational challenges and emerging therapeutic strategies. Trends Pharmacol Sci. 2010;31:596–604.
23. Yu Wai Man P, Griffiths PG. Surgery for traumatic optic neuropathy. Cochrane Database Syst. Rev. CD005024 (2005). Doi:10.1002/14651858.CD005024.pub2.
24. Lee V, Ford RL, Xing W, Bunce C, Foot B. Surveillance of traumatic optic neuropathy in the UK. Eye Lond Engl. 2010;24:240–50.
25. Mahapatra AK, Tandon DA. Traumatic optic neuropathy in children: a prospective study. Pediatr Neurosurg. 1993;19:34–9.
26. Goldenberg-Cohen N, Miller NR, Repka MX. Traumatic optic neuropathy in children and adolescents. J AAPOS Off Publ Am Assoc Pediatr Ophthalmol Strabismus Am Assoc Pediatr Ophthalmol. 2004;8:20–7.
27. Pirouzmand F. Epidemiological trends of traumatic optic nerve injuries in the largest Canadian adult trauma center. J Craniofac Surg. 2012;23:516–20.
28. Levin LA, Beck RW, Joseph MP, Seiff S, Kraker R. The treatment of traumatic optic neuropathy: the international optic nerve trauma study. Ophthalmology. 1999;106:1268–77.
29. Lessell S. Indirect optic nerve trauma. Arch Ophthalmol Chic Ill. 1989;1960(107):382–6.

30. al-Qurainy IA, Stassen LF, Dutton GN, Moos KF, el-Attar A. The characteristics of midfacial fractures and the association with ocular injury: a prospective study. Br. J. Oral Maxillofac. Surg. 1991; 29, 291–301.
31. Jamal BT, et al. Ophthalmic injuries in patients with zygomaticomaxillary complex fractures requiring surgical repair. J Oral Maxillofac Surg Off J Am AssocOral Maxillofac Surg. 2009;67:986–9.
32. Urolagin SB, Kotrashetti SM, Kale TP, Balihallimath LJ. Traumatic optic neuropathy after maxillofacial trauma: a review of 8 cases. J Oral Maxillofac Surg Off J Am Assoc Oral Maxillofac Surg. 2012;70:1123–30.
33. Bonavolontà G. Postoperative blindness following orbital surgery. Orbit Amst Neth. 2005;24:195–200.
34. Cruz AAV, dos Santos AC. Blindness after Le Fort I osteotomy: a possible complication associated with pterygomaxillary separation. J Cranio-Maxillo-fac Surg Off Publ Eur Assoc Cranio-Maxillo-fac Surg. 2006;34:210–6.
35. Kim JJ, Gean AD. Imaging for the diagnosis and management of traumatic brain injury. Neurother J Am Soc Exp Neurother. 2011;8:39–53.
36. Shibuya TY, et al. Visual risks of facial fracture repair in the setting of traumatic optic neuropathy. Arch Otolaryngol Head Neck Surg. 2006;132:258–64.
37. Roccia F, et al. Role of the maxillofacial surgeon in the management of severe ocular injuries after maxillofacial fractures. J Emerg Trauma Shock. 2011;4:188–93.
38. Kim JY, Kim HJ, Kim C-H, Lee J-G, Yoon J-H. Optic nerve injury secondary to endoscopic sinus surgery: an analysis of three cases. Yonsei Med J. 2005;46:300–4.
39. Nau HE, et al. Optic nerve trauma: clinical, electrophysiological and histological remarks. Acta Neurochir (Wien). 1987;89:16–27.
40. Lübben B, Stoll W, Grenzebach U. Optic nerve decompression in the comatose and conscious patients after trauma. Laryngoscope. 2001;111:320–8.
41. Kountakis SE, Maillard AA, El-Harazi SM, Longhini L, Urso RG. Endoscopic optic nerve decompression for traumatic blindness. Otolaryngol.–Head Neck Surg. Off. J. Am. Acad. Otolaryngol.-Head Neck Surg. 2000; 123, 34–7.
42. Joseph MP, Lessell S, Rizzo J, Momose KJ. Extracranial optic nerve decompression for traumatic optic neuropathy. Arch Ophthalmol Chic Ill. 1990;1960(108):1091–3.
43. Seiff SR. High dose corticosteroids for treatment of vision loss due to indirect injury to the optic nerve. Ophthalmic Surg. 1990;21:389–95.
44. Spoor TC, Hartel WC, Lensink DB, Wilkinson MJ. Treatment of traumatic optic neuropathy with corticosteroids. Am J Ophthalmol. 1990;110:665–9.
45. Millesi W, Hollmann K, Funder J. Traumatic lesion of the optic nerve. Acta Neurochir. (Wien) 1988; 93:50–4.
46. Matsuzaki H, Kunita M, Kawai K. Optic nerve damage in head trauma: clinical and experimental studies. Jpn J Ophthalmol. 1982;26:447–61.
47. Bodian M. Transient loss of vision following head trauma. NY State J Med. 1964;64:916–20.
48. Robinson D, Wilcsek G, Sacks R. Orbit and orbital apex. Otolaryngol. Clin. North Am. 2011; 44:903–22, viii.
49. Kallela I, Hyrkäs T, Paukku P, Iizuka T, Lindqvist C. Blindness after maxillofacial blunt trauma. Evaluation of candidates for optic nerve decompression surgery. J. Cranio-Maxillo-fac. Surg. Off. Publ. Eur. Assoc. Cranio-Maxillo-fac. Surg. 1994; 22:220–5.
50. Sabates NR, Gonce MA, Farris BK. Neuro-ophthalmological findings in closed head trauma. J Clin Neuroophthalmol. 1991;11:273–7.
51. Suchoff IB, et al. The frequency of occurrence, types, and characteristics of visual field defects in acquired brain injury: a retrospective analysis. Optom St Louis Mo. 2008;79:259–65.
52. Ciuffreda KJ, et al. Occurrence of oculomotor dysfunctions in acquired brain injury: a retrospective analysis. Optom St Louis Mo. 2007;78:155–61.
53. Rutner D, et al. Occurrence of ocular disease in traumatic brain injury in a selected sample: a retrospective analysis. Brain Inj. 2006;20:1079–86.
54. Sawhney R, Kochhar S, Gupta R, Jain R, Sood S. Traumatic optic nerve avulsion: role of ultrasonography. Eye Lond Engl. 2003;17:667–70.
55. Holmes MD, Sires BS. Flash visual evoked potentials predict visual outcome in traumatic optic neuropathy. Ophthal Plast Reconstr Surg. 2004;20:342–6.
56. Roberts SP, Schaumberg DA, Thompson P. Traumatic avulsion of the optic nerve. Optom Vis Sci Off Publ Am Acad Optom. 1992;69:721–7.
57. Hillman JS, Myska V, Nissim S. Complete avulsion of the optic nerve. A clinical, angiographic, and electrodiagnostic study. Br J Ophthalmol. 1975;59:503–9.
58. Entezari M, Rajavi Z, Sedighi N, Daftarian N, Sanagoo M. High-dose intravenous methylprednisolone in recent traumatic optic neuropathy; a randomized double-masked placebo-controlled clinical trial. Graefes Arch. Clin. Exp. Ophthalmol. Albrecht Von Graefes Arch. Für Klin. Exp. Ophthalmol. 2007; 245:1267–71.
59. Carta A, et al. Visual prognosis after indirect traumatic optic neuropathy. J Neurol Neurosurg Psychiatry. 2003;74:246–8.
60. Levin LA, Joseph MP, Rizzo JF, Lessell S. Optic canal decompression in indirect optic nerve trauma. Ophthalmology. 1994;101:566–9.
61. Alford MA, Nerad JA, Carter KD. Predictive value of the initial quantified relative afferent pupillary defect in 19 consecutive patients with traumatic

optic neuropathy. Ophthal Plast Reconstr Surg. 2001;17:323–7.
62. Cook MW, Levin LA, Joseph MP, Pinczower EF. Traumatic optic neuropathy. A meta-analysis. Arch Otolaryngol Head Neck Surg. 1996;122:389–92.
63. Zimmerer R, Rana M, Schumann P, Gellrich N-C. Diagnosis and treatment of optic nerve trauma. Facial Plast Surg FPS. 2014;30:518–27.
64. Feist RM, Kline LB, Morris RE, Witherspoon CD, Michelson MA. Recovery of vision after presumed direct optic nerve injury. Ophthalmology. 1987;94:1567–9.
65. Simsek T, et al. Traumatic optic nerve avulsion. J Pediatr Ophthalmol Strabismus. 2006;43:367–9.
66. Corrales G, Curreri A. Eye trauma in boxing. Clin. Sports Med. 2009; 28:591–607, vi.
67. Foster BS, March GA, Lucarelli MJ, Samiy N, Lessell S. Optic nerve avulsion. Arch Ophthalmol Chic Ill. 1997;1960(115):623–30.
68. Friedman SM. Optic nerve avulsion secondary to a basketball injury. Ophthalmic Surg Lasers. 1999;30:676–7.
69. Chong CCW, Chang AA. Traumatic optic nerve avulsion and central retinal artery occlusion following rugby injury. Clin Exp Ophthalmol. 2006;34:88–9.
70. Talwar D, Kumar A, Verma L, Tewari HK, Khosla PK. Ultrasonography in optic nerve head avulsion. Acta Ophthalmol (Copenh). 1991;69:121–3.
71. Parver LM, et al. Characteristics and causes of penetrating eye injuries reported to the national eye Trauma system registry, 1985-91. Public Health Rep Wash DC. 1993;1974(108):625–32.
72. Luo P, Fei Z. Twisted steel-induced penetrating head injury. Neurology. 2015;84:1909.
73. Mauriello JA, DeLuca J, Krieger A, Schulder M, Frohman L. Management of traumatic optic neuropathy–a study of 23 patients. Br J Ophthalmol. 1992;76:349–52.
74. Muthukumar N. Traumatic haemorrhagic optic neuropathy: case report. Br J Neurosurg. 1997;11:166–7.
75. Stonecipher KG, Conway MD, Karcioglu ZA, Haik BG. Hematoma of the optic nerve sheath after penetrating trauma. South Med J. 1990;83:1230–1.
76. Crowe NW, Nickles TP, Troost BT, Elster AD. Intrachiasmal hemorrhage: a cause of delayed post-traumatic blindness. Neurology. 1989;39:863–5.
77. Guy J, Sherwood M, Day AL. Surgical treatment of progressive visual loss in traumatic optic neuropathy. Report of two cases. J Neurosurg. 1989;70:799–801.
78. Jordan DR, White GL, Anderson RL, Thiese SM. Orbital emphysema: a potentially blinding complication following orbital fractures. Ann Emerg Med. 1988;17:853–5.
79. Skorek A, et al. Posttraumatic orbital emphysema: a numerical model. J Ophthalmol. 2014;2014: 231436.
80. Satyarthee GD, Sharma BS. Posttraumatic orbital emphysema in a 7-year-old girl associated with bilateral raccoon eyes: revisit of rare clinical emergency, with potential for rapid visual deterioration. J Pediatr Neurosci. 2015;10:166–8.
81. Sun MT, Chan WO, Selva D. Traumatic orbital compartment syndrome: importance of the lateral canthomy and cantholysis. Emerg Med Australas EMA. 2014;26:274–8.
82. Carrim ZI, Anderson IWR, Kyle PM. Traumatic orbital compartment syndrome: importance of prompt recognition and management. Eur J Emerg Med Off J Eur Soc Emerg Med. 2007;14:174–6.
83. Wu M, Yip JLY, Kuper H. Rapid assessment of avoidable blindness in Kunming, china. Ophthalmology. 2008;115:969–74.
84. Wolin MJ, Lavin PJ. Spontaneous visual recovery from traumatic optic neuropathy after blunt head injury. Am J Ophthalmol. 1990;109:430–5.
85. Bracken MB, et al. A randomized, controlled trial of methylprednisolone or naloxone in the treatment of acute spinal-cord injury. Results of the second national acute spinal cord injury study. N Engl J Med. 1990;322:1405–11.
86. Bracken MB, et al. Administration of methylprednisolone for 24 or 48 hours or tirilazad mesylate for 48 hours in the treatment of acute spinal cord injury. Results of the third national acute spinal cord injury randomized controlled trial. National acute spinal cord injury study. JAMA. 1997;277:1597–604.
87. Roberts I, et al. Effect of intravenous corticosteroids on death within 14 days in 10008 adults with clinically significant head injury (MRC CRASH trial): randomised placebo-controlled trial. Lancet Lond Engl. 2004;364:1321–8.
88. Edwards P, et al. Final results of MRC CRASH, a randomised placebo-controlled trial of intravenous corticosteroid in adults with head injury-outcomes at 6 months. Lancet Lond Engl. 2005;365:1957–9.
89. Steinsapir KD, Goldberg RA, Sinha S, Hovda DA. Methylprednisolone exacerbates axonal loss following optic nerve trauma in rats. Restor Neurol Neurosci. 2000;17:157–63.
90. Goldberg RA, Steinsapir KD. Extracranial optic canal decompression: indications and technique. Ophthal Plast Reconstr Surg. 1996;12:163–70.
91. Maurer J, Hinni M, Mann W, Pfeiffer N. Optic nerve decompression in trauma and tumor patients. Eur Arch Oto-Rhino-Laryngol Off J Eur Fed Oto-Rhino-Laryngol Soc EUFOS Affil Ger Soc Oto-Rhino-Laryngol-Head Neck Surg. 1999;256:341–5.
92. Chou PI, et al. Clinical experiences in the management of traumatic optic neuropathy. Neuro-Ophthalmol. 1996;16:325–36.
93. Walsh FB. Pathological-clinical correlations. I. Indirect trauma to the optic nerves and chiasm. II. Certain cerebral involvements associated with defective blood supply. Invest. Ophthalmol. 1966; 5:433–9.

94. Kuppersmith RB, et al. Combined transconjunctival/intranasal endoscopic approach to the optic canal in traumatic optic neuropathy. Laryngoscope. 1997;107:311–5.
95. Hughes B. Indirect injury of the optic nerves and chiasma. Bull Johns Hopkins Hosp. 1962;111:98–126.
96. Li H, et al. Treatment of traumatic optic neuropathy: our experience of endoscopic optic nerve decompression. J Laryngol Otol. 2008;122:1325–9.
97. Guyer DR, Miller NR, Long DM, Allen GS. Visual function following optic canal decompression via craniotomy. J Neurosurg. 1985;62:631–8.
98. Chen C-T, et al. Endoscopically assisted transconjunctival decompression of traumatic optic neuropathy. J. Craniofac. Surg. 2007; 18:19-26-28.
99. Girard BC, Bouzas EA, Lamas G, Soudant J. Visual improvement after transethmoid-sphenoid decompression in optic nerve injuries. J Clin Neuroophthalmol. 1992;12:142–8.
100. Nayak SR, Kirtane MV, Ingle MV. Transethmoid decompression of the optic nerve in head injuries: an update. J Laryngol Otol. 1991;105:205–6.
101. Knox BE, Gates GA, Berry SM. Optic nerve decompression via the lateral facial approach. Laryngoscope. 1990;100:458–62.
102. Kong D-S, et al. Endoscopic optic canal decompression for compressive optic neuropathy. J Clin Neurosci Off J Neurosurg Soc Australas. 2011;18:1541–5.
103. Horiguchi K, et al. Endoscopic endonasal trans-sphenoidal optic nerve decompression for traumatic optic neuropathy–technical note. Neurol Med Chir (Tokyo). 2010;50:518–22.
104. Wang D, Zheng C, Qian J, Barr JJ, Anderson AG. Endoscopic optic nerve decompression for the treatment of traumatic optic nerve neuropathy. ORL J Oto-Rhino-Laryngol Its Relat Spec. 2008;70:130–3.
105. Onofrey CB, et al. Optic canal decompression: a cadaveric study of the effects of surgery. Ophthal Plast Reconstr Surg. 2007;23:261–6.
106. WoldeMussie E, Yoles E, Schwartz M, Ruiz G, Wheeler LA. Neuroprotective effect of memantine in different retinal injury models in rats. J Glaucoma. 2002;11:474–80.
107. Sapieha PS, Peltier M, Rendahl KG, Manning WC, Di Polo A. Fibroblast growth factor-2 gene delivery stimulates axon growth by adult retinal ganglion cells after acute optic nerve injury. Mol Cell Neurosci. 2003;24:656–72.
108. Chen H, Weber AJ. BDNF enhances retinal ganglion cell survival in cats with optic nerve damage. Invest Ophthalmol Vis Sci. 2001;42:966–74.
109. Di Polo A, Aigner LJ, Dunn RJ, Bray GM, Aguayo AJ. Prolonged delivery of brain-derived neurotrophic factor by adenovirus-infected Müller cells temporarily rescues injured retinal ganglion cells. Proc Natl Acad Sci USA. 1998;95:3978–83.
110. Als CNTF. Treatment Study Group. A double-blind placebo-controlled clinical trial of subcutaneous recombinant human ciliary neurotrophic factor (rHCNTF) in amyotrophic lateral sclerosis. Neurology. 1996;46:1244–9.
111. Müller A, Hauk TG, Fischer D. Astrocyte-derived CNTF switches mature RGCs to a regenerative state following inflammatory stimulation. Brain J Neurol. 2007;130:3308–20.
112. Fischer D, Hauk TG, Müller A, Thanos S. Crystallins of the beta/gamma-superfamily mimic the effects of lens injury and promote axon regeneration. Mol Cell Neurosci. 2008;37:471–9.
113. Lam TT, Tso MO. Nitric oxide synthase (NOS) inhibitors ameliorate retinal damage induced by ischemia in rats. Res Commun Mol Pathol Pharmacol. 1996;92:329–40.
114. Tezel G, Yang X, Yang J, Wax MB. Role of tumor necrosis factor receptor-1 in the death of retinal ganglion cells following optic nerve crush injury in mice. Brain Res. 2004;996:202–12.
115. Karim Z, Sawada A, Kawakami H, Yamamoto T, Taniguchi T. A new calcium channel antagonist, lomerizine, alleviates secondary retinal ganglion cell death after optic nerve injury in the rat. Curr Eye Res. 2006;31:273–83.
116. Sarikcioglu L, Demir N, Akar Y, Demirtop A. Effect of intrathecal FK506 administration on intraorbital optic nerve crush: an ultrastructural study. Can J Ophthalmol J Can Ophtalmol. 2009;44:427–30.
117. King CE, et al. Erythropoietin is both neuroprotective and neuroregenerative following optic nerve transection. Exp Neurol. 2007;205:48–55.
118. Kardon RH, Corbett JJ, Thompson HS. Segmental denervation and reinnervation of the iris sphincter as shown by infrared videographic transillumination. Ophthalmology. 1998;105:313–21.
119. Osama H, Ababneh AAK. Classic triad of ross syndrome with diffuse autonomic dysfunction and positive antinuclear antibody titre. Neuro-Ophthalmol. 2012; 36.
120. Thompson HS. Adie's syndrome: some new observations. Trans Am Ophthalmol Soc. 1977;75:587–626.
121. Felten D, Shetty A. Netter's Atlas Of Neuroscience. Saunders; 2010.
122. Stead RE, Dineen RA, Dua HS, Mathew MRK. Multidetector computed tomographic angiography in horner syndrome. Neuro-Ophthalmol. 2009;33:62–4.
123. Borgman CJ. Horner syndrome secondary to internal carotid artery dissection after a short-distance endurance run: a case study and review. J Optom. 2012;5:209–16.
124. Ventura RE, Balcer LJ, Galetta SL. The neuro-ophthalmology of head trauma. Lancet Neurol. 2014;13:1006–16.
125. Lin Y-C, Chuang M-T, Hsu C-H, Tailor A-RA, Lee J-S. First rib fracture resulting in Horner's syndrome. J Emerg Med. 2015;49:868–70.

126. Meng K, Tian W, Lv Z, Song X. Horner's syndrome subsequent to minimally invasive video-assisted thyroidectomy in two patients. Oncol Lett. 2015;10:459–62.
127. Smith SJ, Diehl N, Leavitt JA, Mohney BG. Incidence of pediatric Horner syndrome and the risk of neuroblastoma: a population-based study. Arch Ophthalmol Chic Ill. 2010;1960(128):324–9.
128. Lazar I, Cavari Y, Rosenberg E, Knyazer B. Horner's syndrome in patients admitted to the paediatric intensive care unit: epidemiology, diagnosis and clinical practice. Anaesth Intensive Care. 2013;41:20–3.
129. Weichel ED, Colyer MH, Ludlow SE, Bower KS, Eiseman AS. Combat ocular trauma visual outcomes during operations iraqi and enduring freedom. Ophthalmology. 2008;115:2235–45.
130. de Silva WDD, de Soysa MSM, Perera BL. Iatrogenic Horner's syndrome: a rare complication of thyroid surgery. Ceylon Med J. 2010;55:136.
131. Bayhan Gİ, Karaca M, Yazici Ü, Tanir GA. Case of Horner's syndrome after the surgical treatment of pulmonary hydatid cyst. Türkiye Parazitolojii Derg. Türkiye Parazitoloji Derneği Acta Parasitol. Turc. Turk. Soc. Parasitol. (2010); 34:196–9.
132. The CADISS trial investigators. Antiplatelet treatment compared with anticoagulation treatment for cervical artery dissection (CADISS): a randomised trial. Lancet Neurol. 2015;14:361–7.
133. Baugnon KL, Hudgins PA. Skull base fractures and their complications. Neuroimaging Clin. N. Am. 2014; 24: 439–65, vii–viii.
134. Karasu A, et al. Traumatic epidural hematomas of the posterior cranial fossa. Surg. Neurol. 2008; 69:247-51-52.
135. Odebode TO, Ademola-Popoola DS, Ojo TA, Ayanniyi AA. Ocular and visual complications of head injury. Eye Lond Engl. 2005;19:561–6.
136. Lin DT, Lin AC. Surgical treatment of traumatic injuries of the cranial base. Otolaryngol Clin North Am. 2013;46:749–57.
137. Samii M, Tatagiba M. Skull base trauma: diagnosis and management. Neurol Res. 2002;24:147–56.
138. Stephens JR, Holmes S, Evans BT. Applied anatomy of the anterior cranial fossa: what can fracture patterns tell us? Int J Oral Maxillofac Surg. 2016;45:275–8.
139. Piek J. Surgical treatment of complex traumatic frontobasal lesions: personal experience in 74 patients. Neurosurg Focus. 2000;9:e2.
140. Yilmazlar S, et al. Cerebrospinal fluid leakage complicating skull base fractures: analysis of 81 cases. Neurosurg Rev. 2006;29:64–71.
141. Kienstra MA, Van Loveren H. Anterior skull base fractures. Facial Plast Surg FPS. 2005;21:180–6.
142. Schuknecht B, Graetz K. Radiologic assessment of maxillofacial, mandibular, and skull base trauma. Eur Radiol. 2005;15:560–8.
143. Schlosser RJ, Bolger WE. Nasal cerebrospinal fluid leaks: critical review and surgical considerations. Laryngoscope. 2004;114:255–65.
144. Bumm K, Heupel J, Bozzato A, Iro H, Hornung J. Localization and infliction pattern of iatrogenic skull base defects following endoscopic sinus surgery at a teaching hospital. Auris Nasus Larynx. 2009;36:671–6.
145. Lloyd KM, DelGaudio JM, Hudgins PA. Imaging of skull base cerebrospinal fluid leaks in adults. Radiology. 2008;248:725–36.
146. Savva A, Taylor MJ, Beatty CW. Management of cerebrospinal fluid leaks involving the temporal bone: report on 92 patients. Laryngoscope. 2003;113:50–6.
147. Manson PN, et al. Frontobasal fractures: anatomical classification and clinical significance. Plast Reconstr Surg. 2009;124:2096–106.
148. Arjun S, Joshi MD. Skull base anatomy: overview. Middle, Skull Base: Anterior Skull Base; 2015.
149. Ziu M, Savage JG, Jimenez DF. Diagnosis and treatment of cerebrospinal fluid rhinorrhea following accidental traumatic anterior skull base fractures. Neurosurg Focus. 2012;32:E3.
150. Schievink WI. Spontaneous spinal cerebrospinal fluid leaks and intracranial hypotension. JAMA. 2006;295:2286–96.
151. Mohindra S, Sharma M, Mohindra S. Traumatic chiasmal syndrome. Br J Neurosurg. 2012;26:872–4.
152. Heinz GW, Nunery WR, Grossman CB. Traumatic chiasmal syndrome associated with midline basilar skull fractures. Am J Ophthalmol. 1994;117:90–6.
153. Sharma R, Goyal M, Sharma A, Dada VK, Berry M. Traumatic transection of the optic chiasm: magnetic resonance evaluation. Australas Radiol. 1998;42:80–2.
154. Hassan A, Lanzino G, Wijdicks EFM, Rabinstein AA, Flemming KD. Terson's syndrome. Neurocrit Care. 2011;15:554–8.
155. Worthington JP, Snape L. Horner's syndrome secondary to a basilar skull fracture after maxillofacial trauma. J Oral Maxillofac Surg Off J Am Assoc Oral Maxillofac Surg. 1998;56:996–1000.
156. Fattahi TT, Brandt MT, Jenkins WS, Steinberg B. Traumatic carotid-cavernous fistula: pathophysiology and treatment. J Craniofac Surg. 2003;14:240–6.
157. York G, Barboriak D, Petrella J, DeLong D, Provenzale JM. Association of internal carotid artery injury with carotid canal fractures in patients with head trauma. AJR Am J Roentgenol. 2005;184:1672–8.
158. Antoniades K, Karakasis D, Taskos N. Abducent nerve palsy following transverse fracture of the middle cranial fossa. J Cranio-Maxillo-fac Surg Off Publ Eur Assoc Cranio-Maxillo-fac Surg. 1993;21:172–5.
159. Lehn AC, Lettieri J, Grimley R. A case of bilateral lower cranial nerve palsies after base of skull

trauma with complex management issues: case report and review of the literature. Neurol. 2012;18:152–4.
160. Winkler-Schwartz A, Correa JA, Marcoux J. Clival fractures in a level I trauma center. J Neurosurg. 2015;122:227–35.
161. Connor SEJ, Flis C. The contribution of high-resolution multiplanar reformats of the skull base to the detection of skull-base fractures. Clin Radiol. 2005;60:878–85.
162. Stone JA, Castillo M, Neelon B, Mukherji SK. Evaluation of CSF leaks: high-resolution CT compared with contrast-enhanced CT and radionuclide cisternography. AJNR Am J Neuroradiol. 1999;20:706–12.
163. Warnecke A, et al. Diagnostic relevance of beta2-transferrin for the detection of cerebrospinal fluid fistulas. Arch Otolaryngol Head Neck Surg. 2004;130:1178–84.
164. Bell RB, Dierks EJ, Homer L, Potter BE. Management of cerebrospinal fluid leak associated with craniomaxillofacial trauma. J Oral Maxillofac Surg Off J Am Assoc Oral Maxillofac Surg. 2004;62:676–84.
165. Rocchi G, et al. Severe craniofacial fractures with frontobasal involvement and cerebrospinal fluid fistula: indications for surgical repair. Surg. Neurol. 2005; 63:559-563-564.
166. Ratilal BO, Costa J, Pappamikail L, Sampaio C. Antibiotic prophylaxis for preventing meningitis in patients with basilar skull fractures. Cochrane Database Syst. Rev.2015; 4 CD004884.
167. Sakas DE, et al. Compound anterior cranial base fractures: classification using computerized tomography scanning as a basis for selection of patients for dural repair. J Neurosurg. 1998;88:471–7.
168. Nolte J. Nolte's the human brain: an introduction to its functional anatomy. Mosby Elsevier; 2009.
169. Santos G, Lima T, Pereira S, Machado E. Traumatic middle cerebral artery aneurysm secondary to a gunshot wound. J Neuroimaging Off J Am Soc Neuroimaging 2013; 23:115–7.
170. Buckingham MJ, et al. Traumatic intracranial aneurysms in childhood: two cases and a review of the literature. Neurosurgery. 1988;22:398–408.
171. Wewel J, Mangubat EZ, Muñoz L. Iatrogenic traumatic intracranial aneurysm after endoscopic sinus surgery. J Clin Neurosci Off J Neurosurg Soc Australas. 2014;21:2072–6.
172. Larson PS, Reisner A, Morassutti DJ, Abdulhadi B, Harpring JE. Traumatic intracranial aneurysms. Neurosurg Focus. 2000;8:e4.
173. Kieck CF, de Villiers JC. Vascular lesions due to transcranial stab wounds. J Neurosurg. 1984;60:42–6.
174. Zangbar B, et al. Traumatic intracranial aneurysm in blunt trauma. Brain Inj. 2015;29:601–6.
175. Zhang C, Chen H, Bai R. Traumatic aneurysm on the posterior cerebral artery following blunt trauma in a 14-year-old girl: case report. Neuropediatrics. 2011;42:204–6.
176. Horowitz MB, et al. Multidisciplinary approach to traumatic intracranial aneurysms secondary to shotgun and handgun wounds. Surg Neurol. 1999; 51:31-41-42.
177. Pülhorn H, Chandran A, Nahser H, McMahon C. Case report: traumatic carotid-cavernous fistula. J Trauma Nurs Off J Soc Trauma Nurses. 2016; 23:42–4.
178. Schütz P, Bosnjakovic P, Abulhasan YB, Al-Sheikh T. Traumatic carotid-cavernous fistula in a multiple facial fractures patient: case report and literature review. Dent Traumatol Off Publ Int Assoc Dent Traumatol. 2014;30:488–92.
179. Barrow DL, et al. Classification and treatment of spontaneous carotid-cavernous sinus fistulas. J Neurosurg. 1985;62:248–56.
180. Gallucci GM. Carotid-cavernous sinus fistula: a case study. J Neurosci Nurs J Am Assoc Neurosci. Nurses. 2005; 37:200–2, 210.
181. Corradino G, Gellad FE, Salcman M. Traumatic carotid-cavernous fistula. South Med J. 1988;81:660–3.
182. Ellis JA, Goldstein H, Connolly ES, Meyers PM. Carotid-cavernous fistulas. Neurosurg Focus. 2012;32:E9.
183. Chaudhry IA, Elkhamry SM, Al-Rashed W, Bosley TM. Carotid cavernous fistula: ophthalmological implications. Middle East Afr J Ophthalmol. 2009;16:57–63.
184. Liu Y-C, et al. The recovery time of traumatic carotid-cavernous fistula-induced oculomotor nerve paresis after endovascular treatment with detachable balloons. J Neuroradiol J Neuroradiol. 2014;41:329–35.
185. Wang W-H, et al. Early diagnosis and management of cerebral venous flow obstruction secondary to transsinus fracture after traumatic brain injury. J Clin Neurol Seoul Korea. 2013;9:259–68.
186. Li J, Wei L, Xu B, Zhang X, Wang S. Risk factors and early diagnosis of cerebral venous sinus occlusion secondary to traumatic brain injury. Neurol India. 2015;63:881–8.
187. Connor SEJ, Jarosz JM. Magnetic resonance imaging of cerebral venous sinus thrombosis. Clin Radiol. 2002;57:449–61.
188. van Gijn J. Cerebral venous thrombosis: pathogenesis, presentation and prognosis. J R Soc Med. 2000;93:230–3.
189. Kuehnen J, Schwartz A, Neff W, Hennerici M. Cranial nerve syndrome in thrombosis of the transverse/sigmoid sinuses. Brain J Neurol. 1998;121(Pt 2):381–8.
190. Bousser MG, Chiras J, Bories J, Castaigne P. Cerebral venous thrombosis–a review of 38 cases. Stroke J Cereb Circ. 1985;16:199–213.
191. Freeman WD, Aguilar MI. Intracranial hemorrhage: diagnosis and management. Neurol Clin. 2012; 30:211–40, ix.
192. Parchani A, et al. Traumatic subarachnoid hemorrhage due to motor vehicle crash versus fall from

height: a 4-year epidemiologic study. World Neurosurg. 2014;82:e639–44.
193. Choi JH, et al. Multimodal early rehabilitation and predictors of outcome in survivors of severe traumatic brain injury. J Trauma. 2008;65:1028–35.
194. Servadei F, et al. Traumatic subarachnoid hemorrhage: demographic and clinical study of 750 patients from the European brain injury consortium survey of head injuries. Neurosurgery 2002; 50:261-67-69.
195. Greene KA, et al. Impact of traumatic subarachnoid hemorrhage on outcome in nonpenetrating head injury. Part I: a proposed computerized tomography grading scale. J Neurosurg. 1995;83:445–52.
196. Eisenberg HM, et al. Initial CT findings in 753 patients with severe head injury. A report from the NIH Traumatic Coma Data Bank. J Neurosurg. 1990;73:688–98.
197. Mattioli C, et al. Traumatic subarachnoid hemorrhage on the computerized tomography scan obtained at admission: a multicenter assessment of the accuracy of diagnosis and the potential impact on patient outcome. J Neurosurg. 2003;98:37–42.
198. A multicenter trial of the efficacy of nimodipine on outcome after severe head injury. The European study group on nimodipine in severe head injury. J. Neurosurg. 1994; 80:797–804.
199. Compagnone C, et al. Patients with moderate head injury: a prospective multicenter study of 315 patients. Neurosurgery 2009; 64:690-96-97.
200. Murray GD, et al. The European brain injury consortium survey of head injuries. Acta Neurochir (Wien). 1999;141:223–36.
201. Kakarieka A, Braakman R, Schakel EH. Clinical significance of the finding of subarachnoid blood on CT scan after head injury. Acta Neurochir (Wien). 1994;129:1–5.
202. Moynihan G, Robinson K. Terson's syndrome: subarachnoid haemorrhage presenting as sudden visual loss. Emerg Med Australas EMA. 2012;24:454–6.
203. Armin SS, Colohan ART, Zhang JH. Traumatic subarachnoid hemorrhage: our current understanding and its evolution over the past half century. Neurol Res. 2006;28:445–52.
204. Garfinkle AM, Danys IR, Nicolle DA, Colohan AR, Brem S. Terson's syndrome: a reversible cause of blindness following subarachnoid hemorrhage. J Neurosurg. 1992;76:766–71.
205. Medele RJ, Stummer W, Mueller AJ, Steiger HJ, Reulen HJ. Terson's syndrome in subarachnoid hemorrhage and severe brain injury accompanied by acutely raised intracranial pressure. J Neurosurg. 1998;88:851–4.
206. Stienen MN, Lücke S, Gautschi OP, Harders A. Terson haemorrhage in patients suffering aneurysmal subarachnoid haemorrhage: a prospective analysis of 60 consecutive patients. Clin Neurol Neurosurg. 2012;114:535–8.
207. Czorlich P, et al. Terson syndrome in subarachnoid hemorrhage, intracerebral hemorrhage, and traumatic brain injury. Neurosurg Rev. 2015; 38: 129–36; discussion 136.
208. Lee S-H, Seo J-H, Park S-H, Won YH, Ko M-H. Terson syndrome in aneurysmal subarachnoid hemorrhage: a case report. Ann Rehabil Med. 2015;39:640–4.
209. Kuhn F, Morris R, Witherspoon CD, Mester V. Terson syndrome. Results of vitrectomy and the significance of vitreous hemorrhage in patients with subarachnoid hemorrhage. Ophthalmology. 1998;105:472–7.
210. Srinivasan S, Kyle G. Subinternal limiting membrane and subhyaloid haemorrhage in Terson syndrome: the macular 'double ring' sign. Eye Lond Engl. 2006;20:1099–101.
211. Boesiger BM, Shiber JR. Subarachnoid hemorrhage diagnosis by computed tomography and lumbar puncture: are fifth generation CT scanners better at identifying subarachnoid hemorrhage? J Emerg Med. 2005;29:23–7.
212. Ropper AH, Davis KR. Lobar cerebral hemorrhages: acute clinical syndromes in 26 cases. Ann Neurol. 1980;8:141–7.
213. Dirim BV, Orük C, Erdoğan N, Gelal F, Uluç E. Traumatic posterior fossa hematomas. Diagn Interv Radiol Ank Turk. 2005;11:14–8.
214. Araujo JLV, Aguiar Udo P, Todeschini AB, Saade N, Veiga JCE. Epidemiological analysis of 210 cases of surgically treated traumatic extradural hematoma. Rev Colégio Bras Cir. 2012; 39:268–71.
215. Bor-Seng-Shu E, et al. Epidural hematomas of the posterior cranial fossa. Neurosurg Focus 2004; 16 ECP1.
216. Takeuchi S, et al. Traumatic posterior fossa subdural hematomas. J Trauma Acute Care Surg. 2012;72:480–6.
217. D'Amato L, et al. Prognosis of isolated acute post-traumatic subdural haematoma. J Neurosurg Sci. 2007;51:107–11.
218. Tallon JM, Ackroyd-Stolarz S, Karim SA, Clarke DB. The epidemiology of surgically treated acute subdural and epidural hematomas in patients with head injuries: a population-based study. Can J Surg J Can Chir. 2008;51:339–45.
219. Leitgeb J, et al. Outcome after severe brain trauma due to acute subdural hematoma. J Neurosurg. 2012;117:324–33.
220. Koç RK, Akdemir H, Oktem IS, Meral M, Menkü A. Acute subdural hematoma: outcome and outcome prediction. Neurosurg Rev. 1997;20:239–44.
221. Bullock MR, et al. Surgical management of acute epidural hematomas. Neurosurgery 2006; 58:S7–15; discussion Si–iv.
222. Bullock MR, et al. Surgical management of acute subdural hematomas. Neurosurgery 2006; 58:S16–24; discussion Si–iv.

223. Haselsberger K, Pucher R, Auer LM. Prognosis after acute subdural or epidural haemorrhage. Acta Neurochir (Wien). 1988;90:111–6.
224. Seelig JM, et al. Traumatic acute subdural hematoma: major mortality reduction in comatose patients treated within four hours. N Engl J Med. 1981;304:1511–8.
225. Wilberger JE, Harris M, Diamond DL. Acute subdural hematoma: morbidity, mortality, and operative timing. J Neurosurg. 1991;74:212–8.
226. Tien HCN, et al. Reducing time-to-treatment decreases mortality of trauma patients with acute subdural hematoma. Ann Surg. 2011;253:1178–83.
227. Cohen JE, Montero A, Israel ZH. Prognosis and clinical relevance of anisocoria-craniotomy latency for epidural hematoma in comatose patients. J Trauma. 1996;41:120–2.
228. Poon WS, Li AK. Comparison of management outcome of primary and secondary referred patients with traumatic extradural haematoma in a neurosurgical unit. Injury. 1991;22:323–5.
229. Karibe H, et al. Surgical management of traumatic acute subdural hematoma in adults: a review. Neurol Med Chir (Tokyo). 2014;54:887–94.
230. Zacharia BE, et al. Predictors of long-term shunt-dependent hydrocephalus in patients with intracerebral hemorrhage requiring emergency cerebrospinal fluid diversion. Neurosurg Focus. 2012;32:E5.
231. Faul 2010. Traumatic brain injury in the United States—Emergency Department Visits, hospitalizations and deaths 2002–2006. Available at http://www.cdc.gov/traumaticbraininjury/pdf/blue_book.pdf. Accessed 9th Mar 2016.
232. Capó-Aponte JE, Urosevich TG, Temme LA, Tarbett AK, Sanghera NK. Visual dysfunctions and symptoms during the subacute stage of blast-induced mild traumatic brain injury. Mil Med. 2012;177:804–13.
233. Ryan LM, Warden DL. Post concussion syndrome. Int Rev Psychiatry Abingdon Engl. 2003;15:310–6.
234. Kraus JF, Hsu P, Schafer K, Afifi AA. Sustained outcomes following mild traumatic brain injury: results of a five-emergency department longitudinal study. Brain Inj. 2014;28:1248–56.
235. Dawodu ST. Traumatic brain injury (TBI)—Definition and pathophysiology: overview, epidemiology, primary injury. 2015.
236. Currie S, et al. Imaging assessment of traumatic brain injury. Postgrad Med J. 2016;92:41–50.
237. Perunovic B, Quilty RD, Athanasiou A, Love S. Damage to intracranial optic pathways in fatal closed head injury in man. J Neurol Sci. 2001;185:55–62.
238. Hammoud DA, Wasserman BA. Diffuse axonal injuries: pathophysiology and imaging. Neuroimaging Clin N Am. 2002;12:205–16.
239. Meythaler JM, Peduzzi JD, Eleftheriou E, Novack TA. Current concepts: diffuse axonal injury-associated traumatic brain injury. Arch Phys Med Rehabil. 2001;82:1461–71.
240. Adams ME, Linn J, Yousry I. Pathology of the ocular motor nerves III, IV, and VI. Neuroimaging Clin N Am. 2008; 18:261–82, preceding x–x.
241. Bazarian JJ, Blyth B, Cimpello L. Bench to bedside: evidence for brain injury after concussion–looking beyond the computed tomography scan. Acad Emerg Med Off J Soc Acad Emerg Med. 2006;13:199–214.
242. Li X-Y, Feng D-F. Diffuse axonal injury: novel insights into detection and treatment. J Clin Neurosci Off J Neurosurg Soc Australas. 2009;16:614–9.
243. Mittenberg W, Canyock EM, Condit D, Patton C. Treatment of post-concussion syndrome following mild head injury. J Clin Exp Neuropsychol. 2001;23:829–36.
244. Gentry LR, Godersky JC, Thompson B, Dunn VD. Prospective comparative study of intermediate-field MR and CT in the evaluation of closed head trauma. AJR Am J Roentgenol. 1988;150:673–82.
245. Ogawa T, et al. Comparative study of magnetic resonance and CT scan imaging in cases of severe head injury. Acta Neurochir Suppl (Wien). 1992;55:8–10.
246. Mittl RL, et al. Prevalence of MR evidence of diffuse axonal injury in patients with mild head injury and normal head CT findings. AJNR Am J Neuroradiol. 1994;15:1583–9.
247. Takayama H, Kobayashi M, Sugishita M, Mihara B. Diffusion-weighted imaging demonstrates transient cytotoxic edema involving the corpus callosum in a patient with diffuse brain injury. Clin Neurol Neurosurg. 2000;102:135–9.
248. Hadley DM, et al. Magnetic resonance imaging in acute head injury. Clin Radiol. 1988;39:131–9.
249. Johnston KM, Ptito A, Chankowsky J, Chen JK. New frontiers in diagnostic imaging in concussive head injury. Clin J Sport Med Off J Can Acad Sport Med 2001; 11:166–75.
250. Akiyama Y, et al. Susceptibility-weighted magnetic resonance imaging for the detection of cerebral microhemorrhage in patients with traumatic brain injury. Neurol Med Chir (Tokyo) 2009; 49:97–9; discussion 99.
251. Goodrich GL, Flyg HM, Kirby JE, Chang C-Y, Martinsen GL. Mechanisms of TBI and visual consequences in military and veteran populations. Optom Vis Sci Off Publ Am Acad Optom. 2013;90:105–12.
252. Magone MT, Kwon E, Shin SY. Chronic visual dysfunction after blast-induced mild traumatic brain injury. J Rehabil Res Dev. 2014;51:71–80.
253. Truong JQ, Ciuffreda KJ, Han MHE, Suchoff IB. Photosensitivity in mild traumatic brain injury (mTBI): a retrospective analysis. Brain Inj. 2014;28:1283–7.
254. Katz BJ, Digre KB. Diagnosis, pathophysiology and treatment of photophobia. Surv Ophthalmol. 2016. doi:10.1016/j.survophthal.2016.02.001.
255. Lebensohn JE, Bellows J. The nature of photophobia. Arch Ophthalmol. 1934;12:380–90.

256. Heitger MH, et al. Motor deficits and recovery during the first year following mild closed head injury. Brain Inj. 2006;20:807–24.
257. Keane JR. Neurologic eye signs following motorcycle accidents. Arch Neurol. 1989;46:761–2.
258. Brahm KD, et al. Visual impairment and dysfunction in combat-injured servicemembers with traumatic brain injury. Optom Vis Sci Off Publ Am Acad Optom. 2009;86:817–25.
259. Alvarez TL, et al. Concurrent vision dysfunctions in convergence insufficiency with traumatic brain injury. Optom Vis Sci Off Publ Am Acad Optom. 2012;89:1740–51.
260. Linnau KF, Hallam DK, Lomoschitz FM, Mann FA. Orbital apex injury: trauma at the junction between the face and the cranium. Eur J Radiol. 2003;48:5–16.
261. Dhaliwal A, West AL, Trobe JD, Musch DC. Third, fourth, and sixth cranial nerve palsies following closed head injury. J Neuro-Ophthalmol Off J North Am Neuro-Ophthalmol Soc. 2006; 26:4–10.
262. Ferreira T, Verbist B, van Buchem M, van Osch T, Webb A. Imaging the ocular motor nerves. Eur J Radiol. 2010;74:314–22.
263. Kim E, Chang H. Isolated oculomotor nerve palsy following minor head trauma: case illustration and literature review. J Korean Neurosurg Soc. 2013;54:434–6.
264. Varnamkhasti M, Thomas A. Brain and facial trauma: a neuroradiology perspective. Trauma. 2011;13:317–33.
265. Clusmann H, Schaller C, Schramm J. Fixed and dilated pupils after trauma, stroke, and previous intracranial surgery: management and outcome. J Neurol Neurosurg Psychiatry. 2001;71:175–81.
266. Keane JR. Third nerve palsy: analysis of 1400 personally-examined inpatients. Can J Neurol Sci J Can Sci Neurol. 2010;37:662–70.
267. Young GB. Impaired consciousness and herniation syndromes. Neurol Clin. 2011;29:765–72.
268. ELKammash TH, Enaba MM, Awadalla AM. Variability in sphenoid sinus pneumatization and its impact upon reduction of complications following sellar region surgeries. Egyption J Radiol Nucl Med. 2014; 45:705–14.
269. Cappabianca P, et al. Endoscopic endonasal surgery for pituitary adenomas. World Neurosurg. 2014;82:S3–11.
270. Chin BM, Orlandi RR, Wiggins RH. Evaluation of the sellar and parasellar regions. Magn Reson Imaging Clin N Am. 2012;20:515–43.
271. Bai S, et al. Intraoperative high-field magnetic resonance imaging combined with functional neuronavigation in resection of low-grade temporal lobe tumors. World J Surg Oncol. 2015;13:286.
272. Kaspera W, Adamczyk P, Ślaska-Kaspera A, Ładziński P. Usefulness of intraoperative monitoring of oculomotor and abducens nerves during surgical treatment of the cavernous sinus meningiomas. Adv Med Sci. 2015;60:25–30.
273. Kung NH, Van Stavern GP. Isolated Ocular Motor Nerve Palsies. Semin Neurol. 2015;35:539–48.
274. Hanson RA, Ghosh S, Gonzalez-Gomez I, Levy ML, Gilles FH. Abducens length and vulnerability? Neurology. 2004;62:33–6.
275. Wong AMF, Colpa L, Chandrakumar M. Ability of an upright-supine test to differentiate skew deviation from other vertical strabismus causes. Arch Ophthalmol Chic Ill. 2011;1960(129):1570–5.
276. Kim M-S, Cho M-S, Kim S-H. Delayed bilateral abducens nerve palsy after head trauma. J Korean Neurosurg Soc. 2008;44:396–8.

13 Pediatric Ocular Trauma

Charles D. McCanna and James A. Deutsch

Introduction

Eye injuries in children can cause fear and trepidation even for the most experienced ophthalmologist or emergency room physician. There are several good reasons for this. Young children are much more difficult to examine than adults: they cry, they sometimes do not cooperate, or refuse to open their eyes. This makes performing a good exam much more difficult. Often, it is difficult to obtain a good history of the injury—communication is challenging in the very young, and even older children may not tell the truth about an injury in an attempt to avoid blame or punishment. Additionally, the consequences of an eye injury can be greater in children, as clear vision is required for normal ocular development—amblyopia can occur if visual impairment is not corrected in a timely manner.

Unfortunately, eye injuries in children are not rare; it is the leading cause of acquired monocular blindness in children [1]. Looked at another way, children represent between 29 and 35% of all ocular trauma cases [2, 3]. Children have increased vulnerability because they frequently indulge in high-risk behavior due to their lack of awareness of the possibility of harm. Additionally, children are at increased risk for non-accidental trauma, often inflicted by supposed caregivers. All physicians must be alert to the possibility of intentionally inflicted injuries.

Examination of Pediatric Patients

Examining an injured child is a daunting task. There are some common sense approaches that can help the examiner determine the extent of a child's eye injury.

A calm, soothing manner of speech can go a long way toward gaining the cooperation of a child. Ask the child for their help, and for their permission to examine the eye. Children are fearful of things being done to them, but are more willing to join in a cooperative venture with an authority figure like a doctor. Do not be afraid to use a local anesthetic such as proparacaine. Relieving pain in an eye often enables the child to open the eye, allowing the examiner access to view the injury. No harm will ensue from a topical anesthetic eyedrop, even in the setting of an open globe eye injury.

Use toys or other interesting objects to get the child to move the eye so the doctor can see the full extent of an injury. The child can be seated on the parent's lap. Even an older child will be calmed in the most comfortable of all seats with a parent.

C.D. McCanna · J.A. Deutsch (✉)
Department of Ophthalmology, The State University of New York (SUNY) Downstate Medical Center, 541 Clarkson Ave, E Bldg, 8th Fl, Suite C, Brooklyn, NY 11203, USA
e-mail: jadeutschmd@yahoo.com

C.D. McCanna
e-mail: charles.d.mccanna@gmail.com

C.D. McCanna · J.A. Deutsch
Kings County Hospital Center, Brooklyn, USA

S.C. Kaufman and D.R. Lazzaro (eds.), *Textbook of Ocular Trauma*,
DOI 10.1007/978-3-319-47633-9_13

Occasionally, a screaming, uncontrollable younger child may need to be restrained so that an exam can be done. Professionally built restraints like a papoose wrap can be used so that the eye can be seen. A majority of infants will not be able to be examined at a slit lamp and therefore penlight and portable slit lamp examinations may be necessary. An eyelid speculum can aid the exam, but one should be careful not to apply too much pressure to a potentially open eye.

In cases where severe ocular injury is suspected, an exam under general anesthesia may be necessary. While current literature suggests that early anesthetic exposure may have a link to injury to the developing brain, general anesthesia may be the only method to diagnose and treat a ruptured globe in a child [4]. Risks and benefits of exams under anesthesia should be thoroughly evaluated and discussed with the parents before proceeding.

Epidemiological Causation of Eye Injuries in Children

Armstrong et al. [5] analyzed pediatric eye injuries presenting to US emergency departments from 2001–2007 and found that males accounted for 62% of visits. The most common diagnosis was contusion/abrasion in 54% of the 1,048,500 visits. Being struck by or against an object was the most common cause of eye injury. Most ocular injuries occurred at home and during the spring and summer months.

In 2011, Acar et al. [6] developed a modified version of the Ocular Trauma Scale (OTS) called the Pediatric Ocular Trauma Scale (POTS). This rating system was created due to possible inflation of OTS scores in pediatric patients. Due to high probability of obtaining false initial visual acuity scores or inability to obtain visual acuity in children less than 15 years of age, the new scoring system placed less emphasis on these criteria. Relative afferent pupillary defect was also not included in scoring. Age and zone of injury surrounding the orbit were included in the POTS scoring system. The authors found that the score was strongly correlated with predictability of final visual acuity. It is currently debated whether OTS or POTS is superior in assessing the prognosis after pediatric open globe injury.

Approaches to Common Pediatric Ocular Injuries

Eyelid Lacerations

An essential understanding of eyelid anatomy and nearby structures is essential for eyelid laceration management in the pediatric patient. Examiners must obtain a detailed examination looking for often-misdiagnosed orbital trauma. Ruling out occult injuries, such as open globe injuries, should be the number one priority of the provider.

The examiner must be diligent during the examination to recognize involvement of the orbital septum and lid margin in addition to the lacrimal drainage system (Fig. 13.1). Dog bites, handlebar injuries, and sharp objects cause the majority of eyelid lacerations. In a retrospective record-based analysis, Hwang et al. found that a majority of facial lacerations in children over 10 years old involved the eyelid [7]. Adolescents acquire eyelid injuries more through blunt trauma. Animal bites should be cleaned superficially and surgically repaired if necessary. Prophylactic antibiotics should be given in these cases.

Violation of the orbital septum in laceration may often result in fat prolapse. In this instance, CT scan can be helpful in terms of identifying the extent of the pathology. If the eyelid margin is involved, an effective surgical repair requires good anatomical knowledge to reapproximate the lid margin.

The most common etiology of pediatric canalicular-involving lacerations is a dogbite injury [8]. As with most orbital trauma, boys are affected at higher rates than girls. Goals of laceration repair involving the tear drainage system are to prevent permanent tearing (epiphora) of the pediatric patient. These lacerations are diagnosed with probing and irrigation by an ophthalmologist. Silicone tubes are placed which help maintain patency of the drainage system.

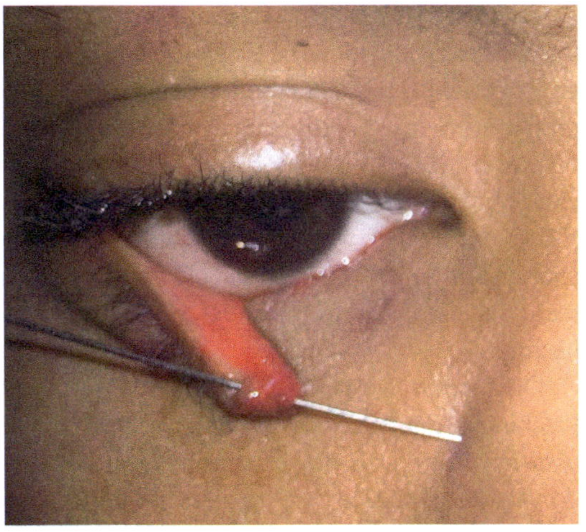

Fig. 13.1 Right lower canalicular-involving eyelid avulsion in a 16-year-old male

When approaching the laceration in pediatric patient, cooperation will likely be an issue. Monitored sedation in the emergency department (ED) or closure in the operating room may be necessary. Canalicular-involving lacerations have better outcomes when repaired in the operating room rather than a minor procedure room [8].

For further information regarding eyelid laceration management, please see Chapter involving the *Eyelids and The Lacrimal System*.

Many children will have favorable cosmetic and functional outcomes if lacerations are repaired in a timely and strategic manner.

Open Globe Injury

The management of an open globe injury in the pediatric patient is of utmost importance. Delay in taking these patients to the operative suite can result in significant visual sequelae. Open globe injury is a full thickness mechanical injury to the cornea and/or sclera. The injury can be classified as a rupture or a laceration of the globe. A laceration of the globe can be further subcategorized into penetrating or perforating injury.

In a 17-year review of open globe injury in the Canadian pediatric population, open globe injuries were three times as prevalent in males than females [9]. Around half of those included in the review were under the age of five.

An open globe injury should be suspected when low intraocular pressure, hemorrhagic chemosis, shallow anterior chamber, and peaked pupil are found during the ocular examination [10]. If an open globe injury is obvious, intraocular pressure measurements and dilation should be avoided.

Patients should be kept *nil per os* (NPO) or nothing by mouth prior to surgery. Treatment involves IV antibiotics and antiemetic agents intended to decrease the chance of expulsion of intraocular contents with increased intraocular pressure. A shield should be placed over a suspected open globe injury until the patient is brought to the operating suite. Timely surgical treatment of the affected structures in the anterior and posterior segments is essential. Closure of primary wounds along with repositioning of prolapsed ocular contents should be accomplished.

Pediatric open globe injuries can result in specific late complications from surgical repair (secondary glaucoma, secondary strabismus, leukoma cornea and phthisis bulbi) that can produce significant visual consequences [11]. Lee et al. [12] reviewed 62 patients with open globe injury under the age of 16 and found that best visual outcomes occurred in those with only corneal injury. Poor prognostic indicators in open globe injury included location of injury, extent of injury, initial presentation of hyphema, vitreous hemorrhage, retinal detachment, central corneal wound, and endophthalmitis [13]. Low visual acuity at initial presentation in addition to subsequent number of surgeries also carries a guarded visual prognosis [14]. Risks of endophthalmitis increased with delayed repair of these penetrating injuries, thus surgical repair in a timely manner is critical [15].

Corneal Abrasions

Corneal abrasions are the most common eye injury in children presenting to the emergency department [16]. A corneal abrasion is a corneal epithelial defect related to trauma. They are usually caused by blunt trauma to the eye, foreign body, or contact lens use. In a study of random newborn subjects from 1 to 12 weeks of age, corneal abrasions were present in 49% of patients [17].

Symptoms include increased tearing, foreign body sensation, sharp pain, and photophobia. Preverbal patients with corneal abrasion may have unexplained inconsolable crying. Rubbing the eye may also be a sign of abrasion in the pediatric patient.

In patients wearing contact lenses, lenses should be removed prior to examination. Following topical anesthesia of proparicaine, topical fluorescein should be applied to the eye. Using a Wood's lamp or Cobalt-blue light under the slit lamp, the epithelial defect will appear yellow-green (Fig. 13.2).

If vertical linear abrasions are observed, the examiner should be suspicious of retained foreign body in the superior palpebral conjunctiva. Eversion of the upper eyelid can be accomplished with aid of a cotton tip applicator, and a foreign body can be removed with a sterile cotton swab which has been soaked in proparicaine, a lens loop, a forceps, or a 30-gauge needle. Special care must be taken when using a needle.

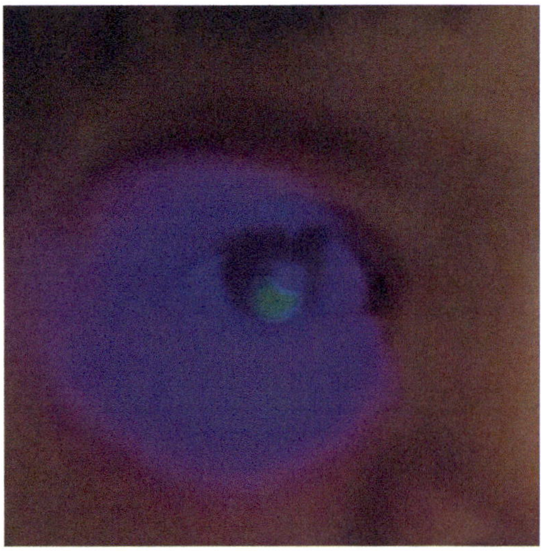

Fig. 13.2 Corneal abrasion with fluorescein staining in a 2-year-old female

Pharmacologic therapy in noncontact lens wearing pediatric patients can be erythromycin, bacitracin or polymyxin B/bacitracin, or topical antibiotic drops such as polymyxcin B/trimethoprim or ofloxacin [18]. Antipseudomonal coverage is necessary in contact lens wearers. These abrasions should be treated with a topical fluoroquinolone antibiotic. Topical steroids should be avoided in these patients due to potential delay in wound healing.

Oral acetaminophen can be used for pain relief. Patching is not necessary for a majority of corneal abrasions. However, for a larger corneal abrasion, do not be afraid to use a pressure patch. In a non-compliant child, a patch can prevent rubbing and promote healing. Evidence for NSAID use for treatment of pain from corneal abrasions is currently lacking. If topical NSAIDs are prescribed, patients should have close follow-up.

Secondary complications of corneal abrasion include corneal ulceration, secondary bacterial infection, corneal scarring, uveitis, and iritis. Recurrent corneal erosions can occur following the initial abrasion due to improper healing of the original epithelial defect.

Resolution often occurs with the above treatments within 1–5 days. Contact lens wearers and those with history of ocular herpes simplex should have particularly close follow-up.

Traumatic Hyphema and Traumatic Iridocyclitis

Blunt trauma to the eye can cause rupture of the vascular supply of the iris and ciliary body resulting in blood in the anterior chamber or a hyphema (see Fig. 13.3). Up to 70% of hyphemas occur in children [19]. Lasting effects of pediatric traumatic hyphema are serious and therefore proper diagnosis and management are of utmost importance in the pediatric patient. A careful examination and identification of associated orbital and ocular injuries is necessary. The most common ocular lesions associated with pediatric traumatic hyphema are corneal abrasions [20].

Patients often present with history of blunt trauma, vision loss, and eye pain. Anisocoria can be present due to a torn iris sphincter muscle in the traumatized eye. Hyphemas are classified by amount of blood in the anterior chamber. A grade I hyphema occurs when there is pooled, layered blood, occupying less than one-third of the anterior chamber; whereas an 8-ball hyphema, or total hyphema, is a grade IV hyphema. Plasmin activates the fibrinolytic system that will break down the clot and allow for filtration of the material through the trabecular meshwork. In a prospective case series of 35 children treated as outpatients for traumatic hyphema, Rocha et al. found that visual prognosis is correlated with the grade of hyphema and posterior segment involvement in the trauma. A microhyphema is defined as red blood cells in the anterior chamber of the eye without layering of blood.

Rebleeding, corneal blood staining, secondary glaucoma and ischemic optic neuropathy are all possible secondary complications of hyphema. Risk of rebleeding, or secondary hemorrhage is increased in the African-American pediatric population [21]. Those patients who are of African-American decent should have a sickle cell screen laboratory analysis at the time of presentation to help rule out sickle cell disease. Patients with sickle cell hemoglobinopathy, who present with hyphema, should be monitored very closely. Mechanical obstruction of the trabecular meshwork from sickled cells can result in increased intraocular pressure. Carbonic anhydrase inhibitors have been shown to increase sickling of cells. In a study of 40 children from the United States with hyphema, sickle cell hemoglobinopathy was associated with increased intraocular pressure but not rebleeding [21].

Treatments for hyphema are often debated, but the general consensus is that topical steroid and topical cycloplegics should be given. Children's dosing of acetaminophen can be given to patients for pain control. Strict bed rest should be encouraged. The head of the bed can be elevated to layer out the hyphema and precipitate clot absorption. Blood thinning agents should not be given. Evidence for use of antifibrinolytic agents including transexamic acid and aminocaproic acid for prevention of rebleeding in pediatric patients is currently lacking [22]. Children should be instructed to limit activity and wear eye shields, protecting them from further injury that may result in rebleed. Otherwise, rebleeding tends to occur posttrauma at day 4 or 5, when the clot contracts.

In hyphemas presenting without trauma, important underlying pathology should always be entertained. Non-accidental trauma should always be in the differential. Causes of spontaneous hyphema in the pediatric population include retinoblastoma, medulloepithelioma, juvenile xanthogranuloma, leukemia, melanoma, and other causes of rubiosis.

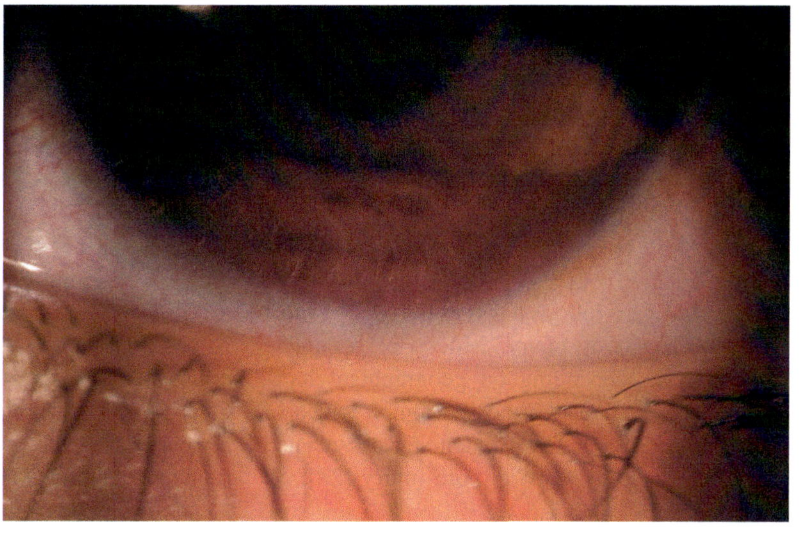

Fig. 13.3 Traumatic Hyphema from soccer ball injury in a 12-year-old male

With blunt trauma to the eye, damage to the iris and ciliary body can occur resulting in anterior chamber inflammation, termed traumatic iridocyclitis. Traumatic iritis accounts for 20% of all iritis [23]. Necrotic blood products released from damage of the structures result in inflammation in the anterior chamber. Traumatic iridocyclitis can present with eye pain, redness, photophobia, and frequently miosis. Conjunctiva may also be injected. Diagnosis is made on slit lamp biomicroscopy with white blood cells present in the anterior chamber of the eye. Inflammatory mediators cause leak of proteinaceous material in the anterior chamber resulting in flare. No clinical trials exist for treatment of traumatic iridocyclitis [24]. Treatment involves topical steroids and topical cycloplegica. If severe, traumatic iridocyclitis can lead to posterior synechiae, keratic precipitates of the cornea, corneal edema and increased IOP potentially causing glaucoma and cystoid macular edema. Topical steroids are usually slowly tapered to prevent rebound iritis. Prognosis with proper treatment is excellent.

Traumatic Cataract and Lens Dislocation

Pediatric traumatic cataract is a major cause of monocular blindness in children and accounts for a majority of pediatric cataract extraction surgical cases [25]. Without proper removal of a cataract, loss of binocular vision along with amblyopia, low vision, strabismus, or even blindness may ensue [26]. Cataract formation can be accompanied by other ocular morbidity resulting in further detriment to visual potential. A retrospective review of 25 children with unilateral cataracts showed that a majority of injuries were caused by paintball and BB gun injuries [27]. Injury from pencils and pens followed this as the second most common mode of injury. Modes of traumatic cataract vary depending on geographical location. In rural India, the most common cause of pediatric cataract was a wooden stick associated injury followed by a sharp thorn injury [28].

Poor visual outcome was seen by a greater majority of patients who were younger (5.25 years) than older (7.5 years). Penetrating injuries resulting in pediatric cataract were more often associated with penetrating injuries compared to blunt trauma [29].

Intervention in these cases involves cataract extraction. Surgical complications are usually minor [30]. However, posterior capsular opacification occurs in roughly 90% of patients, and a YAG capsulotomy procedure is required in the majority of cases. An IOL is placed in pediatric patients with a lens power that should take into account their eventual myopic shift. The main goal of cataract extraction and lens placement is to create a clear axis for proper visual development.

Lens dislocation can also occur with trauma. It may be associated with other types of ocular injury mentioned in this chapter. Underlying ocular and systemic conditions should be considered when minor trauma causes lens dislocation. These include simple ectopia lentis, *ectopia lentis et pupillae*, aniridia, Marfan Syndrome, Homocystinuria, Sulfite Oxidase Deficiency, and Weill–Marchesani syndrome. Lensectomy and vitrectomy are standard treatment for traumatic ectopia lentis. Over 90% of these surgical interventions result in vision or 20/40 or better [31].

Traumatic Retinal Detachment

Traumatic retinal detachments in the pediatric population likely occur as a result of secondary indirect impact from globe deformation [32]. They tend to form in adolescent years due to the protective support of well-formed vitreous earlier in life. Several factors can predispose patients to traumatic rhegmatogenous retinal detachments (RRDs), including inherited syndromes (Stickler syndrome, Wagner syndrome, Marfan syndrome, Knobloch syndrome), prior surgery and past trauma. Myopia is also a risk factor [33]. Most detachments are rhegmatogenous. In a German review of 259 patients under 20 years of age with retinal detachment, 72% were male [34]. 52% of the patient's had disorders predisposing to retinal detachments such as myopia. In a review of RRDs in the pediatric population, Wenick and Baranano found that roughly 40% of RRDs were related to trauma.

With longstanding RRDs, proliferative vitreoretinopathy can ensue and lead to tractional retinal detachments. With communication often lacking in the pediatric patient, children are less likely to report symptoms of retinal detachment. Those who present with macula-on retinal detachments have a better visual prognosis than those who present with macula-off detachments [32].

Blunt Trauma Injuries to the Retina

Traumatic Macular Hole

Full thickness defects in the central macula caused by trauma, termed traumatic macular holes, are likely caused by vitreoretinal forces in the pediatric patient. Mechanism for traumatic macular holes is a contrecoup mechanism that occurs with axial compression of the globe [35]. This causes equatorial outpouching that can cause significant vitreomacular traction and result in hole formation.

Limited data is available on traumatic macular holes in terms of treatment due to their rarity. Possibility of spontaneous closure exists. If surgical repair occurs, traumatic macular holes are usually repaired with pars-plana vitrectomy, with removal of posterior hyaloid. Adherence of the posterior hyaloid is often problematic for retinal surgeons. Autogenous plasmin has been injected in the vitreous cavity to induce posterior vitreous detachments in patients. Concentrated platelet drop placement in the hole has been attempted with promising results showing improvement of visual acuity [36]. There is no concensus on ideal intraocular tamponade if PPV is chosen for treatment of the traumatic macular hole.

Vitreous Hemorrhage

Trauma is the most common cause of vitreous hemorrhage in children. In a review of 261 pediatric eyes from India with vitreous hemorrhage, trauma was the cause of vitreous hemorrhage in 69% of eyes with blunt trauma, accounting for the majority of these cases [37]. These data are supported by other reviews [38].

Younger patients may present with strabismus and/or nystagmus, while older patients will present with decreased visual acuity. Similar to the mechanism of a macular hole, blunt force in the anterior–posterior direction can cause the equatorial region of the eye to bulge and create traction on the retina. Traction on retinal vessels can cause rupture of the vessels resulting in vitreous hemorrhage. Evaluation with ultrasonography is key in identifying integrity of structures posterior to the blood.

Sequelae of vitreous hemorrhage in children include tractional retinal detachment and deprivational amblyopia. Visual acuity at presentation is the most important predictor of visual outcome [39].

Commotio Retinae and RPE Contusions

Commotio retinae is a term used to describe whitening of the retina caused by damage to the outer segments of the photoreceptors within the retina. This is thought to be due to shock waves transmitted throughout the retina from blunt trauma. *Commotio retinale* of the macula is called Berlin's Edema. Occasionally blunt trauma can cause retinal pigment epithelial (RPE) cell contusion with resulting loss of the RPE cells. If present in or surrounding the macula, significant vision loss can ensue.

Prognosis for the pediatric patient is very good and vision usually recovers to baseline in 3–4 weeks [40]. No leakage of fluid is seen on fluorescein angiography and therefore it is not true edema. No treatment to *commotio retinae* has proven beneficial.

Optic Nerve Injury

Traumatic Optic Neuropathy (TON) is another cause of visual dysfunction following trauma in pediatric patients. TON can be divided into direct or indirect causation. Penetration or injury from fractured bony fragments can cause avulsion and direct trauma to the optic nerve. More commonly, the injury is indirect, thought to be the result of shock from orbital impact to the intracanalicular portion of the optic nerve. These mechanisms for pediatric patients are similar to mechanisms of TON in adults [41]. Many cases in the pediatric population present following a fall from a height [42, 43]. Pediatric males are more likely to be affected than females. Patients typically present with a relative afferent pupillary defect, decreased visual acuity, decreased color vision, visual field loss, and normal fundoscopic exam. Optic atrophy with nerve pallor can develop 4–6 weeks following the injury [44]. CT scan of the orbits is necessary to determine the mechanism of TON present. Visual acuity on presentation is highly correlated to visual prognosis [45].

There are no randomized controlled trials for treatment of TON in the pediatric population. The International Optic Nerve Trauma Study, a hallmark randomized control trial that evaluated treatment options for adults with TON, did not include children or adolescents [46]. In a prospective case series of thirty-one children with TON from India, 13 pediatric patients with fracture of the optic canal underwent transnasal trans-sphenoidal optic nerve decompression [42]. Smaller immature boney fragments in the optic canal indicated these patients may benefit from surgery. Seven of these thirteen patients showed visual improvement. The authors argue that due to the relatively small diameter of the pediatric optic nerve canal, there is lesser volume for the traumatized nerve to expand and thus surgical intervention is necessary. No standard protocol currently exists for treatment of optic neuropathy in the pediatric patient. Please see Fig. 13.4.

Non-accidental Pediatric Ocular Trauma

Non-accidental pediatric trauma can often involve ocular structures. When trauma to the head or neck is present, ophthalmic consultation is critical. It is possible that ocular findings present in the infant are the only physical exam findings of abuse in children.

Abusive Head Trauma (AHT), or Shaken Baby Syndrome (SBS), is a form of non-accidental head trauma that can present with ocular findings. In 2009, Christian and Block recommended that the use of the term Abusive Head Trauma be used to replace SBS [47]. The authors argue that in addition to shaking, blunt injury to the brain and spinal cord can also cause injury, thus the term AHT is all-encompassing.

(a) (b)

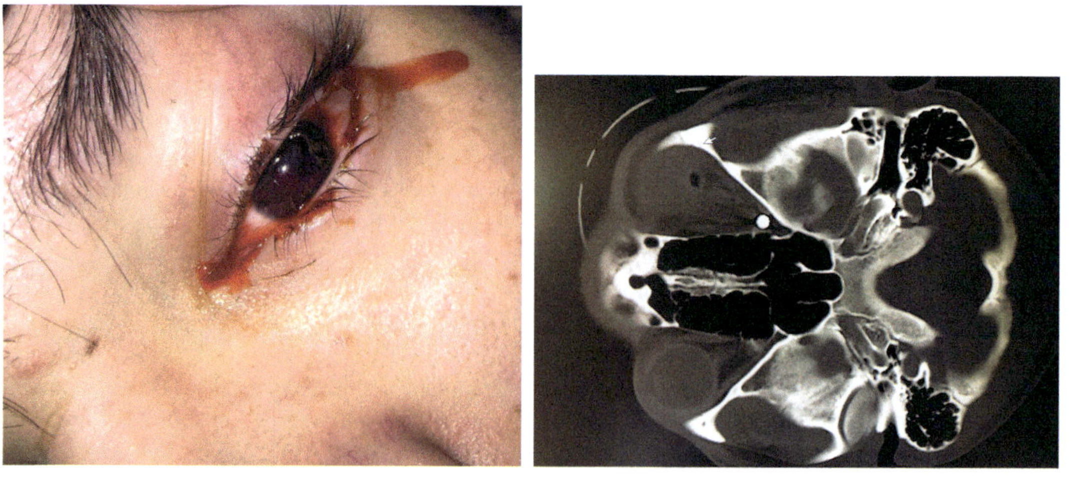

Fig. 13.4 **a** BB gun injury causing ruptured globe-note the hyphema. **b** BB pellet in the orbital apex

The two terms are currently used interchangeably. In addition to multiple bilateral retinal hemorrhages in multiple layers of the retina, subdural hemorrhage and anoxic encephalopathy make up the triad of AHT.

In patients with AHT, there is a high risk of mortality. Those that survive are more difficult to rear, have chronic medical problems and developmental delay [48]. It is thought that the repetitive acceleration–deceleration forces cause damage via vitreomacular traction [49]. This has recently been supported by animal and computer models that show shearing forces between the retinal blood vessels and firmly attached posterior hyaloid [50]. Eighty-five percent of AHT patients present with multiple layered retinal hemorrhages. Dense vitreous hemorrhage is a poor prognostic indicator of visual and neurological outcome [51]. Late neovascularization can occur in these patients in areas of peripheral retinal ischemia and non-perfusion. Laser photocoagulation can be considered to treat these areas.

Findings of non-accidental trauma can include adnexal changes such as ecchymosis, lid edema, and orbital fractures. Anterior segment findings including hyphema, iris prolapse, and corneal laceration can also be seen. Major manifestations occur in the posterior segment with vitreous hemorrhage, retinal detachment, and optic nerve avulsion.

Child Protective Services should be immediately notified if non-accidental trauma is suspected. Careful physician documentation is critical and can be very helpful in a court of law as children age and have visual sequelae. Fundus photography can be important to document trauma. Public health campaigns, and education and support systems for parents can ease stresses of parenthood.

Conclusion

As highlighted in this chapter, a majority of pediatric ocular trauma is preventable, particularly sports-related trauma. Harrison and Tellander showed that over 90% of sport-related eye injuries are preventable. Of the 42,000 sports and recreation-related eye injuries in 2000, 43% occurred in individuals younger than 15 years old [52].

It is in the best interest of the practitioner, patient, and patient's family to have monocular patients identified. Patients who are monocular are especially vulnerable and should wear polycarbonate lenses for ocular protection of the functioning eye. In addition to those that are monocular, pediatric patients involved in high-risk activities such as sporting activities should also wear protective lenses.

Successful campaigns encouraging and at times requiring athletes to wear protective headgear and face protection have been shown to decrease ocular trauma. Kriz et al. [53] in a study published in 2015 observed the before and after implications of mandated protective eyewear (MPE) in high school female field hockey. The group demonstrated that eye/orbital injuries were statistically high in states without MPE (0.080 per 1000 athletic exposures) compared with states implementing MPE (0.025 injuries per 1000 athletic exposures). After induction of MPE, severe eye/orbital injuries were reduced by 67%.

Eye injuries in hockey players in Canada were quantified by a survey of members of the Canadian Ophthalmological Society [54]. Of all injuries, 14% of injured players became legally blind. Groups of 11–15 year olds had the highest number of ocular injuries. Since the mandatory use of face protectors certified by the Canadian Standards Association was enacted, the incidence of eye injury in Canadian amateur hockey has decreased by 50% [55].

Specific protective eyewear recommended by the American Academy of Pediatrics and the American Academy of Ophthalmology should be used during sports where ocular injury is probable. The American Society for Testing and Materials (ASTM) and American National Standards Institute (ANSI) have stringent performance standards for eye protection and have approved protective equipment for recreational activities.

The American Academy of Ophthalmology has designated April as Sports Eye Safety Month in effort to increase awareness of the great majority of sports-related eye injuries that can be avoided by simply wearing the proper protection. Healthcare professionals should properly educate patients concerning eye protection and safety, especially in the setting of monocular patients and those participating in athletics. With more global awareness of the importance of physical protection from ocular injuries, this type of vision-threatening trauma can be reduced or eliminated in the future.

References

1. Strahlman E, Elman M, Daub E, Baker S. Causes of paediatric eye injuries. A population-based study. Arch Ophthalmol. 1990;108:603–6.
2. Maltzman BA, Pruzon H, Mund ML. A survey of ocular trauma. Surv Ophthalmol. 1976;21:285–90.
3. Niiranen M, Raivio I. Eye injuries in children. Br J Ophthalmol. 1981;65:436–8.
4. Ing C, et al. Long-term differences in language and cognitive function after childhood exposure to anesthesia. Pediatrics. 2012;130(3):e476–85.
5. Armstrong GW, et al. Pediatric eye injuries presenting to United States emergency departments: 2001–2007. Graefe's Arch Clin Exp Ophthalmol. 2013;251 (3):629–36.
6. Acar U, et al. A new ocular trauma score in pediatric penetrating eye injuries. Eye. 2011;25(3):370–4.
7. Hwang K, et al. Facial lacerations in children. J Craniofac Surg. 2013;24(2):671–5.
8. Murchison AP, Bilyk JR. Pediatric canalicular lacerations: epidemiology and variables affecting repair success. J Pediatr Ophthalmol Strabismus. 2014;51 (4):242–8.
9. Bunting H, Stephens D, Mireskandari K. Prediction of visual outcomes after open globe injury in children: a 17-year Canadian experience. J AAPOS. 2013;17:43–8.
10. Li X, Zarbin MA, Bhagat N. Pediatric open globe injury: a review of the literature. J Emergencies Trauma Shock. 2015;8(4):216.
11. Meier Petra. Combined anterior and posterior segment injuries in children: a review. Graefe's Arch Clin Exp Ophthalmol. 2010;248(9):1207–19.
12. Lee C-H, et al. Prognostic indicators of open globe injuries in children. Am J Emerg Med. 2009;27 (5):530–5.
13. Bunting H, Stephens D, Mireskandari K. Prediction of visual outcomes after open globe injury in children: a 17-year Canadian experience. J Am Assoc Pediatr Ophthalmol Strabismus. 2013;17(1):43–8.
14. Gupta A, Rahman I, Leatherbarrow B. Open globe injuries in children: factors predictive of a poor final visual acuity. Eye. 2009;23(3):621–5.
15. Narang S, et al. Paediatric open globe injuries. Visual outcome and risk factors for endophthalmitis. Indian J Ophthalmol. 2004;52(1):29.
16. Michael JG, Hug D, Dowd MD. Management of corneal abrasion in children: a randomized clinical trial. Ann Emerg Med. 2002;40(1):67–72.
17. Shope TR, Rieg TS, Kathiria NN. Corneal abrasions in young infants. Pediatrics. 2010;125(3):e565–9.
18. Browner EA. Corneal abrasions. Pediatrics. 2010;125:e565.
19. Kennedy RH, Brubaker RF. Traumatic hyphema in a defined population. Am J Ophthalmol. 1988;106:123.
20. Rocha KM, et al. Outpatient management of traumatic hyphema in children: prospective evaluation. J Am Assoc Pediatr Ophthalmol Strabismus. 2004;8 (4):357–61.
21. Lai JC, et al. Traumatic hyphema in children: risk factors for complications. Arch Ophthalmol. 2001;119(1):64–70.
22. Teboul BK, et al. Clinical evaluation of aminocaproic, acid for managing traumatic hyphema in children. Ophthalmology. 1995;102(11):1646–53.
23. Gutteridge IF, Hall AJ. Acute anterior uveitis in primary care. Clin Exp Optom. 2007;90(2):70–82.
24. Dargin JM, Lowenstein RA. The painful eye. Emerg Clin N Am. 2008;26(1):199–216.
25. Tomkins O, Ben-Zion I, Moore DB, Helveston EE. Outcomes of pediatric cataract surgery at a tertiary care center in rural southern Ethiopia. Arch Ophthalmol. 2011;129(10):1293–7.
26. Acuna OM, Yen KG. Outcome and prognosis of pediatric patients with delayed diagnosis of open-globe injuries. J Pediatr Ophthalmol Strabismus. 2009;46(4):202–7 (quiz 208–9).
27. Reddy AK, Ray R, Yen KG. Surgical intervention for traumatic cataracts in children: epidemiology, complications, and outcomes. J Am Assoc Pediatr Ophthalmol Strabismus. 2009;13(2):170–4.
28. Gogate P, et al. Causes, epidemiology, and long-term outcome of traumatic cataracts in children in rural India. Indian J Ophthalmol. 2012;60(5):481.
29. Brar GS, et al. Postoperative complications and visual results in uniocular pediatric traumatic cataract. Ophthalmic Surg Lasers Imaging Retina. 2001;32(3):233–8.
30. Eckstein M, et al. Use of intraocular lenses in children with traumatic cataract in south India. Br J Ophthalmol. 1998;82(8):911–5.
31. Plager DA, et al. Surgical treatment of subluxated lenses in children. Ophthalmology. 1992;99 (7):1018–23.
32. Sarrazin L, et al. Traumatic pediatric retinal detachment: a comparison between open and closed globe injuries. Am J Ophthalmol. 2004;137(6):1042–9.

33. Wang N-K, et al. Pediatric rhegmatogenous retinal detachment in East Asians. Ophthalmology. 2005;112(11):1890–5.
34. Bier C, et al. [Retinal detachment in pediatrics: etiology and risk factors]. Der Ophthalmologe: Zeitschrift der Deutschen Ophthalmologischen Gesellschaft. 2010;107(2):165–74.
35. Johnson RN, McDonald R, Lewis H, et al. Traumatic macular hole: observations, pathogenesis, and results of vitrectomy surgery. Ophthalmology. 2001;108:853–7.
36. Wachtlin J, Jandeck C, Potthofer S, et al. Long-term results following pars plana vitrectomy with platelet concentrate in pediatric patients with traumatic macular hole. Am J Ophthalmol. 2003;136:197–9.
37. Rishi P, et al. Vitreous hemorrhage in children and adolescents in India. J Am Assoc Pediatr Ophthalmol Strabismus. 2013;17(1):64–9.
38. Spirn MJ, Lynn MJ, Hubbard GB. Vitreous hemorrhage in children. Ophthalmology. 2006;113(5):848–52.
39. AlHarkan DH, et al. Vitreous hemorrhage in pediatric age group. J Ophthalmol 2014. 2014.
40. Ahn SJ, Woo SJ, Kim KE, Jo DH, Ahn J, Park KH. Optical coherence tomography morphologic grading of macular commotio retinae and its association with anatomic and visual outcomes. Am J Ophthalmol. 2013;156(5):994–1001 (e1001).
41. Goldenberg-Cohen N, Miller NR, Repka MX. Traumatic optic neuropathy in children and adolescents. J Am Assoc Pediatr Ophthalmol Strabismus. 2004;8(1):20–7.
42. Gupta AK, et al. Traumatic optic neuropathy in pediatric population: early intervention or delayed intervention? Int J Pediatr Otorhinolaryngol. 2007;71(4):559–62.
43. Zahavi A, et al. Severe cranial neuropathies caused by falls from heights in children. Graefe's Arch Clin Exp Ophthalmol. 2015;1–8.
44. Sarkies N. Traumatic optic neuropathy. Eye. 2004;18(11):1122–5.
45. Ford RL, et al. A 2-year prospective surveillance of pediatric traumatic optic neuropathy in the United Kingdom. J AAPOS. 2012;16(5):413–7.
46. Levin LA, et al. The treatment of traumatic optic neuropathy: the International optic nerve trauma study. Ophthalmology. 1999;106:1268–77.
47. Christian CW, Block R. Abusive head trauma in infants and children. Pediatrics. 2009;123(5):1409–11.
48. Kivlin JD, et al. Shaken baby syndrome. Ophthalmology. 2000;107(7):1246–54.
49. Levin A. Retinal hemorrhage in abusive head trauma. Pediatrics. 2010;126:961.
50. Nadarasa J, Deck C, Meyer F, et al. Update on injury mechanisms in abusive head trauma—shaken baby syndrome. Pediatr Radiol. 2014;44(Supp 4):s565–70.
51. Matthews GP, Das A. Dense vitreous hemorrhages predict poor visual and neurological prognosis in infants with shaken baby syndrome. J Pediatr Ophthalmol Strabismus. 1996;33(4):260–5.
52. US Consumer Product Safety Commission. Sports and recreational eye injuries. Washington, DC: US Consumer Product Safety Commission; 2000.
53. Kriz PK, et al. Eye protection and risk of eye injuries in high school field hockey. Pediatrics. 2015;136(3):521–7.
54. Pashby TJ. Eye injuries in Canadian amateur hockey. Am J Sports Med. 1979;7(4):254–7.
55. Pashby T. Eye injuries in Canadian amateur hockey. Can J Ophthalmol (Journal canadien d'ophtalmologie). 1985;20(1):2–4.

European Perspective of Ocular Trauma Management: Diagnostic and Therapeutic Considerations Based on Our Experience

14

Alessandro Meduri, Mario Urso, Marco Zagari, Alessandro Arrigo and Pasquale Aragona

Introduction

Ocular traumas represent a complex and heterogeneous nosological entity showing high variability both in terms of etiology and clinical expression. The most affected patient categories are children and workers; this data has important implications in terms of long-term prognosis, posttraumatic deficits as well as healthcare and economic cost. Indeed, ocular trauma may cause severe permanent alterations of ocular anatomy as well as visual loss. These patients may show the involvement of all ocular structures, thus requiring the intervention of an experienced surgeon in the pole to pole surgery. Moreover, multidisciplinary intervention may be required, e.g., in cases of the polytraumatized patient, making management and treatment of these cases complex and tricky. It is worth noting that often emergency care units are not able to deal with such events, thus making it necessary to refer the patient to specialized facilities for complex trauma management. However, posttraumatic visual deficits or blindness cannot always be prevented.

Clinical History and Physical Examination

When the patient comes to the physician's attention, the first step is to evaluate the general conditions. Eye trauma management may change according to the pathogenesis of the traumatic event and to ocular structures involved. Careful assessment of the trauma provides primarily the score calculation and analysis of wounds requiring immediate suturing in order to avoid any superinfection. If an ultrasound device is available, it may be used (**when a ruptured globe is not suspected)** to evaluate posterior structures and the presence of any intraocular foreign body (IOFB). The management of an injured eye requires meticulous history collection, measurement of visual acuity, and detection of relative pupillary defects, as well as a careful inspection of the eyes, using anesthetic if needed. A lateral canthotomy with cantholysis should be immediately performed in the case of a sight-threatening retrobulbar hemorrhage. A ruptured globe should be protected by an eye shield. A skull X-ray may be performed to exclude cranial and facial fractures as well as to visualize radio-opaque foreign bodies. Magnetic resonance imaging is contraindicated in cases of metallic IOFB. The magnetic field may cause metallic body dislocation within the eye thus perpetuating further intraocular damage. The vision should be assessed

A. Meduri (✉) · M. Urso · A. Arrigo · P. Aragona
Department of Biomedical, Dental Sciences and Morphofunctional Imaging, University of Messina, Messina, Italy
e-mail: alexmeduri@hotmail.com

M. Urso
e-mail: mariourso@tiscali.it

A. Arrigo
e-mail: alessandro.arrigo@hotmail.com

M. Zagari
Clinic "Centro Europeo", Acicastello, Italy

S.C. Kaufman and D.R. Lazzaro (eds.), *Textbook of Ocular Trauma*,
DOI 10.1007/978-3-319-47633-9_14

using a Snellen chart. If letters cannot be read, the ability to count fingers, detect hand movements, and to perceive light are recorded in that order as CF, HM, PL, and NPL (nil perception of light), respectively. Extraocular muscle assessment is then performed in all nine positions of gaze by asking the patient to follow a pen light or other target. Pupil examination is performed by checking shape, symmetry, red reflex, and reaction to light. The eyelids are examined for lacerations and everted to detect any foreign bodies. If globe rupture is suspected, the lid must not be everted because it could apply undue pressure to the ruptured globe, thus causing extrusion of intraocular contents. Lid wound assessment includes an estimation of thickness, tissue loss, and lacrimal canalicular involvement. An estimation of the anterior chamber depth should be performed. Pupil dilatation is useful for examining the posterior segment, but it must be performed after the evaluation of pupil reactivity and only if the anterior chamber is not found shallow. Systemic and/or local antibiotic therapy (aminoglycoside, fluoroquinolone, and atropine) as well as IOP compensation may be required.

At this point, the patient can be sent to a specialized trauma center for complex management who have the capability to address severe trauma, be supported with appropriate therapy including: removal of any foreign body, restoration of anatomic spaces, anterior chamber cleaning, IOL implantation, vitrectomy, and/or laser treatment.

Workflow Management of Injured Eye

The proper recognition and classification of traumatic eye injury is a fundamental step when approaching the patient. It is known that a number of mechanisms of eye injury exist, including mechanical, chemical, thermal, and combination ones; related eye damage needs specific treatments according to the pathophysiology of trauma [1]. First of all, the use of proper eye trauma terminology is important both for understanding which structures are involved as well as for determining the prognosis. Birmingham Eye Trauma Terminology (BETT) [2, 3] is an internationally standardized terminology allowing a fine description of eye injuries. Following BETT, it is possible to describe clinical features of a given eye trauma (Fig. 14.1).

In particular, "contusion" is used when the eye wall is not injured whereas "lamellar laceration" refers to a partially damaged eye wall. "Laceration" and "Rupture" are used when a full thickness injury of eye wall occurs; these terms differ according to traumatic mechanism, respectively, determined by a sharp or a blunt

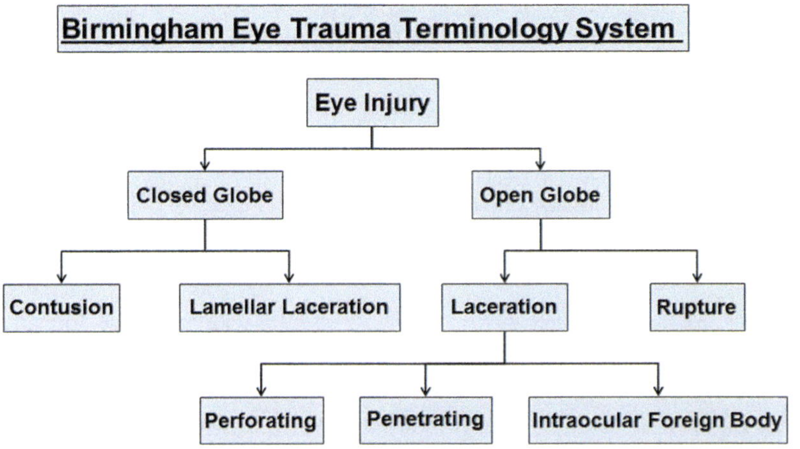

Fig. 14.1 BETT system

object [2, 3]. Once the type of injury is determined, the patient may undergo clinical and instrumental evaluations. In this context, both general and specific exams may be adopted in order to obtain a global description of the patient's clinical conditions. A list of useful examinations, including both conventional ophthalmologic and more specific exams, is provided in Fig. 14.2.

It is worth noting that an eye may be involved alone, thus requiring only ophthalmologic treatment. On the other hand, ocular damage may only be one part of a multi-system trauma, i.e., in the polytraumatized patient; in the latter case, the ophthalmologist is involved secondarily, after the patient's stabilization following the ABCDE rule assessment (airway, breathing, circulation, disability, and exposition) [4].

After clinical and instrumental evaluation of the ocular damage, an important step is to quantify visual prognosis. The Ocular Trauma Score (OTS) [2, 3] is a set of six factors, which provide a prediction of the patient's visual acuity recovery at 6 months follow-up. OTS scores range between 1 (worst prognosis) and 5 (good prognosis). OTS predictive factors and associated scores are shown in Fig. 14.3. The clinical usefulness of OTS has been verified by a number of studies showing the utility of OTS for the evaluation of an injured eye [5–7].

OTS score is a reliable predictor of visual prognosis when assessing an open globe injury. Conversely, a deeper investigation is required when other serious conditions, such as endophthalmitis and retinal detachment, occur in the trauma patient [8].

Clinical and Instrumental Examination

- **Clinical ispection of eye and orbital structures:**
    - **Lids examination;**
    - **Globe examination (cornea, sclera, conjunctiva, pupil, iris, lacrimal system);**
- **Visual Acuity Test;**
- **Pupillary reflexes;**
- **Direct ophthalmoscopy of anterior and posterior chambers;**
- **Extra-ocular muscles motility.**

- **Cranial nerves examination (e.g. in case of ptosis);**
- **Optical Coherence Tomography (OCT) (e.g. in case of retinal injury);**
- **Angiography (e.g. in case of choroidal injury);**
- **Ultrasonography (e.g. in case of suspected foreign body);**
- **Computerized Tomography (TC) (e.g. in case of suspected orbital cavity fracture);**
- **Magnetic Resonance Imaging (MRI) (e.g. in case of suspected optic nerve damage).**

- **Multidisciplinary evaluation (e.g. Plastic Surgery and Maxillo-Facial Surgery).**

Fig. 14.2 Clinical and instrumental evaluation of eye trauma. Ophthalmologic assessment of ocular damage includes the tests showed in *pink box*. This first evaluation may be followed by more specific exams (*orange box*), according to the clinical picture. If larger involvement of extraocular structures occurs, multidisciplinary evaluation may be considered (*violet box*)

Fig. 14.3 Predictive factors and computation of OTS score

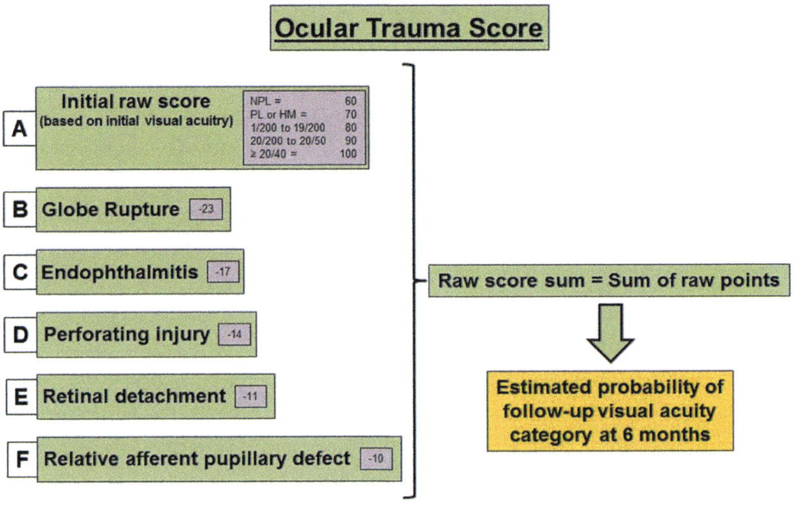

Imaging of the Injured Eye

Imaging of the injured eye (see Fig. 14.2) consists of a number of techniques, which permits a deeper study of the effects of trauma on ocular as well as orbital structures. These represent advanced investigations required when conventional clinical approaches are not sufficient to assess structural alterations after trauma, especially when the posterior segment and the optic nerve are involved. The initial clinical evaluation is critical, since the spectrum of alterations induced by trauma can involve, alone or in combination, several structures. Indeed, previous studies conducted in patients with blunt trauma have shown that traumatic manifestations may include the retina, choroid, optic nerve, and vascular compartment [9, 10]. Regarding the anterior segment, a number of injuries might be expected resulting from direct trauma as well as those associated with posttraumatic factors [11–15]. A list of the most frequent ocular injuries is provided in Fig. 14.4. Other authors have emphasized that trauma most commonly occurs in the young [10]; this should be taken into account when deciding proper therapy as well as when evaluating expected prognosis after ocular trauma.

A brief description of the most commonly used approaches and their specifics is provided below.

Optical Coherence Tomography

Optical Coherence Tomography (OCT) is a noninvasive technique providing microstructural evaluations of the eye's components by means of a laser source and allowing an accurate investigation of eye structures; it is largely used for investigating retinal layers [16]. This approach has been found to be useful for assessing the effect of trauma on the posterior segment as well as for posttraumatic follow-up [17–19]. Moreover, OCT has been reported to clearly detect optic nerve avulsion [20]. Furthermore, a number of studies have shown that OCT may provide useful microstructural information regarding traumatic involvement of the anterior segment [21–23].

Angiography

Angiography is a method for the evaluation of the eye's circulation by adopting contrast agents. It is able to evaluate retinal (by means of a fluorescein agent) as well as choroidal circulation (by means of an indocyanine green agent); perfusion alterations are detected as hypofluorescent areas whereas neovascularization processes are shown as hyperfluorescence. Angiography has been reported to be more sensitive for vascular evaluation when compared to conventional ophthalmoscopy [24]. This technique has been found

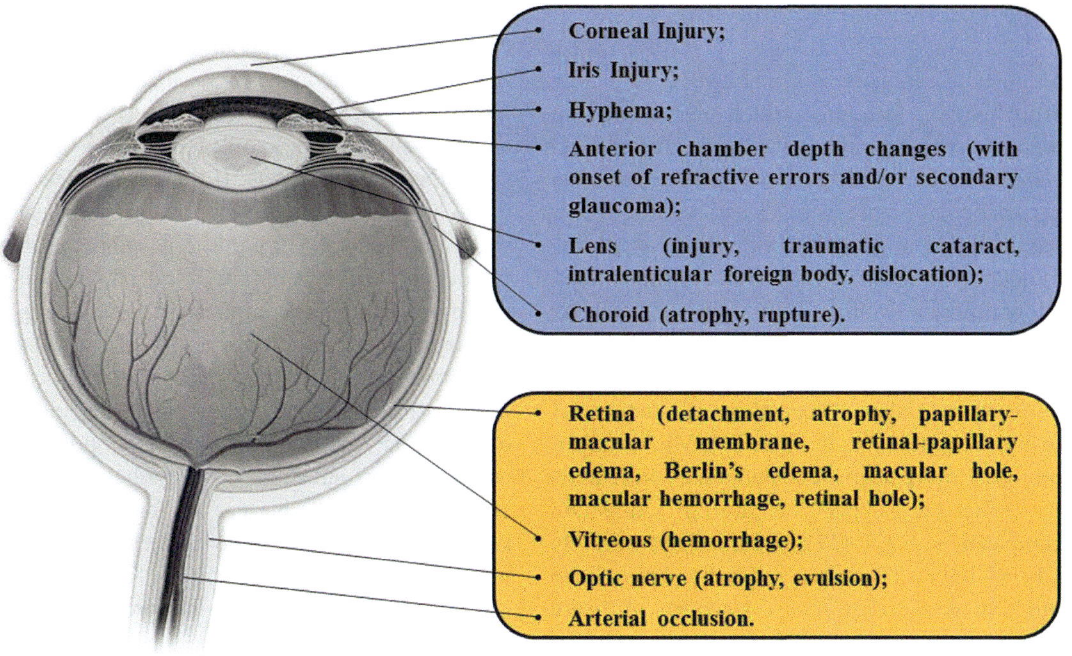

Fig. 14.4 Traumatic injuries of eye's structures

useful especially for assessing traumatic choroidal damage; this can occur with different degrees of alterations which have been clearly detected by indocyanine green angiography [25]. Further, the use of this method has been found to play a role for predicting the visual prognosis in patients with traumatic choroidal involvement [26].

Ultrasonography

Ultrasonography is a noninvasive imaging technique showing morphological images after elaboration of sound echo-ography provided by sound reflection by different tissues. Previous studies have reported its utility for different traumatic injuries, including the evaluation of suspected foreign intraocular body [27], lens damages with phacocele [28] as well as optic nerve involvement [29], thus suggesting a greater utility in different clinical contexts. As stated earlier in the chapter, when rupture of the globe is suspected, ultrasound should not be performed as the pressure from the probe may cause extrusion of intraocular contents.

Computed Tomography

Computed Tomography (CT) is a frequently used imaging technique for structural evaluation of orbital structures and bone-related trauma. It uses radiation to obtain images, based on different tissue densities. CT is the first choice when a bone fracture is suspected; it is useful in cases of orbital perforation as well as foreign body injury [30]. CT is able to detect corneal laceration as well as lens damage [31]; moreover, it can distinguish open globe injuries, extraocular muscle damage, and orbital compartmental syndrome [31–34]. CT can also evaluate vitreous hemorrhage and retinal detachment [35], although its sensitivity is poor [34]. Indeed, it was found that magnetic resonance imaging may be more sensitive when assessing soft tissue involvement, showing detailed images of ocular structures [34, 36].

Magnetic Resonance Imaging

Magnetic Resonance Imaging (MRI) is a powerful imaging technique which allows morphological evaluation of ocular structures through elaboration of signals produced by adopting two perpendicular magnetic fields and radiofrequency pulses. By setting MRI parameters, it is possible to obtain T1 and T2 weighted acquisitions; these allow different evaluations of body tissues. It has been reported that MRI permits detailed evaluations of ocular and orbital structures, especially by using specialized types of scans, such as diffusion weighted imaging [31, 34]. MRI is able to provide a more detailed evaluation of optic nerve by using fat suppression during acquisition, compared with CT [37]. For this kind of study, T1-weighted, T2-weighted Turbo Spin Echo, fluid attenuation inversion recovery, diffusion weighted as well as T1 inversion recovery coronal acquisitions can provide useful information regarding optic nerve involvement in pathological conditions, e.g., optic neuritis and neuromyelitis [38–42]. Although MRI offers several advantages for these kinds of evaluation, especially if adopting advanced postprocessing techniques, its use in ocular trauma is limited when compared to CT because of longer acquisition times, as well as higher costs. Moreover, another MRI limitation is related to the presence of metallic objects (e.g., metallic foreign body) and metallic devices (e.g., cardiac pacemaker), which are contraindicated with MRI, due to magnet induced movement of metallic foreign bodies.

Eye Trauma and Travel

Management of ocular trauma and travel requires careful adoption of appropriate preventive measures in order to avoid worsening of a given ocular injury as well as the onset of "ex novo" complications. After the initial treatment, it is important to reduce the risk of infection through adoption of proper topical and/or systemic antimicrobial therapy, covering both gram+ and gram− pathogen infections [43]. Based on the intraocular pressure (IOP), the use of hypotonic drugs might be required in order to reduce the risk of damage induced by an increase in ocular pressure [44]. In this context, prostaglandin analogs should be avoided because of their pro-inflammatory effects. If the patient needs to travel by plane, a number of preventive measures should be adopted. In particular, stabilization of the ocular surface is required. Indeed, dryness is the most common complication of staying in air-conditioned environments (both transports and closed spaces). Air-conditioning may cause changes in air humidity, thus increasing the risk of infection; for this reason, it is important to consider tear substitutes, re-epithelizing substances, protective lenses, and/or bandages if indicated. In patients who undergo pneumatic retinopexy or vitrectomy, airplane travel must be avoided for 15 days after the procedure. Gas reabsorption must be confirmed in order to avoid the risk of globe explosion caused by gas expansion, induced by high altitude.

Therapy and Long-Term Management

Changes of angle structures induced by chronic inflammation can be observed, producing irido-corneal synechiae or membranes with subsequent trabecular meshwork occlusion and drug resistant ocular hypertension. In order to prevent this complication as well as damage to the retina and optic nerve, an accurate long-term posttraumatic management of ocular inflammation is needed. Angle alterations may occur also in cases of traumatic hyphema; in the latter case, an angle recession can be observed, as well as iridodialysis or cyclodialysis. These changes may cause a secondary glaucoma due to obstructed outflow of trabecular meshwork. A noteworthy condition is iridodialysis, which may create a direct communication between the anterior chamber and choroidal space, thus causing ocular hypotony. If secondary glaucoma surgery fails, due to scarring phenomena interfering with therapeutical process, antimetabolite drugs and tube drainage systems may be necessary [45–51].

Chronic inflammation after vitrectomy and/or foreign body removal usually induces the release of inflammatory factors, with the recruitment of inflammatory cells, fibroblasts, and RPE cells in the retinal layers, thus leading to PVR formation [52]. An optimal management of risk factors combined with particular attention to the onset of emovitreous, inflammation, or infective processes may help to prevent PVR formation; in the case of significant PVR, surgical removal may become necessary.

Despite the careful treatment of ocular trauma, permanent damage can still occur, thus requiring the chronic administration of steroids and immunosuppressant drugs for at least six months or longer. If the involved eye still remains blind or irreversibly damaged, evisceration, or enucleation may represent the only possible therapeutic choice [53].

Postsurgical Pharmacologic Therapy

Postsurgical therapy is mandatory to help anatomical and functional recovery of an injured eye as well as to prevent possible complications [54]. The first priority is to avoid the onset of infection. To achieve this goal, it is important to prescribe broad-spectrum antibiotics, which is often made by using a combination of different medications to optimize coverage. Moreover, the prescription of antibiotics based on wound cultures may be required in order to determine an adequate antibiotic therapy. Culture results are obtained after a number of days. During this wait time, the synergic association of aminoglycosides and fluoroquinolones may help to obtain a good nonspecific antibiotic cover. Another important step is inflammation management; indeed, a traumatic event usually induces the production and release of several inflammatory mediators (e.g., IL1, IL6, PDGF, FGF, and TGFβ). Based on the severity of the trauma, a patient's inflammatory reaction may vary from a slight iritis to a strong reaction with keratic precipitates and irido-corneal angle occlusion with subsequent ocular hypertension. To treat this condition, topical and/or systemic steroids and NSAIDS can be adopted. Furthermore, it is important to identify the risk of ocular hypertension, which may require accurate long-term management.

Conclusion

In this chapter, which provides a European perspective of our management plan of ocular trauma, a comprehensive description of diagnostic procedures and therapeutic choices have been provided. Ocular trauma represents a very heterogeneous condition, sometimes leading to irreversible loss of vision of the involved eye. Anatomical and functional recovery, as well as visual prognosis after ocular trauma, strictly depends upon the traumatic mechanism, ocular structures involved, damage extension, and the patient's visual acuity in the acute phase. Finally, this chapter has underlined how important it is to send patients to specialized trauma centers, after stabilizing the injury, in order to guarantee optimal management as well as to improve the chances of recovery of visual function.

Case Report

A 59 year old patient came to our attention after a perforating injury caused by an iron disk, which involved almost all ocular structures and caused a full thickness corneal wound, aphakia, iris prolapse and tissue loss, vitreous hemorrhage, presence of lenticular fragments in the vitreous, and secondary ocular hypertension. No retinal tears, hemorrhages or detachment were seen. No light perception was measured. After the removal of seven glass foreign bodies (parts of his eyeglasses) dispersed in the anterior chamber, the corneal wound was sutured and the anterior chamber was filled with a viscoelastic substance to restore the anatomical spaces. Then we proceeded with a vitrectomy, and removed many lenticular fragments and clotted blood. The patient developed painful and severe ocular hypertension (40 mm Hg), which required the adoption of strong hypotensive therapy

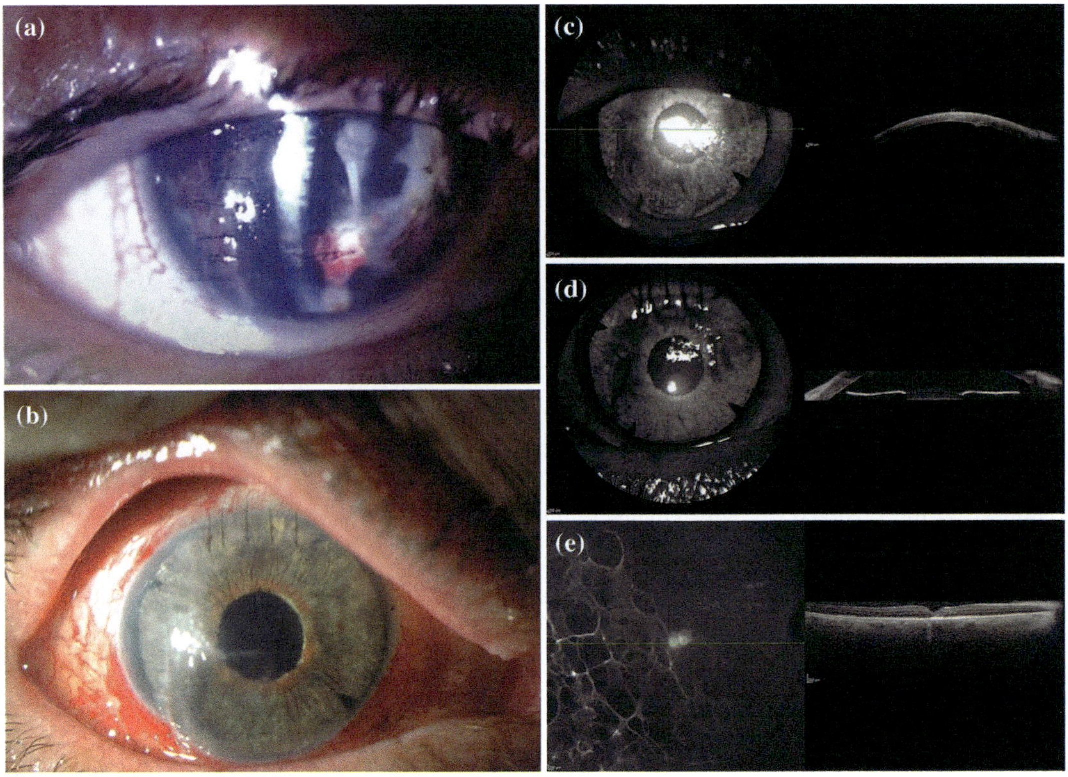

Fig. 14.5 Case report. Injured eye (**a**) showed involvement of several structures at presentation. Postoperative result is shown in (**b**). OCT scans showed posttraumatic structural damages, respectively, of cornea (**c**), anterior chamber (**d**) and retina (**e**)

(brinzolamide, timolol, brimonidine and acetazolamide). The patient was then sent to a specialized trauma center for management. Once assessed and the ocular trauma was stabilized, we proceeded with anterior segment reconstruction, by means of IOL implantation, and iris complex implantation, which was custom designed from an image of the contralateral healthy eye. The patient was then discharged in good conditions with a visual acuity of 5/10, and he did not require any further hypotonic therapy. After one year, a herpetic keratoconjunctivitis caused corneal decompensation; for this reason, the patient underwent an endothelial transplant (DMEK). After one month, ocular hypertension (>40 mm Hg), not responsive to medical therapy, occurred requiring a trabeculectomy with MMC, which failed after two months. An ExPRESS valve was implanted for IOP reduction (10 mm Hg). The patient had final visual acuity of 2/10 (Fig. 14.5).

Conflict of interests

Authors have no conflict of interest to declare.

References

1. Aylward GW. Vitreous management in penetrating trauma: primary repair and secondary intervention. Eye (Lond). 2008;22(10):1366–9. Doi:10.1038/eye.2008.74 (Epub 2008 Apr 18).
2. Kuhn F, Morris R, Witherspoon CD. Birmingham Eye Trauma Terminology (BETT): terminology and classification of mechanical eye injuries. Ophthalmol Clin North Am. 2002;15(2):139–43, v.
3. Kuhn F, Maisiak R, Mann L, Mester V, Morris R, Witherspoon CD. The Ocular Trauma Score (OTS). Ophthalmol Clin North Am. 2002;15(2):163–5, vi.

4. Morris SC. The team approach to management of the polytrauma patient. Virtual Mentor. 2009;11(7):516–20. Doi:10.1001/virtualmentor.2009.11.7.cprl1-0907.
5. Shah MA, Shah SM, Applewar A, Patel C, Shah S, Patel U. Ocular Trauma Score: a useful predictor of visual outcome at six weeks in patients with traumatic cataract. Ophthalmology. 2012;119(7):1336–41. Doi:10.1016/j.ophtha.2012.01.020.
6. Weber SL, Ribeiro LG, Ducca BL, Kasahara N. Prospective validation of the Ocular Trauma Score as a prognostic model to predict vision survival in injured adult patients from a developing country. Eur J Trauma Emerg Surg. 2012;38(6):647–50. Doi:10.1007/s00068-012-0209-7.
7. Turgut B, Kobat SG, Tanyildizi R. The Usage of ocular trauma scoring in the visual prognostic evaluation of traumatic eye injury. Med-Sci. 2014;3(2):1224–33. Doi:10.5455/medscience.2014.03.8123.
8. Rawat P, Rajput S, Gautam M, Tammannavar S. Grading of severity of ocular trauma by various ocular trauma scores and its effect on prognosis. International Journal of Scientific and Research Publications 4(12). 2014. ISSN 2250–3153.
9. Williams DF, Mieler WF, Williams GA. Posterior segment manifestations of ocular trauma. Retina. 1990;10(Suppl 1):S35–44.
10. Atmaca LS, Yilmaz M. Changes in the fundus caused by blunt ocular trauma. Ann Ophthalmol. 1993;25(12):447–52.
11. Tasman W, Jaeger EA. Traumatic cataract. Duane's Clin Ophthalmol. 1997;1:13–4.
12. Kumar A, Kumar V, Dapling RB. Traumatic cataract and intralenticular foreign body. Clin Exp Ophthalmol. 2005;33(6):660–1.
13. Witherspoon CD, Kunh F, Morris R, et al. Anterior and posterior segment trauma. In: Master Techniques in Ophthalmic Surgery. 1995. p. 538–47.
14. Viestenz A, Küchle M. Blunt ocular trauma. Part I: blunt anterior segment trauma. Ophthalmologe. 2004;101(12):1239–57 (quiz 1257–8).
15. Kashiwagi K, Tateno Y, Kashiwagi F, Tsukahara S. Changes in anterior chamber depth due to contusion. Ophthalmic Res. 2009;42(4):193–8. doi:10.1159/000232402.
16. Huang D, Swanson EA, Lin CP, Schuman JS, Stinson WG, et al. Optical coherence tomography. Science. 1991;254(5035):1178–1181.
17. Al Kharousi N, Wali UK, Azeem S. Current applications of optical coherence tomography in ophthalmology. 2013. Doi:http://dx.doi.org/10.5772/53961.
18. Wali UK, Al Kharousi N. Clinical applications of optical coherence tomography in ophthalmology. 2012.
19. Al-Mujaini A, Wali UK, Azeem S. Optical coherence tomography: clinical applications in medical practice. Oman Med J. 2013;28(2):86–91. Doi:10.5001/omj.2013.24.
20. Mumcuoglu T, Durukan HA, Erdurman C, Hurmeric V, Gundogan FC. Functional and structural analysis of partial optic nerve avulsion due to blunt trauma: case report. Indian J Ophthalmol. 2010;58(6):524–6. Doi:10.4103/0301-4738.71705.
21. Madhusudhana KC, Hossain P, Thiagarajan M, Newsom RS. Use of anterior segment optical coherence tomography in a penetrating eye injury. Br J Ophthalmol. 2007;91(7):982–3.
22. Goel N, Pangtey BP, Raina UK, Ghosh B. Anterior segment optical coherence tomography in intracorneal foreign body. Oman J Ophthalmol. 2012;5(2):131–2.
23. Lim SH. Clinical applications of anterior segment optical coherence tomography. J Ophthalmol. 2015;2015:605729. Doi:10.1155/2015/605729.
24. Kempster RC, Green WR, Finkelstein D. Choroidal rupture. Clinicopathologic correlation of an unusual case. Retina. 1996;16(1):57–63.
25. Akman A, Kadayifçilar S, Oto S, Aydin P. Indocyanine green angiographic features of traumatic choroidal ruptures. Eye. 1998;12(Pt 4):646–50 (Lond).
26. Kohno T, Miki T, Hayashi K. Choroidopathy after blunt trauma to the eye: a fluorescein and indocyanine green angiographic study. Am J Ophthalmol. 1998;126(2):248–60.
27. Deramo VA, Shah GK, Baumal CR, Fineman MS, Corrêa ZM, Benson WE, Rapuano CJ, Cohen EJ, Augsburger JJ. Ultrasound biomicroscopy as a tool for detecting and localizing occult foreign bodies after ocular trauma. Ophthalmology. 1999;106(2):301–5.
28. Vodapalli H, Murthy SI, Jalali S, Ali MJ, Rani PK. Comparison of immersion ultrasonography, ultrasound biomicroscopy and anterior segment optical coherence tomography in the evaluation of traumatic phacoceles. Indian J Ophthalmol. 2012;60(1):63–5. Doi:10.4103/0301-4738.91352.
29. Simsek T, Simsek E, Ilhan B, Ozalp S, Sekercioglu B, Zilelioglu O. Traumatic optic nerve avulsion. J Pediatr Ophthalmol Strabismus. 2006;43(6):367–9.
30. Novelline RA, Liebig T, Jordan J, Bilyk JR, Rubin PAD. Computed tomography of ocular trauma. 1994. Emergency Radiology Number 1 American Society of Emergency Radiology.
31. Kubal WS. Imaging of orbital trauma. Radiographics. 2008;28(6):1729–39. Doi:10.1148/rg.286085523.
32. Weissman JL, Beatty RL, Hirsch WL, Curtin HD. Enlarged anterior chamber: CT finding of a ruptured globe. AJNR Am J Neuroradiol. 1995;16(4 Suppl):936–8.
33. Joseph DP, Pieramici DJ, Beauchamp NJ Jr. Computed tomography in the diagnosis and prognosis of open-globe injuries. Ophthalmology. 2000;107(10):1899–906.
34. Lin KY, Ngai P, Echegoyen JC, Tao JP. Imaging in orbital trauma. Saudi J Ophthalmol. 2012;26(4):427–32. Doi:10.1016/j.sjopt.2012.08.002.

35. Imran S, Amin S, Daula MIH. Imaging in ocular trauma optimizing the use of ultrasound and computerised tomography. Pak J Ophthalmol. 2011;27 (3):146–151.
36. Mafee MF, Karimi A, Shah J, Rapoport M, Ansari SA. Anatomy and pathology of the eye: role of MR imaging and CT. Neuroimaging Clin N Am. 2005;15(1):23–47.
37. Barker GJ. Diffusion-weighted imaging of the spinal cord and optic nerve. J Neurol Sci. 2001;186(Suppl 1):S45–9.
38. Mallery RM, Prasad S (2012) Neuroimaging of the afferent visual system. Semin Neurol. 32(4):273–319. Doi:10.1055/s-0032-1331805.
39. Newman N, Biousse V. Diagnostic approach to vision loss. Continuum (Minneap Minn). 2014;20(4 Neuro-ophthalmology):785–815. Doi:10.1212/01. CON.0000453317.67637.46.
40. Kapur R, Sepahdari AR, Mafee MF, Putterman AM, Aakalu V, et al. MR imaging of orbital inflammatory syndrome, orbital cellulitis, and orbital lymphoid lesions: the role of diffusion-weighted imaging. AJNR Am J Neuroradiol. 2009;30(1): 64–70. Doi:10.3174/ajnr.A1315.
41. Al-Shafai LS, Mikulis DJ. Diffusion MR imaging in a case of acute ischemic optic neuropathy. AJNR Am J Neuroradiol. 2006;27(2):255–7.
42. Bender B, Heine C, Danz S, Bischof F, Reimann K, et al. (2014) Diffusion restriction of the optic nerve in patients with acute visual deficit. J Magn Reson Imaging. 40(2):334–40. Doi:10.1002/jmri.24367.
43. Abu El-Asrar AM, Al-Amro SA, Al-Mosallam AA, Al-Obeidan S. Post-traumatic endophthalmitis: causative organisms and visual outcome. Eur J Ophthalmol. 1999;9(1):21–31.
44. Ding C, Zeng J. Clinical study on Hypotony following blunt ocular trauma. Int J Ophthalmol. 2012;5(6):771–3.
45. Dubois L, Steenen SA, Gooris PJ, Mourits MP, Becking AG. Controversies in orbital reconstruction–I. Defect-driven orbital reconstruction: a systematic review. Int J Oral Maxillofac Surg. 2015;44(3):308–15. Doi:10.1016/j.ijom.2014.12.002 (Epub 2014 Dec 24).
46. Dubois L, Steenen SA, Gooris PJ, Mourits MP, Becking AG. Controversies in orbital reconstruction–II. Timing of post-traumatic orbital reconstruction: a systematic review. Int J Oral Maxillofac Surg. 2015;44(4):433–40. Doi:10.1016/j.ijom.2014.12.003 (Epub 2014 Dec 25).
47. Zhang Y, Zhang MN, Jiang CH, Yao Y, Zhang K. Endophthalmitis following open globe injury. Br J Ophthalmol. 2010;94:111–114. Doi:10.1136/bjo. 2009.164913.
48. Keles S, Ondas O, Ekinci M, Sener MT. Paintball-related ocular trauma: paintball or painball? Med Sci Monit. 2014;20:564–8.
49. Dehghani AR, Rezaei L, Salam H, Mohammadi Z, Mahboubi M. Post traumatic endophthalmitis: incidence and risk factors. Glob J Health Sci. 2014;6 (6):68–72. Doi:10.5539/gjhs.v6n6p68.
50. Nobe JR, Gomez DS, Liggett P, Smith RE, Robin JB. Post-traumatic and postoperative endophthalmitis: a comparison of visual outcomes. Br J Ophthalmol. 1987;71(8):614–7.
51. Essex RW, Yi Q, Charles PG, Allen PJ. Post-traumatic endophthalmitis. Ophthalmology. 2004;111(11):2015–22.
52. Cardillo JA, Stout JT, LaBree L, Azen SP, Omphroy L, Cui JZ, Kimura H, Hinton DR, Ryan SJ. Post-traumatic proliferative vitreoretinopathy. The epidemiologic profile, onset, risk factors, and visual outcome. Ophthalmology. 1997;104 (7):1166–73.
53. Atkins EJ, Newman NJ, Biousse V. Post-traumatic visual loss. Rev Neurol Dis. 2008; 5(2):73–81.
54. Scott R. The injured eye. Philos Trans R Soc Lond B Biol Sci. 2011;366(1562):251–260. Doi:10.1098/ rstb.2010.0234.

Erratum to: Textbook of Ocular Trauma

Stephen C. Kaufman and Douglas R. Lazzaro

Erratum to: S.C. Kaufman and D.R. Lazzaro (eds.), *Textbook of Ocular Trauma*, DOI 10.1007/978-3-319-47633-9

The original version of the book was inadvertently published without volume editor name "Stephen C. Kaufman" which has to be included in the "Contributors" list of FM. The erratum book has been updated with the change.

The updated online version of the book can be found at http://dx.doi.org/10.1007/978-3-319-47633-9

S.C. Kaufman and D.R. Lazzaro (eds.), *Textbook of Ocular Trauma*,
DOI 10.1007/978-3-319-47633-9_15

Erratum to: Glaucoma Considerations

Ilan Epstein, Prachi Dua, Edward Chay and Inci Dersu

Erratum to: Chapter 5 in: S.C. Kaufman and D.R. Lazzaro (eds.), *Textbook of Ocular Trauma*, https://doi.org/10.1007/978-3-319-47633-9_5

The captions for Figures 5.9 and 5.10 in Chapter 5 were switched in the initial publication of the volume. The correct captions have been associated with the figures in the updated version of the chapter.

The updated online version of this chapter can be found at https://doi.org/10.1007/978-3-319-47633-9_5

S.C. Kaufman and D.R. Lazzaro (eds.), *Textbook of Ocular Trauma*,
https://doi.org/10.1007/978-3-319-47633-9_16

Index

Note: Page numbers followed by f and t indicate figures and tables respectively.

S.C. Kaufman and D.R. Lazzaro (eds.), *Textbook of Ocular Trauma*,
DOI 10.1007/978-3-319-47633-9

9783319476315